Living with Mental Disorder

This evidence-based text puts a human face on mental disorders, illuminating the lived experience of people with mental health difficulties and their caregivers. Systematically reviewing the qualitative research conducted on living with a mental disorder, this text coalesces a large body of knowledge and centers on those disorders that have sufficient qualitative research to synthesize, including attention-deficit/hyperactivity disorder, autism, intellectual disabilities, mood disorders, schizophrenia, and dementia.

Supported by numerous quotes, the text explores the perspective of those suffering with a mental disorder and their caregivers, discovering their experience of burden, their understanding of and the meaning they give to their disorder, the strengths and coping they have used to manage, as well as their interactions with the formal treatment system and the use of medication.

This book will be of immense value to students, practitioners, and academics that support, study, and treat people in mental distress and their families.

Jacqueline Corcoran is Professor of Social Work at Virginia Commonwealth University, USA. She has published 14 texts and non-fiction books in social work, mental health, and counseling, and over 50 peer-reviewed journal articles, as well as novels. She also maintains a small private practice. For more information, see www.jacquelinecorcoran.com.

Routledge Key Themes in Health and Society

Available titles include:

Turning Troubles into Problems
Clientization in human services
Edited by Jaber F. Gubrium and Margaretha Järvinen

Compassionate Communities
Case studies from Britain and Europe
Edited by Klaus Wegleitner, Katharina Heimerl and Allan Kellehear

Exploring Evidence-based Practice
Debates and challenges in nursing
Edited by Martin Lipscomb

On the Politics of Ignorance in Nursing and Healthcare
Knowing ignorance
Amélie Perron and Trudy Rudge

Empowerment
A critique
Kenneth McLaughlin

The Story of Nursing in British Mental Hospitals
Echoes from the corridors
Niall McCrae and Peter Nolan

Living with Mental Disorder
Insights from qualitative research
Jacqueline Corcoran

Forthcoming titles include:

Social Theory and Nursing
Edited by Martin Lipscomb

Identity, Ageing and Cultural Adaptation
Understanding longevity in crossdisciplinary perspective
Simon Biggs

Living with Mental Disorder

Insights from qualitative research

Jacqueline Corcoran

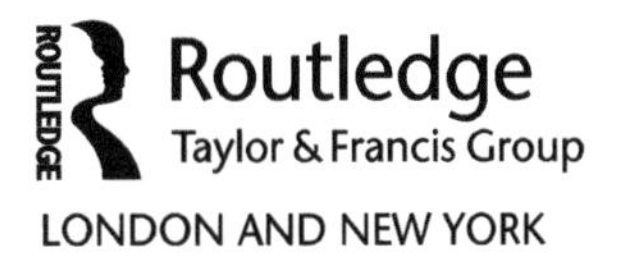

LONDON AND NEW YORK

First published 2016 by Routledge

2 Park Square, Milton Park, Abingdon, Oxfordshire OX14 4RN
52 Vanderbilt Avenue, New York, NY 10017

Routledge is an imprint of the Taylor & Francis Group, an informa business

First issued in paperback 2018

British Library Cataloguing-in-Publication Data
A catalogue record for this book is available from the British Library

Library of Congress Cataloging in Publication Data
Corcoran, Jacqueline, author.
Living with mental disorder : insights from qualitative research /
Jacqueline Corcoran.
p. ; cm. – (Routledge key themes in health and society)
Includes bibliographical references and index.
I. Title. II. Series: Routledge key themes in health and society.
[DNLM: 1. Mental Disorders–Review. 2. Caregivers–psychology–Review. 3. Nursing Research–Review. 4. Qualitative Research–Review. 5. Research Design–Review. WM 140]
RC454
616.89–dc23 2015023818

ISBN: 978-0-415-73944-3 (hbk)
ISBN: 978-0-367-07492-0 (pbk)

Typeset in Goudy
by Wearset Ltd, Boldon, Tyne and Wear

Contents

Tables

Acknowledgments

Meta-synthesis is a complex method that requires detailed attention to many systematic steps. Therefore, no one person could carry out meta-synthesis alone, much less the ten that are represented in this book. And it would not be desirous anyway since a one-person project is susceptible to bias and selectivity. As a result, I was assisted by many people in the implementation of this project. Sincere acknowledgments go to my research assistant Francesca Teixeira who toiled over tedious searches, reference lists, and numerous other details that contributed to this book. My good friend and expert qualitative researcher, Holly Bell, was there at the start to help me make sense of themes and to talk with me about meta-synthesis. My heartfelt thanks also go to colleagues, Matthew Bogenschutz, Joseph Walsh, Heeyhyul Moon, and Masters of Social Work students who provided valuable contributions to chapters, Julia Abell, Amber Berry, Emily Brown, Nathan Crooke, Paula Crooks, Megan Davis, Stephanie Hill, Rebecca Hochbrueckner, Michelle Pineda, Rachel Spence, Thomas Allen Stewart, and Cathleen Surface. I am also very grateful to the following students who contributed data extraction and theme tables: Jessica Bennett, Rachel Brown, Cory Cummings, Sarah Davis, James Gregory, Lindsay Higgenbottham, Olivia Hildebrande, Nicole Peterson, and Brent Schildt. A reference librarian is an essential person on a team devoted to systematic review; Nita Bryant at Virginia Commonwealth University trained many students on the library search process and constructed search strings for the various database searches. Without the assistance of all these people, it would have been impossible to complete this volume.

1 Introduction and overview

In the US, there were 43.7 million adults diagnosed with a mental disorder in the past year, representing 18.6 percent of the population (National Institute of Mental Health, 2012). For children, one in five (about 20 percent) have or will have a mental disorder. Quantitative studies have indicated the toll that mental disorders may take in terms of impaired educational attainment (Mojtabai et al., 2015), employment in terms of days of disability (Bruffaerts et al., 2012), and increased risk of health conditions, such as ulcer (Scott, Alonso, de Jonge, et al., 2013), heart disease (Scott, de Jonge, Alonso, et al., 2013), diabetes (de Jonge et al., 2014), cancer (O'Neill et al., 2014), and hypertension (Stein et al., 2014). Indeed, the burden of impact of mental disorders is seen as more impairing in terms of personal and relationship functioning than physical disorders, although role functioning was viewed as being similarly impaired (Ormel et al., 2008). Further, there is an increased risk of suicidal behavior associated with mental health disorder diagnoses (Nock et al., 2013).

Qualitative research and its synthesis

Along with quantitative research that can tell us about risks associated with mental illness, qualitative research is ideally poised to relay the personal experience, as well as the meaning people give for their suffering, and what has been helpful or not helpful in terms of recovery and adjustment. Qualitative research further allows for the emergence of strengths and resources that people activate to cope with mental disorder. Qualitative research has been defined at its most basic level by asking "open questions about phenomena as they occur in context rather than setting out to test predetermined hypotheses" (Carter and Little, 2007). Data that is generated and analyzed is textual rather than numerical in nature and seeks to comprehend the meaning of human experience (Carter and Little, 2007; Schwandt, 2007; Strauss and Corbin, 1990).

Despite the advantages of qualitative research for the study of mental disorders, there are also limitations, namely the lack of generalizability beyond the small sample that is typically studied. To make up for this limitation and to contribute to knowledge building that qualitative research can so vitally contribute, meta-synthesis has recently developed.

Meta-synthesis is designed to systematically review and integrate results of primary qualitative studies that have been conducted on a similar topic (Finfgeld, 2003; Sandelowski and Barroso, 2006; Paterson et al., 2001). Meta-synthesis is a valuable way to build knowledge in a particular area of study. By drawing on all the relevant studies at once, it may offer new interpretations of findings. Thus, the knowledge of a given subject may become more substantive than if only individual studies were examined (Finfgeld, 2003). Because of its small scope, qualitative research is not as likely to be funded and can be marginalized. However, through the accumulation of such knowledge that can be found through meta-synthesis, qualitative research can contribute to service delivery and policy changes (Finfgeld, 2003).

Meta-synthesis developed in nursing (Paterson et al., 2001; Noblit and Hare, 1988; Sandelowski and Barroso, 2006), and subsequently, health-related topics were the initial focus of study as a result. However, social work has more recently contributed to its perspective (Aguirre and Bolton, 2014; Saini and Shlonsky, 2012), and over the last couple of years meta-syntheses on mental health topics have emerged (e.g., Mollard, 2014).

Evidence-based practice

Several reports have centered on mental health needs in the United States and have suggested the use of "evidence-based practice" (Knitzer, 1982; Cooper et al., 2008; President's New Freedom Commission on Mental Health, 2003). Evidence-based practice (EBP) began in medicine in the early 1990s (Sackett et al., 1991) and was defined as the integration of the best available research knowledge with clinical expertise and consumer values. In other words, evidence-based treatment is a process of using research knowledge to make decisions about particular cases. The process of gathering the available research knowledge involves formulating specific questions, locating the relevant studies, assessing their credibility, and integrating credible results with findings from previous studies (Sackett et al., 1991).

The highest level of evidence is the systematic review and meta-analysis. A *systematic review* aims to comprehensively locate and synthesize the research that bears on a particular question. It uses organized, transparent, and replicable procedures at each step in the process (Littell et al., 2008). Meta-analysis involves the quantitative summary of quantitative studies that have been conducted in an area of knowledge. Meta-synthesis is the qualitative counterpart to meta-analysis, and both are embedded within the systematic review. The Joanna Briggs Institute (2014) recognizes the role of qualitative synthesis in the evidence-based process. The authors of the reviewer manual state that although such synthesis cannot address the effectiveness of interventions, it can offer key information about the impact of having a disorder and the types of intervention that can be helpful. "It also provides a means of giving consumers a voice in the decision-making process through the documentation of their experiences, preferences and priorities" (p. 16). *Living with Mental Disorder: Insights from Qualitative Research* will use meta-synthesis to discover the lived experience of those who suffer from mental health disorders, as well as their caregivers, in managing illness.

Limitations of meta-synthesis

Meta-synthesis is not without controversy (see Finlayson and Dixon, 2008; Jones, 2004; Saini and Shlonsky, 2012). A main limitation is that the meta-synthesist does not have access to the original data (i.e., the transcription of the taped conversations with the individuals that participated in the primary qualitative studies). Instead, he or she relies on the interpretation of these narratives by the author(s) of the particular research. Although researchers of the primary studies typically documented a process for gaining trustworthiness in terms of credibility, transferability, dependability, and confirmability (Lincoln and Guba, 1985), it is unknown the extent to which studies enacted these standards. We rely on the expertise, competence, and ethics of the researcher to carry out the research according to the methods outlined in writing.

Another argument against meta-synthesis is that combining studies together that have a variety of epistemologies, methodologies, methods, and analyses leads to an "apples" and "oranges" approach (Finlayson and Dixon, 2008; Jones, 2004). Despite these objections to meta-synthesis, reviewing comprehensively the qualitative research that has been done on a disorder, and attempting to synthesize some of the dominant findings is, in itself, a contribution, offering "a whole that is more than the sum of its parts." The conceptualization articulated by social workers' researchers Aguirre and Bolton's (2014) involves each study changing "from an individual pocket of knowledge of a phenomenon into part of a web of knowledge about the topic where a synergy among the studies creates a new, deeper and broader understanding" (p. 283). They further argue that the use of various qualitative traditions and data collection methods aids in the process of triangulation, as does the fact that there are multiple perspectives represented across the primary studies.

Format

Each chapter in *Living with Mental Disorder: Insights from Qualitative Research* will address a particular mental health disorder and follow a similar format. First, a brief description of the disorder will be presented, including its prevalence. Second, the relevant quantitative literature, as well as any meta-syntheses that have already been conducted, will be reviewed. The bulk of each chapter will comprise the meta-synthesis that has been undertaken. A summation of the methodology is provided in Chapter 2; each chapter thereafter focuses on the results of the meta-synthesis, with supporting details about the primary studies included and the development of themes in tables. Discussion in each chapter compares and contrasts findings to the quantitative research conducted in the area and any relevant existing meta-syntheses. It will highlight the unique contributions of the qualitative results to practice and policy.

Audience

The use of meta-synthesis as a way to approach the field of mental disorders is unique and cutting-edge. It also offers readers a comprehensive review of qualitative research that has been conducted on mental disorders and covers a vast field, encapsulating it in one volume. The audience for *Living with Mental Disorder* includes graduate students from mental health disciplines (psychiatry, psychology, counseling, nursing, and social work). Practitioners in these fields are another potential audience. *Living with Mental Disorder: Insights from Qualitative Research* puts a human face on mental disorders, illuminates the suffering and the meaning that people make of their disorder, and offers insights into relevant and helpful service provision, all through a replicable and systematic research method. To conclude, *Living with Mental Disorder* will offer the following benefits to readers by:

- providing comprehensive reviews of the qualitative research on each topic of mental health;
- offering a synthesis of the qualitative findings in each area;
- conveying the lived experience of those suffering from mental health disorders and their caregivers;
- offering insights as to perceived contributing factors to mental illness, and what is helpful to recovery;
- offering insight about the strengths and resources that people employ when coping with mental illness;
- offering insights about service delivery systems;
- developing implications for practice and policy from the client perspective

References

Aguirre, R., and Bolton, K. (2014). Qualitative interpretive meta-synthesis in social work research: Uncharted territory. *Journal of Social Work, 14*, 279–294.

Beecher, B. (2009). The medical model, mental health practitioners, and individuals with schizophrenia and their families. *Journal of Social Work Practice, 23*(1), 9–20.

Bruffaerts, R., Vilagut, G., Demyttenaere, K., Alonso, J., Alhamzawi, A., Andrade, L. H., et al. (2012). Role of common mental and physical disorders in partial disability around the world. *The British Journal of Psychiatry: The Journal of Mental Science, 200*(6), 454. doi:10.1192/bjp.bp. 111.097519.

Carter, S., and Little, M. (2007). Justifying knowledge, justifying method, taking action: Epistemologies, methodologies, and methods in qualitative research. *Qualitative Health Research, 17*, 1316–1328.

Cooper, J. L., Aratani, Y., Knitzer, J., Douglas-Hall, A., Masi, R., Banghart, P. L., et al. (2008). Unclaimed children revisited: The status of children's mental health policy in the United States, *Columbia University Academic Commons*. Retrieved from http://hdl.handle.net/10022/AC:P:8917.

de Jonge, P., Alonso, J., Stein, D. J., Kiejna, A., Aguilar-Gaxiola, S., Viana, M. C., et al. (2014). Associations between DSM-IV mental disorders and diabetes mellitus: A role for impulse control disorders and depression. *Diabetologia* 57(4), 699–709.

Finfgeld, D. L. (2003). Metasynthesis: The state of the art – so far. *Qualitative Health Research*, *13*(7), 893–904.

Finlayson, K. W., and Dixon, A. (2008). Qualitative meta-synthesis: A guide for the novice. *Nurse Researcher*, *15*(2), 59–71.

Joanna Briggs Institute. (2014). *The Joanna Briggs Institute Reviewers' Manual. 2014 edition*. University of South Adelaide: Joanna Briggs Institute.

Jones, M. (2004). Application of systematic review methods to qualitative research: Practical issues. *Journal of Advanced Nursing*, *48*(3), 271–278.

Knitzer, J. (1982). *Unclaimed children: The failure of public responsibility to children in need of mental health services*. Washington, DC: Children's Defense Fund.

Lincoln, Y., and Guba, E. (1985). *Naturalistic inquiry*. Newbury Park, CA: Sage Publications.

Littel, J., Corcoran, J., and Pillai, V. (2008). *Systematic reviews and meta-analysis*. New York: Oxford University Press.

Mojtabai, R., Stuart, E., Hwang, I., Eaton, W., Sampson, N., and Kessler, R. (2015). Long-term effects of mental disorders on educational attainment in the national comorbidity survey ten-year follow-up. *Social Psychiatry and Psychiatric Epidemiology*, *50*(10), 1577–1591. doi:10.1007/s00127–015–1083–5.

Mollard, E. (2014). A qualitative meta-synthesis and theory of postpartum depression. *Issues in Mental Health Nursing*, *35*, 656–663.

National Institute of Mental Health. (2012). Any mental disorder (AMI) among adults. Retrieved from www.nimh.nih.gov/health/statistics/prevalence/any-mental-illness-ami-among-adults.shtml.

National Institute of Mental Health. (2012). Any disorder among children. Retrieved from www.nimh.nih.gov/health/statistics/prevalence/any-disorder-among-children.shtml.

Noblit, G. W., and Hare, R. D. (1988). *Meta-ethnography: Synthesizing qualitative studies*. Newbury Park, CA: Sage Publications.

Nock, M. K., Green, J. G., Hwang, I., McLaughlin, K. A., Sampson, N. A., Zaslavsky, A. M., et al. (2013). Prevalence, correlates and treatment of lifetime suicidal behavior among adolescents: Results from the National Comorbidity Survey Replication – Adolescent Supplement (NCS-A). *JAMA Psychiatry*, *70*(3), 300–310.

O'Neill, S., Posada-Villa, J., Medina-Mora, M. E., Al-Hamzawi, A. O., Piazza, M., Tachimori, H., et al. (2014). Associations between DSM-IV mental disorders and subsequent self-reported diagnosis of cancer. *Journal of Psychosomatic Research*, *76*(3), 207–212.

Ormel, J., Petukhova, M., Chatterji, S., Aguilar-Gaxiola, S., Alonso, J., Angermeyer, M., et al. (2008). Disability and treatment of specific mental and physical disorders across the world. *The British Journal of Psychiatry: The Journal of Mental Science*, *192*(5), 368–375. Retrieved from www.ncbi.nlm.nih.gov/pubmed/23303463.

Paterson, B., Thorne, S., Canam, C., and Jillings, C. (2001). *Metastudy of qualitative health research*. Thousand Oaks, CA: Sage Publications.

President's New Freedom Commission on Mental Health. (2003). *Major federal programs supporting and financing mental health care*. Retrieved from www.nsmha.org/reports/PNFCMH/Default.htm.

Sackett, P. R., DuBois, C. L., Cathy, L., and Noe, A. W. (1991). Tokenism in performance evaluation: The effects of work group representation on male-female and white-black differences in performance ratings. *Journal of Applied Psychology*, *76*, 263–267.

Saini, M., and Shlonsky, A. (2012). *Systematic synthesis of qualitative research*. New York: Oxford University Press.

Sandelowski, M., and Barroso, J. (2006). *Handbook of synthesizing qualitative research*. New York: Springer Publishing.

Schwandt, T. (2007). *Dictionary of qualitative inquiry* (3rd edn.). Thousand Oaks, CA: Sage.

Scott, K., Alonso, J., de Jonge, P., Viana, M. C., Liu, Z., O'Neill, S., et al. (2013). Associations between DSM-IV mental disorders and onset of self-reported peptic ulcer in the World Mental Health Surveys. *Journal of Psychosomatic Medicine*, *75*(2), 121–127.

Scott, K. M., de Jonge, P., Alonso, J., Viana, M. C., Liu, Z., O'Neill, S., et al. (2013). Associations between DSM-IV mental disorders and subsequent heart disease onset: Beyond depression. *International Journal of Cardiology*, *168*(6), 5293–5299.

Scott, K. M., Koenen, K. C., Aguilar-Gaxiola, S., Alonso, J., Angermeyer, M. C., Benjet, C., et al. (2013). Associations between lifetime traumatic events and subsequent chronic physical conditions: A cross-national, cross-sectional study. *PLoS One*, *8*(11), e80573.

Stein, D. J., Aguilar-Gaxiola, S., Alonso, J., Bruffaerts, R., de Jonge, P., Liu, Z., et al. (2014). Associations between mental disorders and subsequent onset of hypertension. *General Hospital Psychiatry*, *36*(2), 142–149.

Strauss, A., and Corbin, J. (1990). *Basics of qualitative research: Grounded theory procedures and techniques*. Newbury Park, CA: Sage Publications.

2 Methodology

The main focus of this chapter is the methodology that was followed for each meta-synthesis that is presented in this book. It also includes a discussion of the choices that were made around the inclusion of topics. Although the steps of the methodology are listed below, conducting these studies was not always a straightforward process, and some of the difficulties and conundrums of making particular choices are also included with the following texts seen as particularly useful: Noblit and Hare, 1988; Paterson et al., 2001; and Sandelowski and Barroso, 2007.

Why were certain disorders included and others not?

A comprehensive search was undertaken on the qualitative research of disorders defined by the American Psychiatric Association Diagnostic and Statistical Manual (APA, 2013). Results of the searches varied considerably by disorder; some, such as conduct disorder and oppositional defiant disorder, were topics that were represented very little by the qualitative literature; others had an abundant literature (e.g., child ADHD). Some highly prevalent disorders failed to coalesce around a single topic area that could be synthesized together. For example, despite the fact that anxiety disorders as a class are the most frequent mental disorder diagnosed in the US, there was not a topic for meta-synthesis among the qualitative studies on anxiety. Those tended to involve anxiety about a specific trigger, such as a type of medical condition or revolved around a situation that precipitated anxiety.

A similar pattern in the literature for PTSD was found. Studies were about a wide variety of traumatic events, often physical trauma (e.g., automobile accidents), rather than discussing the experience of living with the after-effects of trauma and the diagnosis of Post-Traumatic Stress Disorder. Surprisingly, substance use disorders did not coalesce around a single topic and remained disparate with a variety of topic areas, represented by a couple of studies each.

Another phenomenon to affect the search process was the more recent adoption of meta-synthesis as a methodology. When the proposal for this book was originally developed, certain topics that were put forward were since studied by other researchers. Secondary trauma for people working in the human services/mental health services field was one such topic, as was post-partum depression in women, which has actually now been the subject of more than one published meta-synthesis.

Another result of doing searches was that some disorders had so much qualitative research accumulated that they could be gathered around several different topics. Intellectual disabilities was the one that most aptly illustrated this. Two Ph.D. level researchers (the author and a research associate) examined each of the qualitative studies separately on intellectual disability and made a determination of topic areas. They started this separately and then worked together collaboratively to come up with the broad themes in the qualitative intellectual disability literature of parents of children with intellectual disabilities (see Chapter 5); adolescents transitioning to adult systems (see Chapter 5); sexuality; health; and people with intellectual disabilities ageing (see Chapter 11).

In other areas, such as depression, there were many qualitative studies, but the only areas left undone by other meta-synthesists were older adults and women's experience of depression. At times, there was such a large area to draw from (e.g., parents of children with autism spectrum disorders), that studies were limited to a certain geographic area. Indeed, Sandelowski and Barroso (2007) advocate for geographic parameters so that compatible studies are synthesized together, although other experts in meta-synthesis have not called for this approach. Rationales for using a geographic parameter were provided in individual chapters (e.g., autism spectrum disorders, bipolar disorder, and women and depression).

Studies that evaluated a specialized program or intervention through qualitative methods were screened out typically since consumer perspectives were so specific to the program rather than the experience of having a mental disorder or caring for a person. However, the experience of treatment was, of course, a theme to develop in most of the studies given the broad topic of mental health.

All types of studies with varying methodological quality were allowed in to the reviews, but studies were screened out if they were missing standard pieces of methodology, such as a sampling and recruitment method, the identified population, and some basic demographic information beyond just the sample size (e.g., Gardner and Harmon, 2002).

Readers will likely find some chapters more or less rich in the findings that are presented. This level of richness has most to do with the findings that were present in the original studies. The aim of the book was to find out, in disorders that had sufficient studies representing them, the major themes that cross-cut through the primary studies. The potential significance and impact of these findings tends to be admittedly variable in nature across topics.

The search and location of studies

Inclusion criteria and search

The general inclusion criteria for studies involved the following: (a) the study employed qualitative methods; (b) participants in the study were people suffering from a particular DSM-defined disorder and generally speaking, it involved their lived experience. However, this was not always an easy, straightforward decision. As an example, in the topic of health for people with intellectual disabilities, there are several studies on people's perceptions of particular types of exercise. Although exercise is clearly health-related, honing in on the experience of each particular type of exercise was seen as going in too specific a direction. However, it is recognized that another researcher might have a different interpretation of what constituted a study on health with people with intellectual disabilities and might have included such studies into the synthesis.

In another example, this one having to do with caregivers of children with ADHD, if a study centered on parents' decision making and experience with their child's receipt of medication, it was included in the meta-synthesis, as one of the main treatments for ADHD is medication, and, indeed, the experience of living with a child with ADHD often includes making a decision about medication.

Search terms initially were very broadly defined. For example, in the initial searches of the topics *older adults with depression* and *intellectual disability*, terms involved the disorder itself (such as intellectual disability/intellectual disorder/mental retardation) with the term "qualitative"). When it became apparent after these searches that the number of studies to screen was unmanageable (totaling in the hundreds for each database), the principal investigator engaged the services of her institution's assigned librarian to help develop more focused search terms. It is also generally accepted now to have a research librarian as a part of team that does systematic review.

Here is a sample that the librarian constructed for the search on substance use disorders, with emphasis on what should be contained in the abstract (AB):

> ("AB personal reflection" OR "AB personal experience" OR AB "lived experience" OR AB phenomenolog* OR AB "qualitative study") AND ((SU substance abuse OR SU chemical dependence OR SU alcohol abuse OR SU drug abuse OR SU addictions OR SU addicts) OR (AB "substance abuse" OR AB "chemical dependence" OR AB "alcohol abuse" OR AB "drug abuse" OR addict OR addictions))

As the process evolved, the search terms involved more possible types of qualitative research with search terms, such as the following that involved women and depression after a preliminary search for depression studies indicated that they coalesced in this area:

> DE "DEPRESSION in women" NOT perinatal NOT postpartum NOT pregnant* AND (ethnography OR "discourse analysis" OR "personal reflection" OR "case study" OR narrative OR "personal experience" OR "lived experience" OR phenomenology* OR qualitative)

Terms were usually applied to the following databases: Academic Search Complete, CINAHL, Medline, Dissertation Abstracts, Psychology and Behavioral Sciences Collection, PsycEXTRA, PsycInfo, PsycNET, PubMed, and Social Work Abstracts. Certain other databases were searched if they were relevant to the topic. For instance, the search for depression in older age relied on AgeLine, as well as the other databases. For autism spectrum disorders and intellectual disabilities, ERIC was consulted. There were no limiters on the search dates. Studies could have been conducted at any point in the past and extended to the present day. The publisher decided against including all the search tables in this volume due to readability, but they are available from the author upon request.

Whenever resources allowed, the database search was completed independently by a doctoral-level and a master-level research assistant; the searches were duplicated for the sake of reliability. All research assistants were trained and supervised by the principal investigator and sought consultation from the reference librarian who provided search terms and strategies for each database and disorder.

Screening studies and selection process

The three-step process of study selection developed by Meade and Richardson (1997) was used to narrow down the results of the search, based first on the title alone, then including the abstract, and last, including the entire text of the study. The research assistants screened to the level of the abstract, and at this point, the principal investigator made the determination based on the abstract and the full-text studies which studies would be included. Common reasons for excluding studies were that they were quantitative rather than qualitative, and the study sample included participants who had various types of disorders rather than just the one disorder that was the focus of the study, or providers of services were the participants.

Studies were conducted at different time periods over the last few years so end-date parameters for stopping a review differed throughout the course of this project. For more detail on screening, data extraction, and theme development, the interested reader should contact the author.

Data extraction and analysis

A data extraction sheet was adapted from Paterson et al. (2001) in order to organize the relevant information on methodologies, descriptions of the sample, and the results of each study. Data extraction was completed by two Masters-level research students per topic and reviewed for accuracy by the author. Tables of the data extraction are provided in each chapter.

The studies were analyzed for themes with the broad framework of Aguirre and Bolton's (2014) conceptualization that each study's themes becomes woven as "part of a web of knowledge about the topic where a synergy among the studies creates a new, deeper and broader understanding" (p. 283). More specifically, the methodological framework provided by Noblit and Hare (1988), which they call "meta-ethnography" was used for the synthesis. Noblit and Hare (1988) suggest making lists and tables of the important phrases, metaphors, and other key findings from each study, and then making comparisons of the main ideas to determine overlap and commonality. Noblit and Hare (1998) discuss the importance of communicating the synthesis through tables and supporting quotes from the original studies, but the creation of lists within tables of themes in each study is also helpful in determining themes. Tables documenting the themes in each study are also presented in each chapter to promote transparency of the process.

Conclusion

The process outlined in this chapter was used for all individual studies presented in this book with the meta-synthesis embedded within a systematic review. A vast body of knowledge generated by qualitative research was reviewed in the course of this project, and the disorders to emerge with sufficient study behind them went through the process of meta-synthesis. These are described in subsequent chapters in this book and represent the state of knowledge of qualitative research on mental disorders at this point in time.

References

Aguirre, R., and Bolton, K. (2014). Qualitative interpretive meta-synthesis in social work research: Uncharted territory. *Journal of Social Work*, *14*, 279–294.

APA (American Psychiatric Association). (2013). *Diagnostic and statistical manual of mental disorders* (5th edn.). Arlington, VA: Author.

Finlayson, K. W. and Dixon, A. (2008). Qualitative meta-synthesis: A guide for the novice. *Nurse Researcher*, *15*(2), 59–71.

Gardner, J., and Harmon, T. (2002). Exploring resilience from a parent's perspective. *Australian Social Work*, *55*, 60–68.

Joanna Briggs Institute. (2014). *The Joanna Briggs Institute Reviewers' Manual. 2014 edition.* University of South Adelaide: Author.

Jones, M. L. (2004) Application of systematic review methods to qualitative research: Practical issues. *Journal of Advanced Nursing*, *48*(3), 271–278.

Meade, M. O., and Richardson, W. S. (1997). Selecting and appraising studies for a systematic review. *Annals of Internal Medicine*, *127*, 531–537.

Noblit, G. W., and Hare, R. D. (1988). *Meta-ethnography: Synthesizing qualitative studies*. Newbury Park, CA: Sage Publications.

Paterson, B., Thorne, S., Canam, C., and Jillings, C. (2001). *Metastudy of qualitative health research*. Thousand Oaks, CA: Sage Publications.

Sandelowski, M. and Barroso, J. (2007). *Handbook for synthesizing qualitative research.* New York: Springer.

Part I

Disorders in children

3 The lived experience of parents of children with ADHD

Attention-deficit/hyperactivity disorder (ADHD) is characterized by a persistent pattern (six months or more) of *inattention* and/or *hyperactivity* and *impulsive behavior* that is more frequent and severe than what is typically observed in others at a comparable developmental level (APA, 2013). Children with ADHD show a lack of self-control and ability to sustain direction. They are distractible, do not often finish what they start, and are irritable and impatient, often interrupting and pestering others. In 2011, 6.4 million children of ages 4–17 years in the United States had a diagnosis of ADHD. The rate of diagnosis is 11 percent, and has increased throughout even recent years – from 7.8 percent in 2003 to 9.5 percent in 2007 and to 11.0 percent in 2011. This involves an increase of 3 percent per year since 1997. Boys are more likely to be diagnosed than girls (13.2 versus 5.6 percent) (Centers for Disease Control and Prevention, 2016).

Pervasive child problems in the way of daily negative interactions and behavioral management difficulties demand considerable parental resources (Coghill et al., 2008). These demands often result in failure, fatigue, demoralization, isolation, strained marital relationships, and neglect or overindulgence of siblings (Whalen and Henker, 1999). A recent systematic review of 22 published and 22 unpublished studies indicated that parenting stress, while greater for parents with children with ADHD compared to "normal" control, was not different from parents of other clinically referred children (Theule, Wiener, Tannock, and Jenkins, 2013). Stress did not differ substantially between mothers and fathers, but the presence of maternal depression, severe ADHD, and conduct problems in children worsened stress, as did having a male child.

In addition to this meta-analysis about parenting stress, a meta-synthesis was also conducted on parenting decisions about treating their children with ADHD medication (Ahmed et al., 2013). Eleven studies involving 335 parents of children were located, and four major themes emerged: (1) confronting the diagnosis; (2) external influences; (3) apprehension regarding therapy; and (4) experience with the healthcare system. Confronting the diagnosis involved coming to terms with the diagnosis itself, often after a period of denial and skepticism about the validity of the disorder, especially considering sensationalized media reports and the brief nature of the initial evaluation that led to a diagnosis. Parental disagreement about these matters was common at this point, and family and friends' opinions – both for and against – weighed in. The school system had an influence on decision making, with parents feeling some pressure from teachers to put their child on medication due to children's poor academic and behavioral performance at school. Parents were worried about side effects of medication, the potential for addiction, the cost of medication, and whether there would be long-term consequences from medication use. For some parents, the noticeably positive impact of medication on children's behavior outweighed these issues, but other parents discontinued their children's medication because of them. The availability of support and information from the healthcare system, which often parents found sketchy, was another influence on treatment decisions. Many parents wanted to exhaust other treatment options first – usually behavioral management programs and natural remedies – before they decided to use medication.

Ahmed et al.'s (2013) meta-synthesis was limited by including only published studies and a focus on treatment decisions. The purpose of this meta-synthesis is to do a comprehensive review of both the published and unpublished studies and to consider the totality of parents' lived experience, not just their choice of whether to medicate their children.

Results

Seventy-three studies, involving 86 reports, fit the inclusion criteria for parental experiences with children diagnosed with ADHD. The majority of parents who participated were married mothers, although fathers were at times the focus of studies (Singh, 2003) and single parents only (Hancock, 2003). The majority of studies were conducted in the US, with other developed countries being represented (UK, Australia, Ireland, Norway), with both published and unpublished studies represented. Most of the studies involved individual interviews (see Table 3.1). The following were the common themes: (1) impact on parents; (2) the process of accepting the diagnosis; and (3) medication (see Table 3.2).

Impact on parenting

The dominant theme was parents' struggle with the emotional burden of caring for a child with ADHD and managing the hyperactive, impulsive, and inattentive behaviors, which were detailed in all studies, including lack of focus, forgetfulness, inability to listen and complete tasks, poor grades, tantrums, aggression, risk-taking, poor social relationships, and running off. Parents talked about the constant mess, and the chaos and conflict that besieged their home life (Kendall, 1998). As a result of this struggle, parents talked about a myriad of feelings:

- exhaustion (Hallberg et al., 2008; Williamset al., 2014; Yuen, 2008):

> I was on extreme exhaustion from fighting, from the sheer exhaustion of just being with [child], even though coming back from school I've

> only got him for about three hours and then he goes to bed ... but you are exhausted.
>
> (McIntyre and Hennessy, 2012, p. 72)

- isolation (Bennett, 2007; Cawley, 2004; Claudius et al., 2011; Klasen, 2000; Lai and Ma, 2014; Morse, 2002; Neophytou and Webber, 2005; Peters and Jackson, 2009; Singh, 2000, 2004; Smith, 2011; Wallace, 2005; Wilder et al., 2009);
- anxiety:

> [I feel] nervous and irritated ... psychologically very tensed and worry about our future life.
>
> (Ho et al., 2011, p. 48)

> My stomach would churn with nerves and I'd think, "He's going to come out in a minute and it will start." I was like that for years. He'd come out and he'd be like a dynamo. I could do nothing with him. I had this constant stress.
>
> (Funes de Hernandez, 2005, p. 114)

- irritation and frustration (Coletti et al., 2012; Cronin, 2004; Ho et al., 2011; Morse, 2002; Peters and Jackson, 2009);
- anger and resentment (Cawley, 2004; Hancock, 2003, p. 63; Morse, 2002; Singh, 2000, 2004; Taylor et al., 2006, 2008):

> I resented Bean terribly, I truly resented him and um my health was not very good because I was like a walking skeleton and I really didn't know how to cope with him at that time and that is when I started getting some ... going to the doctor.
>
> (Hancock, 2003, p. 63)

- embarrassment (Moen et al., 2011);
- despair (Egbert, 1996; Hallberg et al., 2008; Lin et al., 2009; Perry et al., 2005; Smith, 2011);
- desperation (Egbert, 1996):

> I understand the behavior, but sometimes it comes to a moment that I myself feel like I cannot put up with it, you know, like it's too much. And I feel like, "What am I supposed to do?" because it comes to a point, you don't know what else to do.
>
> (Arcia and Fernandez, 1998, p. 344)

- powerlessness and helplessness (Parker, 1994; Villegas, 2007; Williams, 2009):

> I suppose we thought we would tell him what to do and he would obey it. It doesn't work like that.
>
> (Bull and Wheelan, 2006, p. 670)

- grief (Cawley, 2004; DuCharme, 1996; Rice, 1995; Taylor et al., 2006):

  > It's like a death. Nothing is like I expected. Nothing is the same. It's a loss of the nurturing family. Love in this family means being organized and structured and medical, not being easy and laid back and peaceful. Future dreams and day-to-day life is always disrupted. Something is always going wrong. Going to school and having friends and being on a soccer team is always an unpredictable event that, more often than not, ends in criticism or anger or exhaustion.
  >
  > (Kendall, 1998, p. 843)

- guilt for a myriad of reasons, such as being impatient or punitive; not spending more time with children; not knowing about ADHD and starting medications sooner; causing the ADHD in the first place (Coletti et al., 2012; DuCharme, 1996; Gray Brunton et al., 2014; Kendall, 1998; Mills, 2011; Peters and Jackson, 2009; Singh, 2000, 2004; Williams, 2008, 2009):

  > I want to love my child but you feel like there's time when I could almost hate him. You feel like you hate the child because of their behavior and when you find out it's something that they can't help, you feel guiltier.
  >
  > (Funes de Hernandez, 2005, p. 121)

- pressure and stress (Bullard, 1996; Hammerman, 2000; Harborne, Wolpert, and Clare, 2004; Howard, 1993; Mills, 2011; Segal, 2001; Sikirica et al., 2015; Villegas, 2007: Williams et al., 2014):

  > [Mothering] is like an elastic band. It gets stretched so much and then it breaks. There's a breaking point and then you start again. It builds up until it breaks again.
  >
  > (Funes de Hernandez, 2005, p. 121)

Parents found it hard to manage their children's out-of-control behaviors and experienced their child as having the control. In Funes de Hernandez (2005), a parent said: "It's hard to be the mother you want to be because your child doesn't allow it" (Funes de Hernandez, 2005, p. 127). Another mother expressed it as:

> Everything revolves around X for a happy or peaceful household. I feel like he's in charge. Everything he wants he gets. He wears you down and knows exactly which buttons to push to get what he wants. I give in for my peace of mind and then I get angry because I've given in to him. I get angry with myself and angry with everyone because I've done the wrong thing.
>
> (Funes de Hernandez, 2005, p. 127)

Some women became suicidal due to the intense and relentless stress (Hancock, 2003). In Funes de Hernandez (2005), a mother described:

> I thought of suicide a couple of times. I remember once before X started school and he was having a lot of problems I locked myself in the bedroom and all I did was plan and think how I could do away with myself without leaving a mess. I didn't want any one to have to clean up the mess after me. I just thought, "Well if I do that who's going to look after the kids? So go to sleep and think about it and hopefully things will be better in the morning."
>
> (p. 115)

Caregiving was experienced as a "24-hour a day" undertaking (Hallberg et al., 2008). As one mother of a seven-year-old said: "To be a teacher, mother, minder, carer, everything and twenty four [hours] round the clock it's just an exhausting experience" (McIntyre and Hennessy, 2012, p. 72). In Taylor (1999), one parent echoed: "a constant struggle always, always with her, every single day" (p. 22), and another said: "You feel like you are constantly on them all the time, nag-nag-nag. That can be sometimes a terrible feeling" (p. 23). Typical family routines proved to be a daily challenge (Canfield, 2000; Howard et al., 2014; Segal, 1998; Segal and Frank, 1998; Taylor et al., 2008; Wong and Goh, 2014). As one mother reported: "It is very hard for my son to follow the daily routine, such as abiding by the daily rules and finishing his work at hand" (Lin et al., 2009, p. 1679). Certain times of the day presented particular difficulty. One parent stated:

> Nighttime is, is bad because my son doesn't have a high sleep requirement. He, if he doesn't have his nighttime meds, he doesn't go to bed until midnight, one, two, three, four o'clock in the morning. He doesn't sleep without nighttime meds. Um, bedtime is the hardest because it's hard for them to calm down.
>
> (Firmim and Phillips 2009, p. 1165)

Another parent in the same study described difficulties with the morning routine:

> And no matter how early we start, how early they get up, they still end up running out the door. So that's always a battle. So that's how we start our days, just about every day, it drives me insane.
>
> (Firmim and Phillips 2009, p. 1163)

A single mother, speaking about mornings, said: "He's constantly making the whole family late … and we're always mad at him" (Hancock, 2003, p. 90).

Other people found the hours after school very hard as one participant described: "Homework, homework here is 'Lord help us.' … You spend all day at school and then trying to do homework, and then they get distracted, they get frustrated, the anger mounts" (Firmim and Phillips, 2009, p. 1165). Another parent described trying to do routine errands after school:

> Nothing is easy and I'm not only talking about school work, I'm talking about if I need to run an errand after school. If I haven't prepped him for it in advance there can be a meltdown and lot of times, you can't do it. Or, if

> you do it, you pay the consequences of whiny, pain-in-the-ass crying. So I have to think very carefully about what needs to be done when they come home from school, so I can give them time to adjust to what we have to do. Sometimes that doesn't even work.... I always have to be thinking. I always have to be planning.... I have to do even more of that than most mothers. So it's difficult.
>
> (Roosa, 2003, p. 197)

As Moen et al. (2011) summarized participants' responses about how normal routines became disrupted:

> The child with ADHD was described as getting stuck in a rut without being receptive to attempts to correct his or her behavior. Consequently, a normal everyday situation might be turned upside down; hence, joy and expectations the family anticipated were transformed into a sense of failure. As one father explained, 'We were going to find a Christmas tree before Christmas. He sat bickering with his brother in the back seat. We were looking forward to having a nice trip, as you often do before Christmas. He had a massive temper tantrum, a bit extreme, I thought – bad language, behaviour etc.; he just wouldn't calm down, so the trip was completely ruined.
>
> (pp. 447–449)

A subtheme that emerged under the impact on caregivers involved their parenting. Normal behavioral discipline techniques (reinforcing and rewarding positive behaviors and ignoring or punishing undesirable behaviors) only worked in a limited way with these children (Bussing et al., 2006; DuCharme, 1996; Segal, 1994). As one participant said: "There is no easy way to discipline an ADHD child" (Bull and Whelan, 2006, p. 671), and others in Taylor (1999) stated: "It's very frustrating to figure out how to discipline this kid" (p. 21) and "We've tried a lot of different behavior programs" (p. 21). The difficulty with behavioral strategies was echoed in Kendall (1998):

> I get exhausted trying to figure it all out. I know that rewards are supposed to work, but after awhile you run out of rewards and you run out of interest in providing them, especially when it seems it never goes anywhere except just doing the day-to-day stuff one has to do to survive. I mean, do I give him rewards for getting up in the morning, and getting dressed on time and getting to school on time and doing his homework and this and that?
>
> (p. 847)

The challenges of parenting spilled into other areas of the parents' lives. This stress involved threats to health (Bull and Whelan, 2006; Hallberg et al., 2008), and psychological, marital, and social well-being (Peters and Jackson, 2009). In multiple studies, parents changed or quit their jobs to better manage their child's behaviors (e.g., Hallberg et al., 2008; Ho et al., 2011; Moen et al., 2011).

Parents said their children's relentless misbehavior negatively affected their marital relationships (Bullard, 1996; Cawley, 2004; Dennis et al., 2008; Hallberg et al., 2008; Hammerman, 2000; Ho et al., 2011; Howard, 1993; Kilcarr, 1996; Lin et al., 2009; Moen et al., 2011; Okafor, 2006; Roosa, 2003; Squire, 1993): "My marriage nearly split up along the way" (Bull and Whelan, 2006, p. 672). This happened for various reasons.

McIntyre and Hennessy (2012) described that children's need for constant attention meant that children disrupted any time parents had together. As one of the study's participants described:

> From a very young age if myself and [husband] were sitting down to relax he would climb in between us, if you're having a hug he'd climb in between us, if [husband] put his arm around me he'd climb in between us ... every time we were having a conversation we were interrupted.
>
> (p. 72)

Second, mothers often became the primary disciplinarians, again for various reasons. One primary reason was that fathers did not know how to manage the child's unruly behaviors (Chavarela, 2009; Funes de Hernandez, 2005). A mother described: "My husband is very impatient when he deals with my son. He often beats him while taking care of him. Thus, I can't let my husband help me to take care of my son" (Lin et al., 2009, p. 1690). Another participant in Lin et al. (2009) lamented that this led to lack of support: "My son doesn't like to stay with his father because he always ignores him or shouts at him.... You see, no one can give me a hand, not even my husband" (Lin et al., 2009, p. 1698). Because of the effort and finessing involved to manage these children and sometimes cultural reasons (Latino) (Oquendo, 2013; Chavarela, 2009) mothers preferred to handle discipline alone, wanting husbands to offer support and back-up only as needed (Bull and Whelan, 2006). Another reason men were not as involved with their children was because of their own undiagnosed ADHD (Roosa, 2003; Singh, 2003). They were therefore unable to provide the patience, organization, and structure that such a child demands.

Coming to terms with the diagnosis

The process of coming to terms with the diagnosis was often described as a series of stages (Al-Azzam and Daack-Hirsch, 2011; Canfield, 2000; Dennis et al., 2008; dosReis et al., 2007; DuCharme, 1996; Egbert, 1996; Gray Brunton et al., 2014; Hammerman, 2000; Kay, 2007; Kendall, 1998; Mychailyszyn et al., 2008; Okafor, 2006; Parker, 1994; Rice, 1995; Seawell, 2010; Segal, 1994; Sikirica et al., 2015; Taylor et al., 2006; Wilcox et al., 2007; Williams, 2009). Parents struggled to understand their children's behavior, often seeing problems from a very early age (Hancock, 2003; Himmell, 2013; Roosa, 2003; Taylor, 1999), but eventually accepting a biomedical explanation in ADHD (Bull and Whelan, 2006; Perry et al., 2005; Klasen and Goodman, 2000; Lewis-Morton et al., 2014).

For some parents, a "genetic explanation for the ADHD diagnosis was seen as a way of explaining the child's behavior, and the feelings of guilt and frustration were replaced with a sense of relief" (Moen et al., 2011, p. 450). Relief was also named in Kendall (1998), as well as reduced self-blame (Wilcox et al., 2007). However, parents' understanding of the biomedical reasons was often sketchy and superficial (Ahmed et al., 2014; Harborne et al., 2004; Roosa, 2003).

Many parents, as a result, shifted their attributions of the reasons for their children's behaviors, from being ones they *won't* control to ones they *can't* control (Roosa, 2003; Villegas, 2007). As a parent put it in Arcia and Fernandez (1998):

> But the moment comes when you have to say, "Stop." And he can't stop. He can't. I used to think that he didn't want to. That is, could he be deaf? Could he have a problem that he doesn't...? But, the point is that he can't stop. He starts and it is tralalalala. Without being able to, he cannot control himself. That is what I now see.
>
> (p. 342)

Roosa (2003) summarized her participant responses as follows:

> Instead of being a child whose difficulties are caused by willfulness, defiance, or parenting mistakes, he or she comes to be seen as a child who is neurologically disabled, whose behavior is mostly or partially determined by his or her biology.... This new understanding of the child's behavior caused most of these parents to change many specific things about the way they manage difficult behaviors. To begin with, most parents modified their expectations of their child.... Once they set up expectations that were realistic for the individual child, their child's ability to achieve success was enhanced and the parents' frustration at the child was diminished.
>
> (p. 183)

There was a cultural piece found in the Latinas comprising Oquendo's (2013) sample as "bad parenting" was the attribution given to ADHD-type behaviors. As one mother revealed: "I was the type of parent that thought that ADHD was not a valid thing and I thought that it was bad parenting" (p. 95).

Therefore, mothers felt shame when the diagnosis was given: "...well like my parenting skills were not working or, you know I felt like a failure basically. Oh believe me they make you feel like you're the worst person in the world" (Oquendo, 2013, p. 95). These attitudes were not limited to Latino samples. Funes de Hernandez (2005) spoke of mothers not wanting to get help because it would mean they had failed at their parenting role. As one mother said: "I think the main thing is they don't think you can control your children. They think you're putting a label on something that isn't really there and you really don't know what you're talking about" (p. 85).

The "invisible nature" of ADHD was seen as a barrier to people's understanding (Wilder et al., 2009). In Funes de Hernandez (2005), a mother said:

> Saying your child has ADHD is a stigma because people are saying it's just a cop out to excuse his behavior. It's hard to accept that your child sometimes can't help what he's doing. You can see a physical disability like a broken leg but it's hard to accept a child with a disability in the brain.
>
> (p. 85)

As Kendall (1998) explained in the results of their qualitative study:

> Parents constantly were trying to differentiate between normal child behaviors and ADHD behaviors. Because there were no biological markers making diagnosis assured, and because ADHD is so varied in its presentation, making sense of the disorder was an ongoing activity. Parents yearned for more definitive information, and they struggled to understand what was "really going on with their children."
>
> (p. 844)

As another researcher described: "Parents continually spoke of trying to understand and make sense of their sons' ADHD.... 'Maybe that's his personality, maybe that's ADHD, maybe ADHD is personality and vice versa, I genuinely don't know'" (McIntyre and Hennessy, 2012, p. 71).

Some parents struggled with where the line was for "boy behavior" (Himmell, 2013), especially fathers (Singh, 2003) in whom this extended into an internal debate about whether their own boy behavior was symptomatic of ADHD:

> I just thought he was – I had ants in my pants. I remember always being behind. It's just the way it was with me. I did crazy things as a kid. If you had tested me, you'd probably find I had some form of ADD. So I said to [my wife], "Don't worry. He's fine." I just figured [the boy] was the same as me. And I always pulled it out when I had to. I figured he'd do the same.
>
> (p. 312)

A couple of other studies mentioned a parent as having ADHD as children (Kendall, 1998; Roosa, 2003). These parents

> were more understanding and empathic, as well as better able to explain ADHD symptoms to their child and better able to help with homework and other school issues. For these parents, identifying their child's ADHD allowed them to restory their own history, making sense of their own erratic academic paths and odd behavioral traits.
>
> (Roosa, 2003, p. 284)

Medication

Not surprisingly with the topic of ADHD, discussions about medication were common, and indeed, some studies centered on this aspect. There was a considerable amount of ambivalence toward medication, and both positive and negative stances toward it (Bullard, 1996; Canfield, 2000; Charach et al., 2006; Charach et al., 2014; Coletti et al., 2012; Cronin, 1995; Claudius et al., 2011; dosReis et al., 2009; DuCharme, 1996; Egbert, 1996; Hancock, 2003; Jackson and Peters, 2008; Kilcarr, 1996; Klasen, 2000; Larson et al., 2011; Litt, 2004; Martinez, 2015; Mills, 2011; Mychailyszyn et al., 2008; Neophytou and Webber, 2005; Parker, 1994; Rice, 1995; Sikirica et al., 2015; Singh, 2000, 2005; Taylor et al., 2006; Villegas, 2007; Williams, 2008). A common experience seemed to be initial reservations. One parent reported: "I know how difficult it is to decide about medication. I waited 6 months before I allowed my child to try the medication. I didn't want to try the medication before exhausting other options" (Clarke and Lang, 2012, p. 255). Another parent decided to use medication to help her child better manage school and social relationships:

> As she got older it was more apparent that I did really need to treat her symptoms to make her function in the classroom better, to feel better about herself, and more functional in our home and even outside our home, socially with peers or anyone, it had to happen.
>
> (Brinkman et al., 2009, p. 584)

Other parents described medication as "a last resort." One parent explained:

> We wished that we had been able to somehow find a way to manage this without medication, but clearly, that's not the case. We've done our best, given it our best shot, but our son is still suffering. We are gonna give it a trial of medication.
>
> (Brinkman et al., 2009, p. 584)

Some parents reported relief after the child started medication (Singh, 2004). One parent explained: "I wouldn't be without it because he is so difficult without it" (Bull and Whelan, 2006, p. 669). Most participants seemed to like the benefits of medication, particularly the effect it had on school performance, but it was understood not to be a miracle by any means (Bull and Whelan, 2006; Chavarela, 2009; Funes de Hernandez, 2005; Hansen and Hansen, 2006; Ho et al., 2011; Moen et al., 2011; Roosa, 2003). Some parents, however, were not keen on the side effects, causing them to discontinue medication use entirely (Bull and Whelan, 2006; Hansen and Hansen 2006).

Discussion

When results of the qualitative studies on the lived experience of parents with children diagnosed with ADHD were synthesized, it became apparent that parents were under considerable stress trying to manage their children's behavior. The extreme frustration, tension, and exhaustion were clear. Parental descriptions of their experiences deepened the findings from the quantitative literature that speak to the amount of stress that parents with ADHD are under (Theule et al., 2013). This theme was not found in Ahmed et al.'s (2013) meta-synthesis, likely because theirs centered on treatment decisions. Additionally, the current meta-synthesis involved almost twice as many studies and included the unpublished (dissertations) and published literature.

When comparing this meta-synthesis to other child neurodevelopmental disorders, namely intellectual disability and autism spectrum disorders, that are studied in this book, parents of children with ADHD appeared to suffer the most amount of stress. This finding is in contrast to Theule, Wiener, Tannock, and Jenkins (2013), who reported from a meta-analysis that these parents do not have more stress than caregivers of other childhood mental disorders. Our particular finding might have to do with the expectations people had for their children. Parents talked about "the invisible nature" of ADHD and trying to figure out what was wrong with their child, wondering why they were unable to manage and feeling ineffective as parents and inferior in the eyes of others.

An implication for providers is to validate parents' level of stress and the toll it takes on their ability to manage when they are faced with their children's behavior problems. Providing support and helping parents connect with support – family and friends and/or support groups or other formal services – is key for a parent's own mental health, health, and partner relationships. It is key to attend to these areas as deterioration can themselves contribute to worsened outcomes. For instance, maternal depression predicts a worse treatment outcome (Owens et al., 2003), and low parental expressed emotion (criticism and negativity toward the child) may moderate the genetic effect associated with ADHD (Sonuga-Barke et al., 2008). Maternal warmth may protect against ADHD becoming severe or from conduct disorder developing. However, maternal warmth can be difficult to achieve, given the negative affective states expressed in the qualitative studies. Self-care strategies should be a part of work with parents to prevent or ameliorate any possible negative consequences to themselves, as well as their children.

What is notable about this literature is that strengths are lacking. In the chapters on autism spectrum disorders and child intellectual disability, strengths emerged as themes in their meta-syntheses, but none was found here. Neither was there much uniformity about the way parents coped; a parent worn down by caregiving may be unable to spontaneously identify strengths. Practitioners can approach such parents from a strengths-based angle, pointing out personal and environmental resources they are activating to cope and bolstering these.

In the meta-synthesis, parents spoke of their struggle to identify a reason for their children's misbehavior to be able to understand and change it. Although some parents questioned the diagnosis of ADHD, others seemed relieved by being able to affix the label of ADHD on their children's behavior. It now appeared more understandable and reduced parents' self-blame for not being able to manage. A practice implication is that it is important to discuss the meaning of the diagnosis with parents and their beliefs and perceptions rather than accepting the diagnosis as a foregone conclusion.

Four studies had Latino samples (Arcia and Fernandez, 1998; Chavarela, 2009; Hatton et al., 2000; Oquendo, 2013), and two of these indicated the stigma associated with getting an ADHD diagnosis, that it essentially meant parents were ineffective. The possibility of this meaning for Latino clients can be explored, with the understanding that such a stigma belief may not be limited to this cultural group (Funes de Hernandez, 2005).

Another implication from this study is that practitioners can provide parents with appropriate education about the latest working models of ADHD (e.g., Barkley, 2014) so that parents can more fully understand the possible biological basis for ADHD. At the same time, acknowledgment of the controversies about ADHD is important: the fact that although it is hypothesized to be a neuropsychological disorder, substantive evidence is lacking; and the diagnosis is made on the basis of behaviors rather than biological markers.

The treatment outcome literature for ADHD centers on parent training, behavioral management programs (Pelham and Fabiano, 2008). The qualitative literature goes beyond the findings of these studies to glean the difficulties parents have with behavioral management and its limits with children with ADHD. Parents talked about how structured they had to be in their approach to parenting, which seemed to make some parents feel that it sapped the joy out of family life. Practitioners need to understand parents when they complain that some behavioral techniques "don't work." Rather than being seen as a sign of resistance and blaming the parents for their children's behavior, the practitioner should recognize that although behavioral strategies are important for containing the child's behavior, such techniques might have limited impact on these children, leaving parents feeling demoralized in their parenting efforts.

Similar to Ahmed et al.'s (2013) meta-synthesis, this study found that people struggled with the decision about whether to medicate their children given side effects, the classification of the medication as a Schedule II drug, and the admission of defeat it appeared to bring.

Providers should have full exploration with parents around the potential benefits and risks associated with such treatment, taking into account parents' preferences. In order to get general practitioners to engage in this process with parents, Brinkman et al. (2013) created a shared decision making intervention, which shows promise. Parents were provided with information about ADHD and various treatments available, as well as their pros and cons. Parents' experience with behavioral treatment, and their goals, opinions, and values were also elicited in a structured way. In this way, parents selected treatments in a much more informed manner and were more cooperative as a result.

Conclusion

This study synthesized the literature involving qualitative study of parent experiences with a child diagnosed with ADHD. The challenges parents face are poignantly made clear from this review. Such parents need validation, support and education, not blame for being ineffective at their role. The process of coming to terms with the diagnosis and the decision about whether or not to use medication are also crucial themes of parents' experiences, and providers can take an instrumental role in this process.

Table 3.1 Methodological features of primary studies and results from studies of parents of children with ADHD

Author and purpose	*Design*	*Data analysis*	*Sample information*	*Findings*
Ahmed et al. (2014) Study had multiple purposes including: to explore parental knowledge of ADHD and information sources utilized by parents, to explore if parental information needs were being met, and to explore parental views about strategies to meet their information needs.	Focus groups.	Thematic analysis.	N = 16. 56% of participants were males: 9 male participants, 7 female participants. 85% of participants were biological parent of child diagnosed with ADHD.	Prior to their child's diagnosis, the majority of parents expressed that they had very limited knowledge of ADHD. The majority of the parents' primary source of ADHD-related information was the diagnosing HCP (i.e., GP, pediatrician, or child psychologist/psychiatrist). This information was generally verbal. None of the parents received written information from the HCPs during consultations, although many sought such written information from the internet. Parents noted numerous problems with the information they accessed. With regards to the verbal information from HCPs, parents explained that it was too brief ("it was never enough. It opened up more questions than answers"). Strong consensus amongst the parents with regards to wanting access to information in the form of recounts of real-life experiences of other parents with children affected by ADHD: "real information about what kids were going through, rather than just the technical terms."

continued

Table 3.1 Continued

Author and purpose	*Design*	*Data analysis*	*Sample information*	*Findings*
Al-Azzam and Daack-Hirsch (2011) "To elicit (Arab immigrant Muslim) mothers' perceptions of and responses to behavioral problems in children, especially those behaviors associated with ADHD" (p. 1).	Semi-structured interviews, 2 in Arabic, 14 in English.	Qualitative content analysis.	*N* = 16. Purposive sampling. Arab immigrant Muslim mothers with children ages 5–12 in Wisconsin and Iowa. Mothers from Egypt, Jordan, Kuwait, Libya, Oman, Palestine, Sudan, and Syria. Had to have been born and raised in home countries and been living in US for at least a year. Majority unemployed, most had college or graduate degree; average age 36 with 3 children, living in US for 10 years	*Aim 1: Mothers' understanding of behavior problems through theoretical vignettes* 1 Behavior descriptions: • "active child" along with "troublemaker" and "has problems concentrating." 2 Parental responses to behavioral problems if noticed: • punishment, communication, being more involved, using the reward system, and work collaboratively with teachers, with the goal of modifying or eliminating negative behaviors. 3 Causes of behavioral problems: • seeking attention • school difficulties • home environment • parental blame. 4 Triggers for seeking help: • child's developmental stage • consistency/persistence of behavior • mother's inability to control behavior • interference of behavior with child's academic achievement. 5 Sources of help: • family and friends • school services • physicians • professional mental help

Aim 2: Examine Arab immigrant Muslim mothers' understandings and perceptions of an ADHD diagnosis

1 Mothers' understandings and descriptions of ADHD symptoms:
   - inattentive problems
   - hyperactivity behaviors
   - carelessness and lack of motivation
   - anxiety problems
   - rudeness and disrespect
   - normal behaviors.
2 Parental responses to above behavior list:
   - punishment
   - communication
   - being more involved
   - using the reward system
   - work collaboratively with teachers.
3 Causes of behavior.
4 Triggers for seeking help:
   - academic achievement
   - consistency/persistence
   - mothers' inability to control behaviors
   - having all/most of the behaviors together
   - child's developmental stage.
5 Sources of help:
   - family and friends
   - school services
   - seeking professional help.
6 Mothers' information about ADHD.
7 Mothers' attitudes toward treatment modalities.

continued

Table 3.1 Continued

Author and purpose	*Design*	*Data analysis*	*Sample information*	*Findings*
				Aim 3: Compare Arab immigrant Muslim mothers' perceptions of the diagnosis and management of ADHD with Western cultural practices in diagnosis and management 1 Peoples' perceptions of externalizing behavioral problems, including ADHD, in the participants' home countries. 2 Diagnosis and management of behavioral problems, including ADHD, in participants' home countries. 3 Participants' impressions of diagnosis, management, and treatment of ADHD in the US.
Arcia and Fernandez (1998) To explore Cuban American mothers' schemas on ADHD.	Personal interview.	Theme analysis.	N = 7. All Cuban American mothers ages 32–48. All bilingual and bicultural. All participants had one child between ages of 7 and 10 with diagnosis of ADHD.	Mothers had attempted to apply two familiar Cuban labels for children with atypical behavior: *retardado* ("retarded") and *malcriado* ("spoiled, poorly raised"), or *nono* ("pampered"). Active help-seeking occurred only after mothers had developed schemas of ADHD.
Bennett (2007) To explore the extent of medical knowledge of mothers with children with ADHD.	Personal interview.	Foucauldian discourse analysis and discursive psychology.	N = 6. Mothers ages 35–45 in UK. Responded to advertisement in newspaper to be in study.	Experienced strong feelings of isolation, failure, blame, and negative self-esteem: • difficult to identify with normalized accounts of mothering; • all mothers experienced blame but differed in how they negotiated it; • possible to both resist and sustain blame simultaneously.

Brinkman et al. (2009) To understand how parents make decisions about treatment for their child or adolescent with ADHD.	Focus groups.	Theme analysis.	$N = 52$. Parent must have child between ages of 6 and 17. Child must have been seen for ADHD within past 2 years. Random sampling.	Context of decision making, self-doubt, daily struggles at home and school, parental conflict with each other, emotional burden. Factors that influence decision to initiate medication. Factors that support initiation of medication. Factors that delay initiation of medication. Continued doubt and uncertainty. Medication decisions revisited. Trials stopping medication.
Bull and Wheelan (2006) To gain understanding of mothers' experiences of parenting a child with ADHD.	Semi-structured interviews.	Phenomenological analysis.	$N = 10$. Mothers of children with diagnoses of ADHD.	Themes of parental self-doubt, daily struggles at home and school, parental conflict with each other, and emotional burden of decision making impact the process parents experience in making treatment decisions for their children. Parents experience a gamut of emotions when deciding about treatment for their child with ADHD. Emotions include anger, disappointment, desperation, and ambivalence. Multiple factors influenced the decision to initiate medication. Subsequently, revisiting the decision to give their child medicine for ADHD was common. Many parents stated they had been in denial that their child had a problem.

continued

Table 3.1 Continued

Author and purpose	*Design*	*Data analysis*	*Sample information*	*Findings*
Bullard (1996) To explore parents' views on impact of behavior of child with ADHD on them and their families, and their strategies to cope with this behavior and the stress it causes.	Case studies with 3 mothers, focus groups with 13 parents.	Open coding, then theme analysis.	$N = 14$ parents. Parents from southwestern Montana, recruited through critical case sampling. Children ages 6–12, on medication for at least 2 years.	1 The ADHD child's behavior. 2 Reactions to the diagnosis. 3 Medication for treatment of ADHD. 4 Impact upon relationships (marriage, siblings, relatives). 5 Dealing with schools. 6 Dealing with their own emotions. 7 Pervasiveness of ADHD in lives of mothers. 8 Coping: • reducing stress; • parenting techniques; • support from others.
Bussing et al. (2006) To explore "parental self-care strategies for children with hyperactivity or attention problems" (p. 871).	An open-ended question: "How have you changed the way you discipline your child after you became concerned about his/her behavior?"	Mixed method: open coding and then domain analysis.	$N =$ caregivers of 266 children.	1 Prevention of discipline problems. 2 Solution of discipline problems. 3 Parental coping with disciplinary actions.

Canfield (2000) "To gain insight into the parental experience of medication therapy for their ADHD child" (p. 2).	Interview guide approach.	Phenomenological.	$N = 10$. Purposive and criterion sampling, recruited from clinical referrals from 3 southern US states. Parents of male children ages 6–12, taking psychostimulants within past year. Most families middle or working class and white.	*Parental experience* 1 Disappointment at diagnosis of ADHD. 2 Perceive that ADHD is a hoax or misunderstood by others. 3 ADHD cannot be understood until lived with. 4 ADHD does not equal dumb, lazy, or bad. 5 Hiding ADHD from others. 6 Havoc of day-to-day life. 7 Aggravation of simple activities of daily living. 8 ADHD's effect on parent. 9 Adjust life to accommodate ADHD. 10 Hopes, wishes and goals: • hope that he will outgrow it; • wish for a magic cure; • goals for the future. 11 Sources of support and information on ADHD: • books and the internet • faith in God. 12 Concern for what the future will hold: • What will the teen years hold? • Will he be a responsible and productive adult? *Symbolization of the stimulant* 1 Stimulation is an extra something. 2 Stimulant represents that there is a problem: • disappointment that it works; • denial and minimization. 3 You're just doping your child. 4 Realization that stimulant is not a magic cure.

continued

Table 3.1 Continued

Author and purpose	*Design*	*Data analysis*	*Sample information*	*Findings*
				Worth of functional value of stimulants 1 Makes a tremendous difference in child. 2 Helps manage turmoil in the home. 3 Assists parents to modify behavior problems. 4 Helps parent cope with ADHD. *Influences on parental decision making regarding stimulant therapy*
Cawley (2004) To investigate parents' experiences of raising a child diagnosed with ADHD.	In-depth multi-stage semi-structured interviews.	Theme analysis, then content analysis.	$N = 8$. 4 mothers and 4 fathers raising or having raised ADHD child ages 13–23. Parents white, middle- or lower-income; children white male. Child must have 1–4 siblings and live in 2-parent household. Recruited through advertisement and referrals.	• Stress in spousal relationship. • Lack of support from spouse. • Target of abuse from spouse. • Strained relationships with extended family. • Strained relationships with siblings. • Different developmental age at diagnosis. • Optimistic/pessimistic about future of child with ADHD. • Functioning of ADHD child. • Positive aspect from this parenting experience. • Struggles with school system for services. • Comorbidity of the ADHD child. • Disappointed in mental health professionals. • Regret yelling at their child with ADHD. • Fearful about future of child with ADHD. • Unhappy marriage.

Family

- Child with ADHD: appearance, affective behaviors, abuse of parents, criminal behavior, dangerous behaviors, addictive behaviors, child's stressed relationship with siblings.
- Family dynamics: availability of other parent, child with ADHD as focal point, stressed home, social isolation.

Effects

- Affective: loss, grief, depression, embarrassment, shame, guilt, frustration, unsafe, fearful, hypervigilance, alienation, loneliness, struggle, anger, burn-out.
- Behavioral: comparing with other parents, work dysfunction, addictive behaviors, somatic problems, physical/verbal violence.
- Cognitive effects.
- Self-esteem/self-confidence.
- Stressed social relationships.
- Failed expectations.
- Mixed results of therapy.

Coping: what helped?

- Getting a diagnosis.
- Medication.
- Support from spouse.
- Seeking help for own disorders.
- Acknowledgement from others.
- Physical distance.
- Personal traits.
- Work.
- Support groups.
- Sense of humor.
- Faith in God.

continued

Table 3.1 Continued

Author and purpose	*Design*	*Data analysis*	*Sample information*	*Findings*
				Coping: what was needed? • Education about disorder. • Support from professionals. • Support groups. • More effective therapy. • More resources. • More support, empathy, understanding from others. *Coping: what was the most hurtful part of raising a child with ADHD?*
Charach et al. (2006) To understand parents' opinions of ADHD medication.	3 focus groups of parents.	Phenomenology.	*N* = 17 mothers and fathers of 14 children ages 7–14 diagnosed with ADHD and having used stimulant medications	Acceptance of diagnosis and need for treatment is challenging for parents. Conflicting opinions and information on stimulant medications compound the difficulty of decision making concerning medications. Parents' decisions impacted by considerations of side effects, stigma, and child preference.
Charach et al. (2014) To explore parent and young adolescent feelings concerning ADHD medication.	24 in-depth interviews, 12 with teens and 12 with their parents.	Use of interpretist interactionist framework.	*N* = 12 adolescents ages 12–15 with ADHD.	Adolescents' views of ADHD were more complex than that of parents who tended to view ADHD as a disorder requiring treatment. Parent and adolescent feelings about medications were similar in that benefits were generally seen and side effects were a concern. Parents were also concerned with using medication only if needed and wanting children to reach their potential.

Chavarela (2009) To compare and contrast experiences of Mexican and Caucasian mothers raising boys diagnosed with ADHD.	Semi-structured interviews.	Qualitative analysis approach.	N = 6. Mothers of boys with ADHD: 3 Mexican, 3 Caucasian.	Both sets of mothers: • were accepting of the diagnosis; • were just as likely to implement the recommended treatment (they were all wary of using medication and had concerns over side effects); • were involved in assessment and treatment; • were aware of resources and used them to self-educate. *Themes* Both positive and negative experiences with healthcare and educational professionals. Concerns for their children's futures.
Clark and Lang (2012) "set out to examine how mothers describe what they consider to be the responsibilities and duties of mothering a child with ADD/ADHD in conversations with one another on the Internet" (p. 403).	Postings on blogs of mothers with children with ADHD.	Qualitative frame and discourse analysis.	421 posts by 165 posters on 3 blogs or boards on mothering with ADHD.	Mothers were emphatically behind medication.

continued

Table 3.1 Continued

Author and purpose	*Design*	*Data analysis*	*Sample information*	*Findings*
Coletti et al. (2012) To apply "social/cognitive theories to understanding and assessing parent attitudes toward initiating medication" and "factors influencing parent decisions to follow ADHD treatment recommendations" (p. 226).	5 focus groups.	Grounded theory and deductive analytic strategy.	$N = 27$. Parents or legal guardians who had children diagnosed with ADHD by a child psychiatrist in the outpatient clinic, and a recommendation for stimulant treatment.	Shared emotional reactions to living with a child with ADHD and trying to manage behaviors: • frustrating and heartbreaking; • self-blame and guilt; • difficult morning routine. Although claiming to be adherent, parents' narratives described them as being non-adherent with medications. Parents endorsed facilitators of medication (would result in functional gains for children, would help ensure child safety). Fear of side effects, personality changes, social norms that said medication was a cop out. Parents wanted to do everything they could behaviorally and holistically before they went to medication. Parents' perceptions of providers: • Parents liked providers who listened and who allowed collaboration in decision making. • They were adamant that they (parents) were the ultimate decision makers about their children taking medication. They liked providers who were conservative in terms of wanting to take medication slowly and in a sequenced way, and respected other behavioral treatments.

				• In terms of information provision from providers, some wanted a comprehensive approach whereas others wanted a more "comprehensible" (basic) approach. • Empathy and compassion were more important than expertise and experience.
Corimer (2012) To understand parent's medication decisions for their children with ADHD.	Semi-structured interviews.	Grounded theory.	*N* = 16. 13 mothers and 3 fathers of children with ADHD.	Parents turned to medication in an effort to restore stability to their family life. Parents note stress and exhaustion. Author notes parents go through an acceptance process in regards to medication.

Cronin (1995)
"To describe the relationship of the childhood conditions known as ADD and cystic fibrosis with mothers' reports of personal and family stress" (p. 3).
Cronin (2004)
To explore "how the type of hidden impairment in a child influences family routines and occupations" (p. 83).
	Open-ended interviews.	Grounded theory.	*N* = 45
			22 mothers of children with ADHD, 23 mothers of children with cystic fibrosis.
			ADHD mothers recruited from the Morris Center.
			Most mothers middle class.
				• Medication and social perception.
				• Challenges to mother's sense of well-being.
				• ADHD and the health care system.
				• Perception of antagonism by the healthcare establishment.
				• Adolescence and chronic disability.
				• Siblings and chronic disability.
				• Family demands.
				• Family resources:
				  • income;
				  • social-emotional support;
				  • health care support.
				• Family appraisal.
				• Making disability-related problems less visible to outsiders.
				• Maintaining a routine.

continued

Table 3.1 Continued

Author and purpose	*Design*	*Data analysis*	*Sample information*	*Findings*
				Frustrated with controversy around diagnosis, medication, and service for ADHD: • strained relationships with healthcare and school systems due to high demands and social sanctions; • persistently censured and challenged by others. Strong fear of being considered a bad mother. No such thing as a "normal" day – always on alert and didn't have normal routines: • stress of being constantly vigilant to keep child safe and out of trouble. Felt distress because their child didn't conform well to social standards. Expressed exhaustion in their role as mother: • often had to choose between meeting own needs and needs of child.
Claudius et al. (2011) To explore how families deal with and make decisions about treatment and care for their children with ADHD.	Semi-structured interviews.	Grounded theory.	*N* = 28 families with children diagnosed with ADHD.	Families preferred to be in charge of decision making (versus letting a professional make the treatment decisions). Families noted that ADHD caused challenges for child, in family relationships, and in family functioning. Caregivers reported negative effects on their physical and mental health. Increased marital and sibling conflict were noted.

				Also noted were effects on job, social relationships, as well as feelings of isolation within caregivers. Medication: parents initially were hesitant and had mixed feelings, but most were willing to try. Medications in general were felt to be helpful, but parents continued to have mixed feelings due to side effects and limits to benefits.

Dennis et al. (2008)
"To explore parents' and professionals' beliefs regarding the causes of ADHD and their perceptions of service providers" (p. 24).
	Focused groups, semi-structured interviews, and narrative interviews.	Thematic analysis.	Focus groups: $N = 46$.
			Semi-structured interviews: $N = 29$ (25 professionals, 5 volunteers).
			Narrative interviews: $N = 7$.
			Purposive sampling to get range of ages of children (6–14 years old) from two boroughs in north London:
			Borough A: $N = 30$,
			Borough B: $N = 16$ (mainly ethnic minority parents).
				Parents' views
				• Beliefs about ADHD: biological and social causes.
				• Ethnic minority mothers more likely to attribute ADHD to lack of cultural understanding.
				• Communication problems with professionals: lack of continuity of care.
				• Seeking help because of crisis with child.
				• Trial and error in parent management of ADHD: stimulant treatment, alternative strategies.
				• Impact on family:
				  • strain in parent-child relationship;
				  • resentment by siblings;
				  • marital conflict and tension;
				  • financial burden.
				• Support.
				Professionals' views
				• Provision of care.
				• Resources.

continued

Table 3.1 Continued

Author and purpose	*Design*	*Data analysis*	*Sample information*	*Findings*
dosReis et al. (2009) To determine parents' understanding of ADHD medication and how that influences their treatment decisions. dosReis et al. (2010) How do parents and their children experience mental health stigma? How do prior experiences of service use influence treatment of children with ADHD? Mychailyszyn et al. (2008) To examine how the perception of a diagnosis by African American mothers of children with ADHD impacts their use of clinical outpatient services. Larson et al. (2011) dosReis et al. (2007) To understand the process parents go through in recognizing need and seeking treatment for their child's ADHD.	Semi-structured telephone interviews.	Grounded theory used for data analysis.	$N = 48$. Parents of children newly diagnosed with ADHD. Recruited from inner city clinics. $N = 26$ (this was the earlier sample that was built upon in later studies). Parents were recruited from primary care, developmental, and mental health pediatric outpatient clinics affiliated with a large teaching hospital in Baltimore. Of the 26 parents, 22 (85%) were the child's biological parent and 20 (77%) were mothers.	Parents who felt medication was "unacceptable" were less likely to begin and continue medication use than other parents. Stigma: concerns with labeling, feelings of social isolation and rejection, perceptions of a dismissive society, influence of negative public views, exposure to negative media, and mistrust of medical assessments. Parents experienced caregiver strain as result of child's behavior. Range of understanding and acceptance of diagnosis by caregivers: • contemplating the origin: where did ADHD come from? • some thought that was just child's innate personality; • others still attributed behavior to other factors after diagnosis. • re-evaluating ability of child to control behaviors after diagnosis. Perception of responsibility and need to address ADHD varied: • some parents proactive; • some resistant or avoided addressing problems. Treatment beliefs influenced by past experiences/observations with medication: • some encouraged to seek treatment, others discouraged. Parents confused by conflicting societal advice on what course of action to take with child.

	Semi-structured telephone interviews.	Grounded theory.		Descriptions of the behavior: • placing the behavior in context; • making sense of the behavior; • seeing the effect of the behavior; • approaches to seeking information; • managing the behavior; • parents' vision for their child. Many parents identified their child's behavior as out of context for what was expected of peers their child's age. Described children as inattentive, unfocused, and distractible. Parents often experienced immediate resolution, pragmatic management, attributional ambivalence, and coerced conformance, during this phase. *Understanding* Parents reported believing that their children's behavior were due to genetics, medical issues, child development, something within them, prenatal drug or alcohol use, lead exposure, or early parenting practices. *Acceptance* Parents acknowledged their children needed help.

continued

Table 3.1 Continued

Author and purpose	*Design*	*Data analysis*	*Sample information*	*Findings*
DuCharme (1996) To examine parents' perceptions about raising a child with ADHD, including school experience, medical personnel, and family and social issues.	Phenomenological interviews.	Phenomenology.	N = 7. 7 parents selected from pool of 22 based on criteria: had adolescent with ADHD ages 12–19, from different ethnic, socioeconomic, educational, and geographic backgrounds. 5 women and 2 men, with 10 children diagnosed with ADHD (8 boys, 2 girls). Most middle class, 1 Hispanic, 7 white; living near large metro areas in southwest, midwest, and east US.	*Family issues* 1 Parent views regarding identification of ADHD: • initiation of process; • hearing the diagnosis. 2 Parent views of family interactions: • spouses, siblings, extended family members; • family routines. 3 Parent views of community interactions: • social activities, sports activities. *Medical issues* 1 Parent views of medical personnel: • confusion between medical and educational issues; • specialists vs. pediatricians; • difficulties obtaining qualified physicians. 2 Parent views on medication: • medication and dosages; • process of taking medication; • beliefs about medication. *Parenting issues* 1 Frustrations with raising a child with ADHD: • discipline: ability to follow directions, high risk behavior, removal from community; • difference in home and school behavior.

2 Parent views regarding their feelings:
   - helplessness, feeling blamed, fatigue, embarrassment, loneliness, grief.
3 Modifications to family routine:
   - lifestyle changes;
   - management of significant challenges;
   - inflexibility of child's thinking.
4 Parent views regarding their fears:
   - something bad could happen at anytime;
   - fear of the future.

Parent strategies

1 Views regarding child's academic strategies.
2 Personal strategies.
3 Parents' attitudinal and cognitive strategies:
   - maintaining a positive attitude;
   - picking their battles;
   - providing positive modeling;
   - being actively involved in child's life;
   - being proactive;
   - calming their own life;
   - continuing to try;
   - maintaining a long-term perspective;
   - possessing a disability perspective;
   - taking one day at a time.

School issues

1 School placement:
   - retention, service delivery model.
2 Transitions in school.
3 Parents' feelings when interacting with school personnel.

continued

Table 3.1 Continued

Author and purpose	*Design*	*Data analysis*	*Sample information*	*Findings*
Egbert (1996) To describe mothers' perceptions of parenting children with ADHD.	Unstructured interviews.	Thematic analysis.	$N = 6$. Mothers recruited from ADHD support group meetings with snowballing sampling. Mothers were over 30 and had more than 1 child; all white and working outside the home; wide range of socioeconomic levels. 9 ADHD children 6–19 years old: 3 girls, 6 boys.	*Realization something was wrong* • Problem behaviors. • School and academic problems. *Diagnosis gap* • Lack of recognition. • Parental conflict. • Blame. • Desperation. *The adjustment process* • Feelings of grief. • Feelings of regret. • Feelings of guilt. • Feelings of acceptance. *After a diagnosis* • Euphoria. • Behaviors often deteriorate. • Personal understandings. • Parenting strategies. *Feelings about the medication* • Starting the medication. • Adjusting the medication. • Stopping the medication. • Child's feelings about medication. *Frustration* • Misconceptions. • School. • Extended family. • Sibling, parenting, child's frustrations.

				This is forever • Extended parenting. • Worries and fears. *Advice for others* • Schools. • Healthcare providers. • Other mothers.
Firmim and Phillips (2009) (Replicates R. Segal's (1998) study of 17 Canadian families.) To explore the challenges parents face in rearing children with ADHD.	Narrative interviews.	Theme analysis.	*N* = 17 American families with at least one child possessing a clinical diagnosis of ADHD.	Parents showed a high level of involvement in their lives. Afternoon/evening is most difficult time of day for parents and children. Parents become innovative in helping their children complete necessary tasks. Routine is important. Structure is important.
Funes de Hernandez (2005) To understand the perspective of mothers raising children diagnosed with ADHD.	Open-ended interviews.	Hermeneutic phenomenological methodology with feminist perspective.	*N* = 12. Mothers of children with ADHD.	"Eight themes identified included silence, dealing with the 'invisible' disability, isolation, support, dealing with medical professionals, dealing with stressors, self-judgment, and reinventing of the self" (p. 81): • silence was due to stigma, ignorance, being judged as a failure as a mother due to child's ADHD/behavior; • mixed experience with helpfulness of both educational and health care professionals; • support was lacking socially and professionally; • concerns/guilt over medicating child; • "reinventing of the self" had to do with acceptance of the diagnosis and acceptance that having a child with ADHD did not mean that you were failure as a mother.

continued

Table 3.1 Continued

Author and purpose	*Design*	*Data analysis*	*Sample information*	*Findings*
Gerdes et al. (2014) To understand how Latino parents go about getting help for a child with symptoms of ADHD.	Qualitative questions asked after watching a video of a child with typical ADHD behaviors.	Use of grounded theory for data analysis.	*N* = 73 parents of children with ADHD between 5 and 12 years of age. 63% female parents. 90% Mexican descent. 80% annual family income of less than $40,000.	Study found that parents had a lack of knowledge concerning ADHD and found barriers to parents who wanted to access help. After watching video, 75% of parents blamed parents or family for child behaviors. Only 25% recommended use of mental health professional.
Goodwillie (2014) To explore the use of "protective vigilance" in parents of children diagnosed with ADHD.	Interviews.	Interpretive phenomenological analysis.	*N* = 6 families.	Parents reported that children needed "firmer boundaries, greater consistency and required more parental vigilance." The author called this need/behavior "protective vigilance" (p. 260) and stated that it should be considered a normal response to caregiving for an ADHD child. Parents described it as "emotionally and physically exhausting" (p. 264). One father noted: "They are a child that you have to watch all the time; I have to be ahead of him all the time; he doesn't think, he just does" (p. 261). Grandparents could provide important support, but were often unable to keep up with the ADHD child.

Gray Brunton et al. (2014) To explore how UK parents made sense of ADHD and what their own identities were post-diagnosis.	Semi-structured interviews.	Discourse analysis.	$N = 12$. 8 mothers, 4 fathers from UK. Recruited with purposive sampling through advertisement at local charity.	Believed ADHD explained by two repertoires: • biological-genetics; • social environmental/parenting influences. Both repertoires caused parents to experience self-blame and identity problems: • struggled with parental accountability; • uncomfortable with this model but didn't know how to explain ADHD in any other way. Medical diagnosis held limited value: • still viewed skeptically and controversially by others; • parents still struggled with accountability and responsibility for child's behavior.
Hallberg et al. (2008) To explore the main concern of being parents of teenage daughters diagnosed with ADHD.	Semi-structured interviews.	Grounded theory.	$N = 12$. All participants selected lived in western Sweden.	Strained life situation of parents with teenage daughters diagnosed with ADHD. Parents are exposed to long-term stress, which affects their physical and psychological health.
Hammerman (2000) To understand the impact on parents of having a child diagnosed with ADHD.	Semi-structured interviews.	Phenomenology.	$N = 8$ families. Children 5–10 years old, equal number of boys and girls. Snowball sampling. Caucasian families from New York City area, variety of social classes.	1 Parents' views on parenting and expectations. 2 Adjusting to parenthood. 3 Current expectations for child with ADHD: • want child to be happy and fulfill their potential. 4 Recognition of child's difficulties: • knew there was a problem since child's birth; • knew they were different from other children.

continued

Table 3.1 Continued

Author and purpose	*Design*	*Data analysis*	*Sample information*	*Findings*
				5 Getting a diagnosis: • kept trying to find out why child was having so many difficulties; • trying alternate solutions; • diagnosed and undiagnosed ADHD in parents. 6 Response to diagnosis: • difficulty accepting it; • relief and hopeful; • worried about having to use medication; • frustration when medication doesn't work; • confusion from dealing with professionals; • initial guilt and responsibility for diagnosis. 7 Gender of child: • easier because of child's gender; • would be easier if child was different gender; • more difficult because of child's gender; • influence of gender on how parent interacts with child. 8 Child's behavior: • difficulty dealing with extreme behavior; • exhausted and frustrated from dealing with behavior; • behavior becoming more challenging as child gets older.

9 Child's peer relationships and response to authority:
- positive interactions;
- negative interactions;
- difficulty disciplining child.

10 Child's impact on close personal relationships:
- limits relationships;
- hiding that child has ADHD from others;
- no impact or positive impact;
- difficulty finding babysitters.

11 Impact on relationships with extended family:
- more difficult due to family's lack of understanding of ADHD;
- family relationships improve as child's behavior improves.

12 Impact on nuclear family relationship:
- limit family activities and less time for other children.

13 Impact on career choice:
- limits career choice;
- positive impacts on job.

14 Role of mother:
- mother feeling positive or negative about performance;
- mother experiencing effects of ADHD most because of primary caretaking role.

15 Role of father:
- positive or negative;
- not available enough to care for child.

continued

Table 3.1 Continued

Author and purpose	*Design*	*Data analysis*	*Sample information*	*Findings*
				16 Impact on parents' self-perception. 17 Impact on marital relationships: • lack of support from spouse; • strain on marriage, less time for each other. 18 Parental stress: • constant demands; • financial stress. 19 Professional support: • difficulty getting diagnosis; • difficulty finding right provider. 20 Educational planning: • constant need for advocacy and monitoring of child. 21 Need for more services.
Hancock (2003) The primary focus of this study is an examination of effects of a son's ADHD on the mother-son dyad.	Individual interview.	Theme analysis.	*N* = 9. 9 mothers ranging in age from 28 to 45 years. Two terms require definition for present study: "single parent" and "attention deficit hyperactivity disorder." Sons of research participants must have a diagnosis of ADHD in order to participate in the study. Diagnosis must be based on DSM-IV criteria.	*Themes* 1 Pre-treatment years. 2 Receiving help support, and services. 3 Mothers' intrapersonal experience. 4 Mothers' interpersonal experience. 5 Mothers' perceptions of the intrapersonal experience of their sons. 6 Mothers' perceptions of the interpersonal experience of their sons. 7 Parenting issues. 8 Other struggles and issues. 9 Mother/son relationship. 10 Family and role models. 11 Moving forward.

Hansen and Hansen (2006) To explore parent's perceptions of and everyday experiences with medication used to treat ADHD.	Semi-structured interviews.	Theme analysis.	$N = 10$ families. Canadian Parents. Method: convenience sampling. Recruitment: from the Community Research Ethics Board; two cities. Demographics: 10 families, children 8–22 years old, 9 boys, 2 girls, parents (29–56 years old).	Dilemma: balancing act/side effects. Dilemma: termination of treatment. Desirable and undesirable effects. Role of medication in child's future. Everyday experiences/daily life: how medication affects it.
Harborne et al. (2004) To investigate the individual experiences of parents directly affected by having children with ADHD, and how they make sense of different aetiological models.	Semi-structured interviews.	Grounded theory.	$N = 10$. 9 mothers, 1 father of boys 8–11 years old, all British. Participants recruited by letters sent to families selected from a Child Development Centre database.	Discrepancy about disorder: some parents believed it was biologically based, while others considered it due to psychological and social factors. 1 Battled with family members and professionals. 2 Felt blamed by them because of child's behavior. 3 Experienced emotional distress due to differing views they had to battle against.

continued

Table 3.1 Continued

Author and purpose	*Design*	*Data analysis*	*Sample information*	*Findings*
Himmel (2013) To gain insight into parents' perceptions and experiences about their children diagnosed with ADHD, the ADHD diagnosis, and to determine if single sex education has an effect on ADHD symptoms.	Personal interview.	Questionnaire, and field notes.	N = 9. Purposive sampling. Child that that has been medically diagnosed with ADHD and who has participated in the Scouting program in the last two years. Participants were recruited from the Two Bay Scouting organization and sent an email of interest; those who responded were selected based on the inclusion criteria (as above). Demographics of participants: 4 female, 5 male; 7 white, 1 Asian, 1 Native American; all 9 married.	*Common themes* Lack of focus in school (67%). Lack of focus towards simple instruction (100%). Communication problems (33%). Emotional instability (22%). Impaired social skills (44%). *Common themes among diagnoses* Ambiguity (33%). Pressure from educators (22%). Personal guilt (44%). Medication was treatment method used by 100% of participants, with 67% reporting positive results and 22% reporting treatment was ineffective. Common themes of parental experiences of ADHD children within the school system reported: • 22% as feeling the teachers went the extra mile; • 33% reported negative experiences; • 44% were indifferent; • 89% parents reported their children struggled academically, homework was a source of stress for 44%; • 89% reported advantages to single sex education; • 78% felt that the pseudo-educational setting served as a better learning environment; • 44% felt that the male leaders provided an advantage towards engaging the boys of the program.

Ho et al. (2011) To explore Chinese parents' experiences of caregiving to a child with ADHD at home.	Semi-structured interviews.	Theme analysis.	$N = 12$. Purposeful sampling. Parents caring for a child with ADHD residing at home. 2 parents were fathers, 10 were mothers. Ages ranged from 35 to 46, with a median of 38.5 years.	Concept of ADHD: • limited understanding of ADHD; • sources of knowledge about ADHD. Barriers to childcare in ADHD: • great difficulties encountered in childcare; • care-giving burden; • limited resources or means to get support; • ambivalence to follow medication regimen. Psychological effects in care-giving: • a bundle of negative feelings; • feelings of anger and hostility; • feelings of abandonment and discrimination. Positive aspects of care-giving: • gains from care-giving experiences; • personal growth through care-giving process.
Howard (1993) "To explore the parental perception of the impact of an ADD child on the marital and family functioning" (p. vi).	Open-ended interviews.	Thematic analysis.	$N = 30$ couples. Requirement that couple be in an intact marriage and biological parents of child 6–12 years old in public school system; couple has at least 1 other child. Couples from north central Texas, most recruited through child and adolescent psychiatric clinic. Families all white, most middle to upper-middle class. Children: 22 males, 8 females.	1 Effect on marriage: • positive effects; • negative effects; • effect of diagnosis on marriage. 2 View of parenting: • stress and frustration. 3 Sibling relations: • unaffected by ADD. 4 Family interaction. 5 Family schedule: • problems getting ADD child up in morning or to bed at night; • helping ADD child complete homework. 6 Changes in family due to ADD diagnosis of child. 7 Impact on family closeness.

continued

Table 3.1 Continued

Author and purpose	*Design*	*Data analysis*	*Sample information*	*Findings*
Jackson and Peters (2008) To understand the feelings of mothers of children with ADHD in relation to stimulant medication use.	Interviews.	Thematic analysis.	$N = 11$ mothers of children with ADHD	Parents expressed ambivalence in relation to use of stimulant medications. Noted were feelings of confusion and concerns over stigma.
Kay (2007) To look at how parents make decisions about using medication to treat their latency age children diagnosed with ADHD.	Semi-structured interviews.	Grounded theory: dimensional analysis.	$N = 14$ mothers of children who began medication treatment between ages 5 and 12, in California; 12 white, 2 Asian; most upper-middle class. Purposeful convenience sampling. Children: 13 boys, 1 girl; 6 still taking stimulant medication.	*Getting best fit for child specific to school setting* Parental context: • perspective of party of treatment (parents, doctors, teachers); • parents doing what's right for "my" child; • personal qualities of the child; • parental assessment of intellectual abilities; • child not getting along with other kids/not fitting in; • public vs. private school setting. Impact on parental actions: • relationship of parent with teacher; • stigma of diagnosis; • parent having no choice/feeling pressured. Parental treatment processes: • requesting and making modifications; • learning curves; • making tradeoffs.

				Other themes • Cluster of symptomatic behaviors that brought child's problems to adult's attention. • Prompt for evaluation for parents. • Parents' acceptance of/agreement with diagnosis. • Older children "finding their own way": making own decisions about treatment. • Parent perspectives towards treatment varied widely.
Kendall (1998) To understand the process parents of children with ADHD go through from struggling with disorder through accepting.	2 individual and 2 family interviews.	Grounded theory.	*N* = 59 people from 15 families. Purposive sampling from advertisements at clinics, schools, and other community organizations. 1/3 single-parent; most middle or upper-middle socioeconomic status, except for 3 single-parent poor.	Disruptive behaviors described. Constant disruption. Parents maintained control over situation by making sense, recasting biography, and letting go of the good ending. Through this process, they ended up with letting go of the idea of the normal child and recasting biography (considering their own lives in light of ADHD they experienced, grieving, parents individuating from their children instead of remaining in enmeshment).

continued

Table 3.1 Continued

Author and purpose	*Design*	*Data analysis*	*Sample information*	*Findings*
Kilcarr (1996) "To examine the relationship that exists between the father and his son who has ADHD" (Abstract)	Phone interviews.	Thematic and metathematic analysis.	*N* = 16 fathers. Upper-middle class (average income $210,000), 14 white and 2 middle-eastern; recruited through developmental pediatrician's private practice in Washington D.C. area. Half of fathers self-identified own signs of ADHD. Average age of son 8 years, 7 months.	*Metathemes* 1 Difficulty of decision to use medication for father: • continue to question decision and long-term effects of medication even after positive results with it. 2 Impact of father's awareness of son's development: • profound impact on how father interacts and supports son; • correlation between father's knowledge of impact of ADHD on son's development and his emotional support for son. 3 ADHD behavior strategies greatest challenge for fathers: • context of medication use; • context of maturation of father and son; • fathers' agreement about most effective way to limit problematic behaviors. 4 Ability of son to control behavior: • fathers understood sons' ability to control behavior consistently; • still had varying levels of ambivalence about what son could control/not control.

5. School interactions:
   - fathers' recognition of vital role of school and academics in addressing ADHD issues;
   - school important in fostering and developing positive self-esteem in son.
6. Family structure:
   - role of family structure in establishing sense of security and safety in son.
7. Impact of father's family history and development:
   - profound effect on father's interaction with son;
   - fathers' relating with sons' struggles because of feeling of responsibility to work with them.
8. Lack of rational action with ADHD in fathers:
   - despite education about managing ADHD, fathers still reported times of intolerance and impatience;
   - effect on son's emotional eruption.
9. Sons' inability to consistently attend to relevant information:
   - pervasive problem for fathers;
   - creates large amount of stress and worry for fathers.
10. Lack of agreement between couple about how to handle ADHD behaviors:
    - causes stress, poor communication, and increasing difficulties in spouses' relationship.

continued

Table 3.1 Continued

Author and purpose	*Design*	*Data analysis*	*Sample information*	*Findings*
Klasen (2000) To examine "the experience of parents and doctors dealing with hyperactive children, focusing in particular on the process of medicalization" (p. 334). Klasen and Goodman (2000) "To investigate the views that parents and GPs hold about hyperactivity, and to explore how far these views, and clashes between these views, influence access to services" (p. 199).	Semi-structured interviews.	Grounded hermeneutic theory.	$N = 39$. Purposive sampling: to include wide range of parent views about what hyperactivity meant and variety of social groups. 10 general practitioners (GPs). Mothers in all cases, fathers also in 1/3, all from UK.	Created profound sense of alienation for parents. Affects family and social roles and parents' perceptions of their parental and social roles. Medicalization helped to validate and legitimize parents' experiences – gave them more control and improved parent-child relationships. *Theme 1: Is hyperactivity a mental disorder?* • Parents report and GPs seem to confirm that often doctors don't believe it's a real medical problem. • Referrals to specialist often determined by persistence of parents. *Theme 2: Is labeling disabling or enabling?* • Parents generally viewed it positively; relieved guilt and helped connect them to resources; improved parent-child relationships. • Most GPs believed it did more harm than good – attempt by parents to avoid dealing with parenting shortcomings.

				Theme 3: Is hyperactivity the cause or effect of family dysfunction? • Most GPs saw it as result of dysfunctional families. • Parents saw it as the cause of stress and dysfunction in family. Hyperactivity starts earlier in child's life than services are available for. Information on hyperactivity often conflicting and ambiguous: • GPs untrained/unknowledgeable about disorder; • needed specialist backup services not available.
Lai and Ma (2014) To identify subjective experiences of Chinese parents/caregivers of children diagnosed with ADHD.	Focus groups.	Family interviews/ parent narratives.	$N = 24$. All participants were caregivers. 5 fathers, 15 mothers, 1 grandmother, and 3 caregivers from 21 families.	Parents being alarmed by the teacher. Judging by child's defying and inattentive behavior, parents suspected child might have problems, which was later confirmed by teacher's assessment at school. 1 Long waiting period of our mental health service. 2 Insufficient informational and service support. 3 Academically oriented education system. 4 Lack of understanding from service providers as well as teachers. They felt disappointed, depressed, powerless, and socially isolated. They could hardly share their parenting difficulty with parents of non-problem children, their friends, and relatives.

continued

Table 3.1 Continued

Author and purpose	*Design*	*Data analysis*	*Sample information*	*Findings*
Leslie et al. (2007) To examine family perspectives about treatment decision making for their child with ADHD.	Structured in-depth interviews.	Theme analysis.	$N = 8$. Recruited from San Diego ADHD Project (SANDAP). Purposeful sampling. At least 5 families enrolled from each of four racial/ethnic/cultural groups. Distributed range of socioeconomic status. Child recently diagnosed with ADHD or had previous diagnosis and up for re-evaluation. Children between ages of 6 and 15 years. Male children (79%).	Families perspectives on causes of child's ADHD symptoms: • internal factors to child: genetics, cognitive style; • external factors: trauma history, family separation, environmental stressors; • mixed factors: developmental perspective. Impact of child's symptoms: • impact on family (caretakers' well-being, relationships, jobs); • impact on child (school and social functioning, self-esteem, behavior problems); • impact on logistics (access to school/medical services frustrations, frequent driving to doctors). Treatment goals and preferences: • intervention acceptance consistent with ADHD guidelines; • less scientific interventions (nutrition, supportive counseling, faith-based methods).

Lewis-Morton et al. (2014) To explore how 4 families in the process of an ADHD diagnosis negotiated competing explanations of the problem.	Semi-structured interviews.	Discursive analysis: discourse and conversational analysis.	$N = 4$ families. Children had been referred to Child and Adolescent Mental Health Services (CAMHS) for assessment. Families of children 6–18 years old recruited from CAMHS to participate.	Psychosocial explanations: • family dynamics: minimizing problems at home; comparison with siblings; • school context: positive; not cause of problems. Discipline vs. other response: • self-responsibility: illness vs. naughtiness. Biological/genetic explanations: • genetic inheritance. Explorations prior to a diagnosis: • families gradually eliminated other possible causes until arriving at ADHD. Balancing discipline and attachment needs: discipline vs. comfort.
Lin et al. (2009) To understand the experiences of primary caregivers who are raising school-aged children with ADHD.	Individual interviews.	Theme analysis.	$N = 12$. Purposeful sampling. Participants had to be major caregivers of school-aged children with clinically diagnosed ADHD.	Theme 1: Burdens of caring. Theme 2: Lack of sufficient support systems. Theme 3: Mechanisms of coping.

continued

Table 3.1 Continued

Author and purpose	*Design*	*Data analysis*	*Sample information*	*Findings*
Litt 2004 "To explore health related carework of low-income women caregivers of special needs children" (p. 625).	Semi-structured interviews. 3 themes: • medical issues related to child's disability; • interactions with service providers; • effect of carework on caregivers' lives.	Theme analysis.	*N* = 15. Caregivers from central Iowa from households at 200% of poverty line with at least 1 child with special needs. 11 single mothers; 14 white, 1 latino; 10 unemployed; 7 received cash assistance. 24 children with disability, 15 with ADHD. Recruited through letters to Area Education Agency clients and advertisement at Supplemental Security Income (SSI) outreach program	Direct carework challenges. Difficult relationship with service providers: • fear of child being taken away/being charged with child abuse/neglect. Medication: benefits of and intensive level of care to administer/monitor. Challenges of advocacy. Economic challenges: managing care of child with new regulations/requirements to work; cut in public benefits.

Martinez (2015) "To qualitatively examine the extent that culture and acculturation within an ecological system impact the process of obtaining treatment for mothers with children diagnosed with ADHD" (p. 2).	Semi-structured interviews.	Interpretive phenomenological analysis.	N = 10. Recruited through convenience and snowball sampling in Hartford Co., CT. All participants' primary language was Spanish; 8 were single mothers; average education tenth grade; average residency in US 11 years.	1 Maintaining individual cultural identity: • balancing Puerto Rican identity while embracing Euro-American culture to meet needs of children. 2 Preserving familial cultural identity: • ensuring children kept their Puerto Rican identity within Euro-American culture. 3 Assessing ADHD: • teachers' observations contribute to initial contact with professionals to assess child for ADHD. 4 Language barriers: • language can become barrier when seeking treatment. 5 Stigmatization: • having child with ADHD can lead to feelings of being stigmatized for mothers. 6 Support services: • ensuring child receives support services despite obstacles; • impact of cultural differences on services. 7 Treatment utilization: • psychotherapy treatment utilization was prominent in comparison to use of medication to address symptoms of ADHD. 8 Trust in providers: • mental health care providers' Spanish language abilities not a necessity, but a preference that helped to enhance trust.

continued

Table 3.1 Continued

Author and purpose	*Design*	*Data analysis*	*Sample information*	*Findings*
McIntyre and Hennessy (2012) To explore experiences of parents of male children with ADHD in Ireland.	Individual open-ended interviews.	Theme analysis.	*N* = 18. Parents of 7–12-year-old boys with diagnosis of ADHD. 13 mothers, 2 mother–father dyads, and 1 mother–grandmother dyad.	1 Getting your head around ADHD. 2 The child takes over. 3 Emotional impact. 4 Inconsistency of structural supports. 5 Ignorance and discrimination. 6 It's not all bad.
Mills (2011) To investigate the experiences and decision making processes of families deciding about medication treatment for children with ADHD diagnoses.	Semi-structured interviews.	Constant comparative analysis, then open and axial coding.	*N* = 19 families. Randomly selected from convenience sample. 30 children with ADHD: 17 (57%) male, 13 (43%) female; 11 (37%) not medicated, 19 (63%) medicated. 1 father, 16 mothers interviewed individually; 2 couples interviewed together.	No differences in decision making process of families medicating, not medicating, and mixture of both. • Parent guilt and self-blame. • Media influence on decision making. • Hesitation and resistance to medication. • Attempting other interventions before turning to diagnosis. • Difficulty getting a diagnosis. • Diagnosis equivalent to medication. • Effectiveness of medication. • Quality of life for child. • Quality of life-family stress. • Marital/gender issues. • Concerns/doubts about decision. • Feeling judged.

Moen et al. (2011) Moen et al. (2014) To gain insight into Norwegian families lived experiences with children diagnosed with ADHD.	Individual interviews.	Phenomenology.	*N* = 9. 5 mothers, 4 fathers. 3 participants were single parents. Have at least 1 child with ADHD diagnosis for at least 1 year. Members of Norwegian ADHD Association	"Contending and adapting every day – windsurfing in unpredictable waters." "Maintaining the self and parenthood, interacting with the social network." 1 Safeguarding a functioning family: • managing daily life: family life steered by child's difficulties, need for structure and routine, relationship between siblings and ADHD child; • developing special skills: continual process; • becoming an adult. 2 Fighting for acceptance and inclusion: • sharing vs. being alone with responsibility; • when to seek help for problems; • interacting socially: source of conflict for child.
Morse (2002) To explore the experiences and feelings of low-income, minority primary caretakers of children with ADHD.	Structured interviews.	Coding (Miles & Huberman model).	*N* = 7. Caretakers from New York City, recruited through purposive sampling from outpatient child and adolescent local hospital. *N* = 6 black, *N* = 1 Hispanic. *N* = 5 birth mothers, *N* = 1 adoptive father, *N* = 1 adoptive mother. All caretakers currently single; *N* = 4 income under £25,000.	*Themes* 1 Frustration: • child's attention seeking behavior; • routine activities like shopping; • dealing with effects of child's behavior; • difficulty setting limits. 2 Isolation: • parents as outsiders. 3 Acceptance and support of ADHD child: • expressions of love and empathy. 4 Connectedness: • family relationships; • peer relationships. 5 Support received from others: • limited but intense.

continued

Table 3.1 Continued

Author and purpose	*Design*	*Data analysis*	*Sample information*	*Findings*
				6 Anger: • child's behavior; • reactions from others about child's behavior; • interactions with educational community; • intrusion by foster care; • responses of psychiatric community.
	Semi-structured interviews.	Grounded theory.	*N* = 34. Parents of children diagnosed with ADHD within 1 month of study, recruited through clinicians in Baltimore. Children 6–18 years old, 88% black (*N* = 30).	Making sense of diagnosis: • forming opinions about ADHD; • contemplating the origin: where did ADHD come from? • re-evaluating ability of child to control behaviors after diagnosis. Conceptualization of an ADHD diagnosis: • medical label vs. general problem vs. rejecting that it was an illness. Implications for treatment of childhood ADHD: • medical label: viewed origin of problem as biological, more likely to continue treatment; • general problem: mixed view of origins of problem, only one-half continued treatment; • rejected ADHD as an illness: mixed view of origin, all continued to seek treatment.

Neophytou and Webber (2005) "To explore the effects on mothers of boys diagnosed with ADHD" (p. 313).	Personal interviews – 5 over 3-month period with various family members. Teachers interviewed twice.	Thematic analysis.	*N* = 3 families. Male children with recent diagnosis who were being treated with Ritalin, all age 9 at start of study. Convenience sampling from major hospital in Australia. In all families parents separated before diagnosis; mothers were primary caretakers (age late twenties–early thirties).	1 Effects on mother prior to diagnosis: • very difficult time, especially social events; • feelings of confusion, embarrassment, self-doubt; • used isolation and avoidance to cope. 2 The diagnosis process: • initiated by teachers; • medication presented as only solution; • reactions of relief. 3 Medication: • results of medication: boys' behavior improved, alleviated stress and pressure felt by mothers; • 3 reservations: • dosage levels; • parenting confidence/competence; • side effects: caused them to stop using medication at times. 4 Reaction of children: • disliked/felt stigmatized by ADHD label; • negative self-image as result of diagnosis.

continued

Table 3.1 Continued

Author and purpose	*Design*	*Data analysis*	*Sample information*	*Findings*

Okafor (2006)
To explore how Puerto Rican mothers experience having a child with ADHD.
	Focus groups and in-depth interviews.	Thematic and contextual analysis using eco-cultural approach.	$N = 15$.
			Focus groups recruited through Latino parent education and advocacy organization in Hartford, CT; 10 families recruited for in-depth interviews from focus groups.
			All mothers born in Puerto Rico, with family income below 300% of poverty line.
			All children on medication for at least 6 months.
				Focus group themes
				• Mothers' perceptions of child having difficult time behaving.
				• Mothers' challenges and personal sacrifices:
				  • sacrificing jobs, personal relationships, relationships with other children;
				  • separation from spouse;
				  • lack of family cohesiveness;
				  • feelings of depression, guilt, pain, faith, and hope.
				• Mothers see strengths when children behave positively.
				• Mothers see child weaknesses as product of ADHD disability and not their personality.
				• Mothers' belief that child's behaviors are abnormal and greatly affect child's ability to learn and function well.
				• Variety of ways that children were diagnosed.
				Mothers make significant accommodations to:
				• parent child with ADHD;
				• have good and supportive relationships at home;
				• work and keep a job;
				• obtain childcare and/or recreational activities;
				• go to grocery store, church, public events, and to visit families and friends;
				• have their children in school;
				• visit the doctor's office.

Oquendo (2013) To understand the perspective of Latino mothers raising sons with ADHD.	Semi-structured interviews.	Grounded theory.	$N = 11$ Latino mothers of sons with ADHD.	*Themes* • Authoritative, mother-driven parenting style. • Mother/son relationship positive with empathy. • Process of acceptance/some shame involved. • Mothers accepted help and advocated for child. • Support was lacking.
Parker (1994) To reveal meaning of experience of parenting a child with ADHD.	Open-ended interviews.	Hermeneutic phenomenology.	$N = 6$. Purposive sampling of 4 mothers and 2 fathers (5 children male, 1 female) from a parent support group in southern US.	1 Early awareness by parent that something was different/wrong with child: • by age 3 most parents suspected that child was not going to be normal; • struggles coming to terms with awareness that child was disabled. 2 Parenting has been difficult and challenging: • extreme feelings of frustration, anger, disappointment, and fatigue. 3 A wonderful/horrible child with very inconsistent and extreme behavior: • opposite behavior in different settings like home vs. school. 4 Parents feeling helpless, hopeless, and like a failure due to criticism from self and others: • decision to use medication; • resistance of children to taking medication; • stigma for child of taking medication. 5 Parents' fear of what future will hold for child.

continued

Table 3.1 Continued

Author and purpose	*Design*	*Data analysis*	*Sample information*	*Findings*
Perry et al. (2005) To explore how Latino parents managed their child's ADHD within the sociocultural context of their everyday lives.	Semi-structured interviews.	Theme analysis.	$N = 24$. Convenience sampling of Latino parents with a child with ADHD. 13 Latino parents were born in Mexico. Most had lived in the United States for 14 years. All families had a child between 6 and 19 years.	1 Finding out about ADHD. 2 Taking on a biomedical meaning. 3 Living between two cultures. 4 Caring for a child with ADHD. 5 Looking toward the future with ADHD.
Peters and Jackson (2009) To look at experience of mothering a child with ADHD.	In-depth interviews.	Feminist theory.	$N = 11$. Recruited via media release and snowball sampling. Mothers who were primary caretakers of child with ADHD diagnosis from New South Wales, Australia. Children 3–15 years old; 10 male, 1 female. 4 single mothers, 7 in relationship with child's father.	1 Caring responsibility is overwhelming: • demands unrelenting, frustrating, and difficult; • negatively impacted mother's life – social isolation; • lacked care support from partner, school, other professionals. 2 Being stigmatized, scrutinized, criticized: • ADHD diagnosis poorly understood by others; • some mothers concealed diagnosis because of negative perceptions of it, or wished they had concealed it. 3 Guilt and self-blame: • feelings of self-blame exacerbated by perception of others; • feared for social exclusion of child; • alienated from immediate/extended family.

				4 Mother as advocate: • needed to act as advocate for child for medical treatment; • difficult to gain definitive diagnosis and right treatment; • have to work closely with teachers to get needs met in schools.
Rice (1995) "To investigate the impact of ADHD on the psychosocial functioning of three children and their families" (p. 2).	Case studies.	Grounded theory.	N = 3 families. 2 in Australia, 1 in US. Purposive sampling in multi-site settings. David: 7 years old, lived in North Carolina; home-schooled by mother; parents very religious. Kate: lived in Queensland, 7 years old, diagnosed with ADHD but not taking medication. Bruce: lived in Queensland, 14 years old; not yet officially diagnosed with ADHD when study began.	1 Adjustment of family to child with ADHD: • stages of acceptance of condition; • grief/sense of loss at not having a "normal" child; • non-acceptance of condition by family and friends; • misdiagnosis by professionals. 2 Child with ADHD and parenting stress: • coping with hyperactive child; • concern for child being more susceptible to other health problems; • adverse social interactions between parent and child; • unsatisfactory experiences with medical and educational professionals; • professionals' lack of knowledge. 3 Diagnostic assessment process from parents' perspective: • stress of diagnostic process for parents; • impact of parents' values and beliefs in diagnostic process.

continued

Table 3.1 Continued

Author and purpose	*Design*	*Data analysis*	*Sample information*	*Findings*
				4 Parental views of drug intervention: • parents accepted medication under duress; • incomplete information about medication side effects; • short-term effects of medication; • influence of media on parents' perception about medication.
Seawell (2010) "To gain a greater knowledge of how families understand their child once a diagnosis of ADHD has been identified" (p. ii).	Semi-structured interviews.	Grounded theory.	*N* = 6 families. Purposive criterion and maximum variation sampling from large Texas metro area to obtain heterogeneity in sample. 4 single-parent households, 2 children being raised by grandparent/s; 2 families black, 2 white, 1 Jamaican American, 1 Hispanic. Children: 4 boys, 2 girls; 8–12 years old.	*Parent themes* 1 Diagnosis of ADHD provided relief and understanding for families and decreased their sense of guilt, blame and confusion. 2 Diagnosis of ADHD shifted view of their child from that of problem child to child with ADHD. 3 Diagnosis helped families learn and seek knowledge, and find access to intervention: • having name for what was going on helped families learn how to deal with it and know what to do. 4 Prior to diagnosis many families had sense of frustration: • didn't understand or know how to deal with what was happening. 5 Access to treatment and intervention made biggest change. 6 Problems were seen more at school or daycare than at home.

				7 Diagnosis of ADHD not seen as a big deal: • not surprised by diagnosis; • not resistant to ADHD label. *Themes for children* 1 Child's interpretation and description of ADHD as "hyper," "energy," or "crazy." 2 Diagnosis of ADHD helped them understand why they behaved the way they did. 3 People understood or treated them differently after they got the ADHD diagnosis.
Segal, E. (1994) To explore mothers' experiences of parenting a child with ADHD. Segal, E. (2001) To gain understanding of the experience of mothers raising children with ADHD.	Interviews.	Grounded theory.	*N* = 25. Participants recruited from ChADD in Chicago area. All mothers had some college education, 25% had advanced degrees; all white and middle to upper-middle class. 38 children with ADHD (31 males, 7 females): 15 mothers with 1 ADHD child, 7 with 2 ADHD children, 3 with 3 ADHD children	*Pre-diagnosis* 1 Mothers being at their wits end with child: • not being able to discipline child/change child's behavior; • child needing constant attention/ demanding care. 2 Knowledge that something was wrong: • feelings of responsibility for child's behavior. 3 Seeking answers: • no-delay mothers: sought help/diagnosis very quickly; • short-delay mothers: experienced a few years of child's behavior before seeking help; • long-delay mothers: long process of getting diagnosis; • lack of information/professional knowledge about ADHD.

continued

Table 3.1 Continued

Author and purpose	*Design*	*Data analysis*	*Sample information*	*Findings*
				After diagnosis 1 Universal feelings of relief for mothers. 2 Better understanding and acceptance of child's behavior. 3 Feelings of grief and loss for no-delay and short-delay mothers. 4 Diagnosis coming too late to help long-delay mothers. *Learning to mother* 1 A difficult child: affects every facet of family life. 2 Daily living is strained for mothers: • isolation; • tied to the house; • marital stress; • family size limited; • attitudes of extended family. 3 Mothers unknowing: blundering through parenting: • being on their own; • keeping relationship with child. 4 Mothers knowing: doing the "work": • acquiring knowledge/information; • structuring child's activities; • constantly having to monitor child; • battling the schools; • finding the necessary resources. 5 Present feelings about children.

6 Wishing it could have been different.
7 Guarded optimism.

Life has changed

1 Different road of parenting:
- not what mother was planning on/anticipating;
- an invisible handicap;
- always on duty;
- a never ending job;
- the grief doesn't end.

2 Coming to terms:
- managing the burden;
- reframing what life is about;
- these were the cards I was dealt.

3 Being stretched beyond belief:
- changed sense of self;
- it takes a whole village to raise child.

"No-delay" mothers: Had young children who were appropriately diagnosed. Mothers were able to access help and information.

"Long-delay" mothers: Mothers of older children who were raised during a time when less information was available on ADHD. These mothers had increased problems with misinformation and lack of appropriate assistance.

Both groups experienced stress and grief due to the ADHD.

continued

Table 3.1 Continued

Author and purpose	*Design*	*Data analysis*	*Sample information*	*Findings*
Segal, R. (1998) To understand how families with children with ADHD adapt their daily routines to enable child's occupational competence. Segal, R. (2000) To explore strategies used by mothers of children with ADHD to complete daily tasks. Segal and Frank (1998) To examine how families with ADHD children work to construct daily afternoon schedules.	Personal interviews.	Grounded theory.	N = 17 families. Recruited from ADHD support groups in southern California. Had to have ADHD child ages 6–11 and be able to communicate in English. 12 2-parent families (only 3 fathers participated), 5 single-mother families.	Getting to school and work on time: • used enabling strategies; • morning routine adaptations; • difficult time for parents. Doing homework while child can concentrate: • enabling strategies and routine adaptations in afternoon. Three strategies used by mothers to complete tasks while caregiving for child with ADHD: 1 "Enfolding": • multitasking. 2 "Temporal unfolding": • breaking tasks into smaller pieces, some of which can be completed at a later time. 3 "Unfolding by inclusion": • breaking tasks into smaller pieces, some of which can be completed by another individual. Strategies selected based on available funds and help. Mothers using these strategies had to choose which tasks would be completed each day and which would go undone.

				Organizing afternoon schedule: • homework: in relation to child's medication schedule; • dinner: so that family could all eat together regardless of child's schedule; • free time: only after child finishes homework/chores – incentive for child. Similarity of family schedules and effect of shared culture on schedules.
Sikirica et al. (2015) "To explore the unmet needs of children/ adolescents with ADHD and their caregivers in eight European countries" (p. 269).	Semi-structured interviews.	Theme analysis.	N = 66. Caregivers: 74% female; 30% shared caregiver role with partner; 52% employed. Children/adolescents: 66% male; mean age 11.9. 38 caregivers of children ages 6–17, 28 caregivers of adolescents ages 13–17. Recruited from online panels families had signed up for. Families from France, Germany, Italy, Netherlands, Norway, Spain, Sweden, and UK.	*Unmet needs* 1 Difficulties with diagnosis: process was difficult. 2 ADHD symptoms still present even with medication, only partially effective. 3 Difficulties with school and psychosocial functioning. 4 Difficulties with home and family life: very demanding for parents. 5 Treatment concerns with using medication: personality changes and side effects. 6 Impact on caregivers: stressful, worried about child's future.

continued

Table 3.1 Continued

Author and purpose	*Design*	*Data analysis*	*Sample information*	*Findings*
Singh (2000) To explore parents' understanding of what Ritalin does and how it makes a difference their child and for themselves. Singh (2003) To explore fathers' perspectives on perspectives on ADHD behaviors, diagnosis, and drug treatment.	Semi-structured in-depth interviews using version of Zaltman Metaphor Elicitation Technique.	Hermeneutic perspective.	$N = 34$. Purposeful sampling from neurodevelopmental clinic near Boston. 22 mothers and 12 fathers. Parents white and middle to lower-middle class; 85% mothers working full- or part-time, 100% fathers working full-time. Age of sons 7–12 years.	*Themes from mothers* 1 Experiences of disconnection: • the inaccessible boy; • the lost boy literally and figuratively; • the out-of-control boy. 2 Understanding ADHD as a disconnection in brain. 3 Mothers' believing that their own parenting practices to blame for child's behavior. 4 Schools reinforcing blame for mothers. 5 Father's absence in ADHD treatment diagnosis and process. 6 Isolation of mothers and sons. 7 Mothers not living up to what their conception of being a "good mother" was. 8 Mothers' anger and frustration. 9 Accepting scientific explanation for ADHD. *Themes from fathers* 1 Not seeing anything seriously wrong before diagnosis. 2 Fathers' thinking that child is just being a normal boy: • "I was like that too." 3 Believing son's behavior result of mother's actions.

				Themes from both 1 Mothers and fathers polarized in how they viewed diagnosis. 2 Different views of mothers and fathers about how much self-control child has. *Using Ritalin* 1 Mothers' positive views of using Ritalin. 2 Ritalin helping to uncover the real self of the child. 3 Fathers' views on Ritalin: • not believing in using it. 4 Costs and benefits of using Ritalin for mothers. 5 Mothers feel better due to distance Ritalin creates between them and their child. 6 Weekend use of Ritalin: • dilemma to medicate for child in sporting events.
Singh (2004) To explore "the problem of blame in relation to ADHD diagnoses and Ritalin use from the perspective of mothers of boys with ADHD" (p. 1193). Singh (2005) "To investigate parents' use of the moral ideal of authenticity as part of their narrative justifications for dosing decisions and actions" (p. 34).	Auto-driven interviews: How do you think and feel about Ritalin (or other psychostimulant) treatment?	Grounded theory.	$N = 61$. Original sample from Singh 2000 and 2003, as well as 17 mothers and 10 fathers recruited with theoretical sampling. Families white, mostly middle class with boys with ADHD ages 7–12.	1 Mothers' self-blame – "the Good Mother" ideal: • responsibility: mother's ability to solve problems of her child; • connection: relationship between mother and son; • maternal instinct: sacrifice self for child; • anger: driven by feelings of inadequacy, guilt, frustration, isolation. 2 Blame from others: • fathers' attitudes: different perception of sons' behavior; • community settings: everyday experiences in public with son.

continued

Table 3.1 Continued

Author and purpose	*Design*	*Data analysis*	*Sample information*	*Findings*
				3 Absolution from blame for mothers: • son using medication helped dramatically to reduce feelings of guilt/blame; • blaming the brain: after diagnosis mothers understood sons' behavior as not anybody's fault ("no-fault"); • however, mothers still responsible for controlling sons' behavior (medication). Mothers: success vs. freedom: • locating the self: mothers' perceptions of ADHD in sons: part of behavior, or part of self? • using medication to achieve success for sons; • weekend dosing dilemmas; • perception that medication prevented son from being himself. Fathers: alternate view of sons' self: • greater attribution of behavior to "boys will be boys" instead of to ADHD as medical problem; • dilemma with using Ritalin for sons' sports activity; • fathers usually left decision of if/when to use medication to mothers.

Smith (2011) To examine the perceptions of mothers and fathers of children with ADHD in terms of the stressors they have experienced as a result of raising a child with ADHD.	Semi-structured interviews.	Theme analysis.	*N* = 14. 9 female, 5 male. 2 participants, 1 male and 1 female, were aunt and uncle of child diagnosed with ADHD.	*Themes* Diet restrictions as a method of treatment. Decisions to use or not use medications. Homework. Child's relationship with friends. Child's relationship with family members. Child behaviors. Activities avoided. Maternal depression. Impact on marriage/friends. Parental stress relievers.
Squire (1993) "To examine the perceptions of family members regarding the impact of ADHD on their family system" (p. ii).	Semi-structured interviews.	Miles & Huberman data analysis.	*N* = 5 families. Recruited from mid-size midwestern US city through snowball sampling. All families had 2 parents and 2–4 children (1 of whom was diagnosed with ADHD); all family members had to agree to participate in study. All parents white, with at least 2 years higher education, middle class, 4 Catholic; all ADHD children male.	*Family atmosphere* 1 Family together time: • mealtimes, vacation/travel, leisure time. 2 Conflict: • marital, among children, between parents and children. 3 Stress: • fathers' stress, marital stress, ADHD child stress, siblings' stress. *Family coping and adaptation* 1 Parental adaptations. 2 ADHD child adaptations. 3 Sibling adaptations. *Family view of self* 1 Parental view of family. 2 ADHD child's view of family. 3 Family view of siblings of ADHD child.

continued

Table 3.1 Continued

Author and purpose	*Design*	*Data analysis*	*Sample information*	*Findings*
Sullivan (2008) To investigate the coping strategies of single mothers of children with ADHD who receive treatment.	Individual interview.	Theme analysis.	*N* = 10. All mothers ages ranged from 31 to 49 years. Ages of child with ADHD ranged from 9 to 12 years.	All mothers indicated that: • they were using some kind of behavior management technique with their child; • they take privileges away from their child as a form of discipline: such as playing video games, watching television, or playing outside; • they have used a "time-out" as a form of disciplining their child. This usually consisted of the child going to his/her room to calm down.
Taylor et al. (2008) To explore the routines that Western Australian mothers use to get their child with ADHD ready for school on time.	Initially open-ended interviews, then guiding questions used after theme was refocused on mothers' morning routine.	Grounded theory.	*N* = 18 mothers. Sampling for variation used. All were white mothers living in Perth, Australia: 4 from low socioeconomic suburbs, 11 from medium, 3 from high. Children were ages 8–17, only 1 not prescribed medication for ADHD.	*Instilling an awareness of time in child with ADHD* 1 Daily experiences of mothers in dealing with chaos: • some children got up very early, disturbing the sleep patterns of other family members (hyperactive); • some children slow to get up and have no concept that things need to be done in a timely manner in the morning (hypoactive); • mothers experienced large amount of stress getting both types of children ready for school in the morning in a timely manner.

2. Assigning blame:
   - mothers blamed morning difficulties on child's ambivalence about time;
   - perception that child has a self-serving selective awareness of time that is only used when getting ready to do something that they value.
3. Understanding their child's concept of time management:
   - self-reflection by mothers;
   - analyzing their own attitudes;
   - realizing that child usually had different concept.
4. Developing strategies that instill an awareness of time management:
   - manipulative controlling strategies;
   - organizational controlling strategies;
   - directive controlling strategies;
   - pharmacological controlling strategy;
   - self-governing teaching strategies;
   - self-governing negotiation strategies;
   - self-governing prompting strategies;
   - discreet self-governing supervisory strategies.

---

continued

Table 3.1 Continued

Author and purpose	*Design*	*Data analysis*	*Sample information*	*Findings*
Taylor et al. (2006) To examine "the decision-making processes that Western Australian parents utilise when deciding whether to medicate or not to medicate their child diagnosed with Attention Deficit Hyperactivity Disorder" (p. 111).	Semi-structured interviews.	Grounded theory.	*N* = 33. Theoretical sampling. 28 mothers and 5 fathers from Perth, Australia. Recruited from support group and hospital center. 15 single parents; 22 parents of primary aged boys and girls, 11 parents of teenage boys.	1 Parents' grieving over the loss of their child's "normal" status; 7 substages: a denying the diagnosis; b seeking alternate treatment options; c venting anger; d experiencing emotional turmoil; e expressing remorse; f feeling depressed; g guarded acceptance. 2 Parental cynicism of society's dichotomous attitude towards ADHD and the use of medication as the preferred treatment option. 3 "Doing the right thing by my child" – adopting proactive parenting practices: a assuming responsibility for the proactive titration of their child's medication; b educating others.

Villegas (2007) To identify "the experiences and challenges of parents with children diagnosed with ADHD" (p. i).	In-depth interviews.	Grounded theory.	$N = 10$ parents. Theoretical and purposive sampling from outpatient clinic in rural southwest US. 9 females (6 mothers, 3 grandmothers), 1 male (step-father); most with highest education level of high school; all participants Hispanic.	*Challenges with support systems* 1 Internal factors: • insufficient emotional support; • some limited emotional support. 2 External factors: • school; • friends; • local mental health services. *Challenges maintaining safety in the home* 1 Safety issues within the family: • feeling divided (sibling rivalry); • feeling guarded: parents threatened by child's behavior. 2 Lack of self-care. *Stressful challenges raising child* 1 Lack of freedom or control: • sense of powerlessness; • sense of pressure; • sense of helplessness. 2 Lack of respite care. *Experience regarding child's medication* 1 Lack of confidence using medication or in medication's effectiveness. 2 Lack of awareness/information about medication. 3 Sense of hope from using medication. *Perception of future challenges for child* 1 Worries and fears about the future. 2 Hopefulness about the future.

continued

Table 3.1 Continued

Author and purpose	*Design*	*Data analysis*	*Sample information*	*Findings*
Wallace (2005) To describe a mother's report of bringing up a son diagnosed with ADHD.	Semi-structured interview with a topic guide.	Grounded theory.	$N = 10$. Mothers recruited from regional ADHD support groups in New South Wales, Australia.	Nuclear families: • mothers making sense of sole responsibility for care of son through family relationship rationale. Siblings: • greater tension between them than with children outside family. Extended families: • varying levels of support and acceptance of diagnosis. Social network: • mothers' feelings of isolation and alienation. Education system: • teachers: acceptance but continual struggles with son's behavior; • sons being bullied and retaliating. Medical system: • mothers searched until they found support.

Wilcox et al. (2007) To analyze how parents' explanatory models of child's ADHD diagnosis change through seeking help their child's problems.	Semi-structured interviews.	Coding and theme analysis.	$N = 24$. Parents (10 fathers, 14 mothers) recruited from child development center in Goa, India.	Onset and cause of illness: • diagnostic label not accepted readily by parents; • multiple causal attributions common by parents. Impact of illness: • importance of schools: behavior problems major factor for deciding to seek help; • direct adverse effect on parents of child's behavior. Help-seeking behavior and relationship to causal attributions: • most common attempted interventions were educational and religious; • explanatory models affected by help-seeking; • parent causal attributions and impact of problem contributed to help-seeking behavior; • shift in parent self-blame after seeking help; • parents adopted new strategies to deal with child's behavior after seeking help; • change in parent's perception of future and seriousness of child's problem after seeking help.

continued

Table 3.1 Continued

Author and purpose	*Design*	*Data analysis*	*Sample information*	*Findings*
Wilder et al. (2009) "To explore the effects of race, class, and marital status upon identity construction and mothering strategies in eight women caring for children with ADHD" (p. 59).	Weekly reports over 3-month period.	Discourse analysis.	*N* = 8. Experience sampling method: selected children ages 14–16, with equal number diagnosed before and after elementary school, equal number of girls and boys, and equal number of black and white children. No exclusionary criteria applied to mothers of children. 7 mothers, 1 grandmother; 2 lower class, 3 lower-middle, 3 middle; 3 single, 5 married; 4 white, 4 black.	1 Shared discourses of "good" mothering: • every mother presented herself as a "good" mother; • constantly evaluating child's ADHD behavior in reflection of their parenting choices. 2 "Good" mothering as self-reflection and sacrifice: • giving up personal satisfaction to care for child. 3 "Good" mothering as a way to defend and normalize the child with ADHD: • ADHD as an "invisible" disability; • mothers feeling isolated and stigmatized, lacking support, and working to prove ADHD is legitimate; • mothers as advocates. 4 Divergent discourses of mothering practices – attributed to race, class and/or marital status: a class and marital status as mothering capital: • effect of mother's status on amount of aid and resources for parenting ADHD child; b racial differences in discipline; c differentials in academic buffering: • mothers ensuring child's education needs being met through individual and structural buffering.

Williams (2008) "To study parental explanatory models for children's ADHD" (p. ii).	Semi-structured interviews using modified version of Kleinman's questions.	Grounded theory.	*N* = 30. Recruited from Boulder area, Colorado, through clinics and parent support groups. 27 mothers, 1 father, 2 mother and father couples; most post-secondary education or higher; 25 middle class or higher; 25 white, 3 Hispanic, 1 Asian, 1 Middle Eastern.	1 How parents name/label condition. 2 Who saw ADHD first. 3 Belief in causation of ADHD. 4 When it first started. 5 Belief about why it first started. 6 Problems created. 7 Parents' feelings. 8 Parents' fears. 9 Belief about duration of condition. 10 What makes the conditions better. 11 What makes conditions worse. 12 Dreams about child's condition. 13 Belief in treatment. 14 Treatment used for ADHD. 15 Desired results from treatment. 16 Child as gifted/talented. 17 Child engaging in rhythmical activity. 18 Stressors as cause/trigger of ADHD. 19 Learning style differences. 20 Improvement related to child being interested in activities they are doing. 21 Adverse effects of pharmaceuticals. 22 Spirituality or religion as a resource. 23 Parents' own drug regime. 24 Maternal guilt. 25 Child's sensitivity to sensory overload. 26 Age-related improvements.

continued

Table 3.1 Continued

Author and purpose	*Design*	*Data analysis*	*Sample information*	*Findings*
Williams (2009) "To explore the emotions, attitudes, and perceptions of mothers of girls who were late diagnosed with ADD" (p. 9).	Multiple individual interviews.	Grounded theory.	*N* = 8. Mothers of girls with ADD diagnosed in high school, recruited through purposive sampling from a psychiatric clinic in north central Florida. Mothers white, 37–56 years old; 1 with high school degree, 7 college degree or higher.	*Influencing factors for mother-daughter relationship* • Mothers diagnosed with ADD had better understanding of daughters behavior. • Mother's ability to cope with difficult situations. • Mother's outlook for the future. *Understanding daughter's struggle* • Mothers seeing themselves in daughter. • Development of empathy for mothers towards daughters. • Mothers' knowing the facts about ADD: • being uninformed; • feeling powerless. *Coping* • Dealing with personal issues. • Dealing with own chaos. • Carrying the responsibility of dealing with daughter's ADD. • Blaming themselves. • Being able to accommodate. • Changing parenting style. • Shielding daughter. • Finding balance between independence for daughter and support. *Envisioning the future* • Expecting more or expecting less. • Providing reassurance.

Williams et al. (2014) To explore parents' perspectives of parenting a child with ADHD who was unmedicated.	Semi-structured in-depth open-ended interviews – 16 parents twice, 2 parents once.	Grounded theory.	*N* = 18. Recruited in Perth, Australia from various sources: social workers, snowball sampling, email appeals. Parents 32–49 years old, 13 mothers and 5 fathers. Children ages 5–13.	*Development of substantive theory of gaining control* 1 Challenging situations: • parent facing difficult behavior from child and decides they have to respond; • situations direct or indirect. 2 Parental resources: • parents frequently emotionally stressed, physically tired, not knowing what to do, having no option of how to respond. 3 Cognitive pathways: • conscious measured approach to dealing with a challenging situation; • generally associated with more positive outcomes; • hopeful solutions with child; • sharing control: involvement of child in decisions; • optimizing performance: child capable of performing to higher level. 4 Emotional pathway: • parents forcing control in challenging situations; • parents avoiding challenging situations; • protecting the self/justifying behavior after judgement from others.

continued

Table 3.1 Continued

Author and purpose	*Design*	*Data analysis*	*Sample information*	*Findings*
Wong and Goh (2014) To provide "in-depth insights on the biodirectional dynamics between parents and their children with ADHD" (p. 601).	In-depth semi-structured interviews.	Open coding, then theme analysis.	*N* = 13. 8 parents, 5 children, all Chinese in Singapore. Purposive sampling: child must be aged 8–12, in mainstream school, with formal diagnosis of mild ADHD without any known comorbidities.	1 Stressful moments in parent-child dynamics: • everyday life situations: homework, unruly behavior. 2 Parents' strategies to manage the stress: • incentives, threats, physical punishment used as last resort. 3 Children's strategies and responses to parental methods and parents' responses: • children report compliance or noncompliance a result of their mood; • no absolute compliance from children. 4 Positive elements of parent-child relationships despite child's ADHD: • relationships reported to be fairly positive.

Table 3.2 Final themes from studies of parents of children with ADHD

Author	*Theme 1: Impact on parents*	*Theme 2: Process of acceptance of diagnosis*	*Theme 3: Medication*
Ahmed et al. (2014)		X	
Al-Azzam and Daack-Hirsch (2011)	X	X	
Arcia and Fernandez (1998)	X	X	
Bennett (2007)	X		
Brinkman et al. (2009)			X
Bull and Whelan (2006)	X	X	X
Bullard (1996)	X		X
Bussing et al. (2006)	X		
Canfield (2000)	X	X	X
Cawley (2004)	X		
Charach et al. (2006)		X	X
Charach et al. (2014)			X
Chavarela (2009)	X	X	X
Clark and Lang (2012)			X
Coletti et al. (2012)	X		X
Corimer (2012)		X	X
Cronin (1995)	X		
Cronin (2004)	X		
Claudius et al. (2012)	X		X
Dennis et al. (2008)	X		
dosReis et al. (2010); dosReis et al. (2009); dosReis et al. (2007); Mychailyszyn et al. (2008)	X	X	X
DuCharme (1996)		X	
Egbert (1996)	X	X	X
Firmim and Phillips (2009)	X	X	X
Funes de Hernandez (2005)	X		
Gerdes et al. (2014)	X	X	X
Goodwillie (2014)		X	
Gray Brunton et al. (2014)	X		
Hallberg et al. (2008)	X	X	
Hammerman (2000)	X		
Hancock (2003)	X	X	
Hansen and Hansen (2006)	X	X	X
Harborne et al. (2004)			X
Himmel (2013)	X	X	
Ho et al. (2011)	X	X	
Howard (1994)	X		X
Jackson and Peters (2008)	X		
Kay (2007)			X
Kendall (1998)			X
Kilcarr (1996)	X	X	
Klasen (2000)	X		X
Klasen and Goodman (2000)	X	X	
Lai and Ma (2014)		X	

continued

Table 3.2 Continued

Author	*Theme 1: Impact on parents*	*Theme 2: Process of acceptance of diagnosis*	*Theme 3: Medication*
Larson et al. (2011)	X		
Leslie et al. (2007)	X	X	
Lewis-Morton et al. (2014)	X		
Lin, Huang and Hung (2009)		X	
Litt (2004)	X		
Martinez (2015)	X		X
McIntyre and Hennessy (2012)	X		
Mills (2011)	X	X	
Moen et al. (2011, 2014)	X	X	X
Morse (2002)	X		
Neophytou and Webber (2005)	X		
Okafor (2006)	X	X	X
Oquendo (2013)	X		
Parker (1994)	X	X	
Perry et al. (2005)	X	X	X
Peters and Jackson (2009)		X	
Rice (1995)	X		
Roosa (2003)	X	X	X
Seawell (2010)	X	X	X
Segal, E. (1994)	X	X	
Segal, E. (2001)	X	X	
Segal, R. (1998, 2000); Segal and Frank (1998)	X	X	
Sikirica et al. (2015)	X		
Singh (2000); Singh (2003)	X	X	X
Singh (2004); Singh (2005)	X	X	X
Smith (2011)	X	X	X
Squire (1993)	X	X	
Sullivan (2008)	X		
Taylor et al. (2008)	X	X	
Taylor et al. (2006)	X		X
Villegas (2007)	X	X	X
Wallace (2005)	X		X
Wilcox et al. (2007)	X		
Wilder et al. (2009)	X	X	
Williams (2008)	X		
Williams (2009)	X	X	X
Williams et al. (2014)	X		
Wong and Goh (2014)	X		

References

Ahmed, R., Mccaffery, K., and Aslani, P. (2013). Factors influencing parental decision making about stimulant treatment for attention-deficit/hyperactivity disorder. *Journal of Child and Adolescent Psychopharmacology*, *23*(3), 163–178.

APA (American Psychiatric Association). (2013). *Diagnostic and statistical manual of mental disorders* (5th edn.). Arlington, VA: Author.

Barkley, R. A. (Ed.). (2014). *Attention deficit hyperactivity disorder: A handbook for diagnosis and treatment* (4th edn.). New York: Guilford Press.

Brinkman, W. B., and Epstein, J. N. (2011). Treatment planning for children with attention-deficit/hyperactivity disorder: Treatment utilization and family preferences. *Patient Preference and Adherence*, *5*, 45–56. doi:10.2147/PPA.S10647.

Brinkman, W., Hartl Majcher, J., Poling, L., Shi, G., Zender, M., Sucharew, et al. (2013). Shared decision-making to improve attention-deficit hyperactivity disorder care. *Patient Education and Counseling*, *93*, 95–101.

Centers for Disease Control and Prevention. (2016). Attention deficit/hyperactivity disorder: Data and statistics. Retrieved from www.cdc.gov/ncbddd/adhd/data.html.

Coghill, D., Soutullo, C., d'Aubuisson, C., Preuss, U., Lindback, T., Silverberg, M., et al. (2008). Impact of attention-deficit/hyperactivity disorder on the patient and family: Results from a European survey. *Child and Adolescent Psychiatry and Mental Health*, *2*(1), 31.

Kendall, J. (1998). Outlasting disruption: The process of reinvestment in families with ADHD children. *Qualitative Health Research*, *8*, 839–857.

Owens, E. B., Hinshaw, S. P., Kraemer, H. C., Arnold, L. E., Abikoff, H. B., Cantwell, D. P., et al. (2003). Which treatment for whom for ADHD? Moderators of treatment response in the MTA. *Journal of Consulting and Clinical Psychology*, *71*(3), 540–552.

Paterson, B., Thorne, S., Canam, C., and Jillings, C. (2001). *Metastudy of qualitative health research*. Thousand Oaks, CA: Sage Publications.

Pelham, W. E. Jr, and Fabiano, G. A. (2008). Evidence-based psychosocial treatments for attention-deficit/hyperactivity disorder. *Journal of Clinical Child and Adolescent Psychology*, *37*(1), 184–214.

Perry, C. E., Hatton, D., and Kendall, J. (2005). Latino parents' accounts of attention deficit hyperactivity disorder. *Journal of Transcultural Nursing*, *16*(4), 312–321.

Sonuga-Barke, E. J., Lasky-Su, J., Neale, B. M., Oades, R., Chen, W., Franke, B., et al. (2008). Does parental expressed emotion moderate genetic effects in ADHD? An exploration using a genome wide association scan. *American Journal of Medical Genetics Part B: Neuropsychiatric Genetics*, *147B*(8), 1359–1368.

Sonuga-Barke, E. J., Brandeis, D., Cortese, S., Daley, D., Ferrin, M., Holtmann, M., et al. (2013). Nonpharmacological interventions for ADHD: Systematic review and meta-analyses of randomized controlled trials of dietary and psychological treatments. *American Journal of Psychiatry*, *170*(3), 275–289.

Taylor, D. (1999). *Impact of attention deficit hyperactivity disorder (ADHD) on parents and children: What are the lived experiences of a parent with a child with ADHD?* (Order No. 1394492). Available from ProQuest Dissertations and Theses Global. Retrieved from http://search.proquest.com/docview/304851012?accountid=14780.

Theule, J., Wiener, J., Tannock, R., and Jenkins, J. M. (2013). Parenting stress in families of children with ADHD: A meta-analysis. *Journal of Emotional and Behavioral Disorders*, *21*(1), 3–17.

Whalen, C., and Henker, B. (1999). The child with attention-deficit/hyperactivity disorder in family contexts. In H. Quay and A. Hogan (Eds.), *Handbook of disruptive behavior disorders* (pp. 139–155). New York: Kluwer Academic/Plenum.

Williams, C. (2008). *Parental explanatory models of children's attention deficit hyperactivity disorder* (Order No. 3398567). Available from ProQuest Dissertations and Theses Global. Retrieved from http://search.proquest.com/docview/304851012?accountid=14780.

References in systematic review

Ahmed, R., Aslani, P., Boarst, R., and Yong, C. W. (2014). Do parents of children with attention-deficit-hyperactivity disorder (ADHD) receive adequate information about the disease and its treatments? A qualitative study. *Patient Preference and Adherence*. Dove Press Journal. Vol. 8, 661–669.

Al-Azzam, M., and Daack-Hirsch, S. (2011). Arab immigrant Muslim mothers' perceptions of children's attention deficit hyperactivity disorder. *Procedia – Social and Behavioral Sciences*, *185*, 23–34.

Arcia, E., and Fernandez, M. C. (1998). Cuban mothers' schemas of ADHD: Development, characteristics, and help seeking behavior. *Journal of Child and Family Studies*, *7*(3), 333–352.

Bennett, J. A. (2007). *(Dis)ordering motherhood: Experiences of mothering a child with attention deficit hyperactivity disorder (ADHD)* (Order No. U185374). Available from ProQuest Dissertations and Theses Global. Retrieved from http://search.proquest.com.proxy.library.vcu.edu/docview/301638456?accountid=14780.

Brinkman, W., Sherman, S., Zmitrovich, A., Visscher, M., Crosby, L., Phelan, K., et al. (2009). Parental angst making and revisiting decisions about treatment of attention-deficit/hyperactivity disorder. *Pediatrics*, *124*, 2, 580–589. doi: 10.1542/peds.2008–2569.

Bull, C., and Whelan, T. (2006). Parental schemata in the management of children with Attention Deficit-Hyperactivity Disorder. *Qualitative Health Research*, *16*(5), 664–678. doi: 10.1177/1049732305285512.

Bullard, J. A. (1996). *Parent perceptions of the effect of ADHD child behavior on the family: The impact and coping strategies* (Order No. 9717369). Available from ProQuest Dissertations and Theses Global. Retrieved from http://search.proquest.com.proxy.library.vcu.edu/docview/304274502?accountid=14780.

Bussing, R., Koro-Ljungberg, M. E., Williamson, P., Gary, F. A., and Garvan, C. W. (2006). What "Dr. Mom" ordered: A community-based exploratory study of parental self-care responses to children's ADHD symptoms. *Social Science and Medicine*, *63*(4), 871.

Canfield, S. K. (2000). *The lonely journey: Parental decision-making regarding stimulant therapy for ADHD* (Order No. 9989350). Available from ProQuest Dissertations and Theses Global. Retrieved from http://search.proquest.com.proxy.library.vcu.edu/docview/304661030?accountid=14780.

Cawley, P. P. (2004). *The parent's experience of raising a child with attention deficit hyperactivity disorder* (Order No. 3142068). Available from ProQuest Dissertations and Theses Global. Retrieved from http://search.proquest.com.proxy.library.vcu.edu/docview/305072457?accountid=14780.

Charach, A., Skyba, A., Cook, L., and Antle, B. J. (2006). Using stimulant medication for children with ADHD: What do parents say? A Brief Report. *Journal of the Canadian Academy of Child and Adolescent Psychiatry*, *15*(2), 75–83.

Charach, A., Yeung, E., Volpe, T., Goodale, T., and dosReis, S. (2014). *Exploring stimulant treatment in ADHD: Narratives of young adolescents and their parents*. BMC Psychiatry, *14*, 110.

Chavarela, S. (2009). *Cultural differences in the experience of the assessment, diagnosis, and treatment of ADHD in a son: Interviews with three Mexican and three Caucasian American mothers* (Order No. 3377439). Available from ProQuest Dissertations and Theses Global. Retrieved from http://search.proquest.com/docview/305174662?accountid=14780.

Chien, W., Ho, C., and Wang, L. (2011). Parent's perception of care-giving to a child with Attention-Deficit Hyperactivity Disorder: An exploratory study. *Contemporary Nurse*, *40*(1), 41–56.

Clarke, J., and Lang, L. (2012). Mothers whose children have ADD/ADHD discuss their children's medication use: An investigation of blogs. *Social Work in Healthcare*, *51*, 402–416. doi: 10.1080/00981389.2012.660567.

Claudius, M., Palinkas, L. A., Wong, J. B., and Leslie, L. K. (2011). Putting families in the center: Family perspectives on decision making and ADHD and implications for ADHD care. *Journal of Attention Disorders*, 6(8), 675–684.

Coletti, D., Pappadopulos, E., Katsiotas, N., Berest, A., Jensen, P., and Kafantaris, V. (2012). Parent perspectives on the decision to initiate medication treatment of attention-deficit/hyperactivity disorder. *Journal of Child and Adolescent Psychopharmacology*, *22*(3), 226–237.

Corimer, E. (2012). How parents make decisions to use medication to treat their children's ADHD: A grounded theory study. *Journal of the American Psychiatric Nurses Association*, *18*(6), 345–356.

Cronin, A. F. (1995). *The influence of attention deficit disorder on mother's perception of family stress: Or, "Lady, why can't you control your child?"* (Order No. 9607357). Available from ProQuest Dissertations and Theses Global. Retrieved from http://search._ proquest.com.proxy.library.vcu.edu/docview/304202251?accountid=14780.

Cronin, A. (2004). Mothering a child with hidden impairments. *The American Journal of Occupational Therapy: Official Publication of the American Occupational Therapy Association*, 58(1), 83–92.

Dennis, T., Davis, M., Johnson, U., Brooks, H., and Humbi, A. (2008). Attention deficit hyperactivity disorder: Parents' and professionals' perceptions. *Community Practitioner: The Journal of the Community Practitioners' and Health Visitors' Association*, *81*(3), 24–28.

dosReis, S., Barksdale, C., Sherman, A., Maloney, K., and Charach, A. (2010). Stigmatizing experiences of parents of children with a new diagnosis of ADHD. *Psychiatric Services (Washington, D.C.)*, *61*(8), 811–816.

dosReis, S., Mychailyszyn, M. P., Evans-Lacko, S. E., Beltran, A., Riley, A. W., and Myers, M. A. (2009). The meaning of attention-deficit/hyperactivity disorder medication and parents' initiation and continuity of treatment for their child. *Journal of Child and Adolescent Psychopharmacology*, *19*(4), 377–383.

dosReis, S., Mychailyszyn, M., Myers, M., and Riley, A. (2007). Coming to terms with ADHD: How urban African-American families come to seek care for their children. *Psychiatric Services (Washington, D.C.)*, 58(5), 636–641.

DuCharme, S. (1996). *Parents' perceptions of raising a child with attention deficit hyperactivity disorder* (Order No. 9706149). Available from ProQuest Dissertations and Theses Global. Retrieved from http://search.proquest.com.proxy.library.vcu.edu/docview/3043 14626?accountid=14780.

Egbert, M. A. (1996). *Description of the mothers' perceptions of parenting children with attention deficit hyperactivity disorder* (Order No. 1381177). Available from ProQuest Dissertations and Theses Global. Retrieved from http://search.proque.st.com.proxy.library. vcu.edu/docview/304312266?accountid=14780

Firmim, M., and Phillips, A. (2009). A qualitative study of families and children possessing diagnoses of ADHD. *Journal of Family Issues*, 30(9), 1155–1174. doi: 10.1177/ 0192513X09333709.

Funes de Hernandez, A. M. N. (2005). *The everyday world of mothers of children with ADHD: Diverse voices of contemporary mothers* (Order No. 1429256). Available from ProQuest Dissertations and Theses Global. Retrieved from http://search.proquest.com/docview/305367314?accountid=14780.

Gerdes, A., Lawton, K., Haack, L., and Schneider, B. (2014). Latino parental help seeking for childhood ADHD. *Administration and Policy in Mental Health and Mental Health Services Research, 41*(4), 503–513. doi:10.1007/s10488-013-0487-3.

Goodwillie, G. (2014). Protective vigilance: A parental strategy in caring for a child diagnosed with ADHD. *Journal of Family Therapy, 36*(3), 255–267. doi:10.1111/1467-6427.12010.

Gray Brunton, C., McVittie, C., Ellison, M., and Willock, J. (2014). Negotiating parental accountability in the face of uncertainty for attention-deficit hyperactivity disorder. *Qualitative Health Research, 24*(2), 242–253.

Hallberg, U., Klingberg, G., Reichenberg, K., and Moller, A. (2008). Living at the edge of one's capability: Experiences of parents of teenage daughters. *International Journal of Qualitative Studies on Health and Well-being, 3*(1), 52–58.

Hammerman, A. R. (2000). *The effects of attention deficit hyperactivity disorder children on mothers and fathers: A qualitative study* (Order No. 9961167). Available from ProQuest Dissertations and Theses Global. Retrieved from http://search.proquest.com.proxy.library.vcu.edu/docview/304618017?accountid=14780.

Hancock, D. F. (2003). *The lived experience of single mothers with sons with ADHD* (Order No. MQ83789). Available from ProQuest Dissertations and Theses Global. Retrieved from http://search.proquest.com/docview/305251486?accountid=14780.

Hansen, D. L., and Hansen, E. H. (2006). Caught in a balancing act: Parents' dilemmas regarding their ADHD child's treatment with stimulant medication. *Qualitative Health Research, 16*(9), 1267–1285.

Harborne, A., Wolpert, M., and Clare, L. (2004). Making sense of ADHD: A battle for understanding? Parents' views of their children being diagnosed with ADHD. *Clinical Child Psychology and Psychiatry*, 9(3), 327–339.

Himmel, D. R. (2013). *Parents perceptions of raising male children with ADHD* (Order No. 3603732). Available from ProQuest Dissertations and Theses Global. Retrieved from http://search.proquest.com/docview/1471911674?accountid=14780.

Ho, S. W., Chien, W. T., and Lang, L. Q. (2011). Parents' perceptions of care-giving to a child with attention deficit hyperactivity disorder: An exploratory study. *Contemporary Nurse, 40*(1), 41–56.

Howard, B. G. (1993). *Parental perception of the impact on the marital and family functioning of the attention deficit disorder child: A qualitative study* (Order No. 9417390). Available from ProQuest Dissertations and Theses Global. Retrieved from http://search.proquest.com.proxy.library.vcu.edu/docview/304089569?accountid=14780.

Jackson, D., and Peters, K. (2008). Use of drug therapy in children with attention deficit hyperactivity disorder (ADHD): Maternal views and experiences. *Journal of Clinical Nursing, 17*(20), 2725–2732.

Kay, R. (2007). *Parental decision making in the administration of stimulant medication for their latency age children with attention deficit hyperactivity disorder (ADHD)* (Order No. 3301292). Available from ProQuest Dissertations and Theses Global. Retrieved from http://search.proquest.com.proxy.library.vcu.edu/docview/304712597?accountid=14780.

Kendall, J. (1998). Outlasting disruption: The process of reinvestment in families with ADHD children. *Qualitative Health Research*, 8(6), 839–857.

Kilcarr, P. J. (1996). *A self-selected qualitative study examining the relationship between a father and his son who has attention deficit hyperactivity disorder (ADHD)* (Order No. 9707629).

Available from ProQuest Dissertations and Theses Global. Retrieved from http://search.proquest.com.proxy.library.vcu.edu/docview/304314500?accountid=14780.

Klasen, H. (2000). A name, what's in a name? The medicalization of hyperactivity, revisited. *Harvard Review of Psychiatry*, *7*(6), 334–344.

Klasen, H., and Goodman, R. (2000) Parents and GPs at cross-purposes over hyperactivity: A qualitative study of possible barriers to treatment. *British Journal of General Practice*, 50, 199–202.

Lai, K., and Ma, J. (2014) Family engagement in children with mental health needs in a Chinese context: A dream or reality? *Journal of Ethnic and Cultural Diversity in Social Work*, *23* (4), 173–189. doi:10.1080/15313204.2013.838815.

Larson, J., Yoon, Y., Stewart, M., and dosReis, S. (2011). Influence of caregivers' experiences on service use among children with attention-deficit hyperactivity disorder. *Psychiatric Services (Washington, D.C.)*, *62*(7), 734–739.

Leslie, L., Plemmons, D., Monn, A., and Palinkas, L. (2007). Investigating ADHD treatment trajectories: Listening to families' stories about medication use. *Journal of Developmental and Behavioral Pediatrics*, *28*(3), 179–188. doi: 10.1097/DBP.0b013e3180324d9a.

Lewis-Morton, R., Dallos, R., McClelland, L., and Clempson, R. (2014). "There is something not quite right with Brad...": The ways in which families construct ADHD before receiving a diagnosis. *Contemporary Family Therapy*, *36*(2), 260–280.

Lin, M. J., Huang, X. Y., and Hung, B. J. (2009). The experiences of primary caregivers raising school-aged children with attention-deficit hyperactivity disorder. *Journal of Clinical Nursing*, *18*(12), 1693–1702.

Litt, J. (2004). Women's carework in low-income households: The special case of children with attention deficit hyperactivity disorder. *Gender and Society*, *18*(5), 625–644.

Martinez, L. (2015). *Puerto Rican mothers of children diagnosed with attention deficit hyperactivity disorder: Factors that impact the treatment seeking process* (Order No. 3687504). Available from ProQuest Dissertations and Theses Global. Retrieved from http://search.proquest.com.proxy.library.vcu.edu/docview/1669495242?accountid=14780.

McIntyre, R., and Hennessy, E. (2012). "He's just enthusiastic. Is that such a bad thing?" Experiences of parents of children with attention deficit hyperactivity disorder. *Emotional and Behavioral Difficulties*, *17*(1), 65–82.

Mills, Ida. (2011). Understanding parent decision making for treatment of ADHD. *School Social Work Journal*, *36*(1), 41–60.

Moen, O., Hall-Lord, M., and Hedelin, B. (2011). Contending and adapting everyday: Norwegian parents' lived experience of having a child with ADHD. *Journal of Family Nursing*, *17*(4), 441–462. doi:10.1177/1074840711423924.

Moen, O., Hall-Lord, M., and Hedelin, B. (2014). Living in a family with a child with attention deficit hyperactivity disorder: A phenomenographic study. *Journal of Clinical Nursing*, *23*(21/22), 3166–3176.

Morse, E. (2002). *Caretakers of children with ADHD: Issues and experiences* (Order No. 3061992). Available from ProQuest Dissertations and Theses Global. Retrieved from http://search.proquest.com.proxy.library.vcu.edu/docview/305457445?accountid=14780.

Mychailyszyn, M., dosReis, S., and Myers, M. (2008). African American caretakers' views of ADHD and use of outpatient mental health care services for children. *Families, Systems, and Health*, *26*(4), 447–458.

Neophytou, K., and Webber, R. (2005). Attention deficit hyperactivity disorder: The family and social context. *Australian Social Work*, 58(3), 313–325.

Oh, W. O., and Kendall, J. (2009). Patterns of parenting in Korean mothers of children with ADHD: A q-methodology study. *Journal of Family Nursing*, *15*(3), 318–342.

Okafor, M. N. (2006). *Narrating realities of Latino mothers of children with attention deficit hyperactivity disorder ADHD using ecological and cultural approach* (Order No. 3244585). Available from ProQuest Dissertations and Theses Global. Retrieved from http://search.proquest.com.proxy.library.vcu.edu/docview/305321453?accountid=14780.

Oquendo, S. A. (2013). *A qualitative study of parenting styles of mothers within Latino families raising sons with ADHD* (Order No. 3612241). Available from ProQuest Dissertations and Theses Global. Retrieved from http://search.proquest.com/docview/1506155007?accountid=14780.

Parker, R. B. (1994). *The meaning of the experience of parenting a child with attention-deficit hyperactivity disorder* (Order No. 1358453). Available from ProQuest Dissertations and Theses Global. Retrieved from http://search.proquest.com.proxy.library.vcu.edu/docview/230771897?accountid=14780.

Perry, C. E., Hatton, D., and Kendall, J. (2005). Latino parents' accounts of attention deficit hyperactivity disorder. *Journal of Transcultural Nursing, 16*(4), 312–321.

Peters, K., and Jackson, D. (2009). Mothers' experiences of parenting a child with attention deficit hyperactivity disorder. *Journal of Advanced Nursing, 65*(1), 62–71.

Rice, D. N. (1995). *Psychosocial variables operating in families having a child with attention deficit hyperactivity disorder* (Order No. 9538493). Available from ProQuest Dissertations and Theses Global. Retrieved from http://search.proquest.com.proxy.library.vcu.edu/docview/304213142?accountid=14780.

Roosa, N. E. (2003). *Parenting a child with ADHD: Making meaning when the experts disagree* (Order No. 3088244). Available from ProQuest Dissertations and Theses Global. Retrieved from http://search.proquest.com/docview/305228284?accountid=14780.

Seawell, M. (2010). *Family narratives of ADHD: Labels promoting change* (Order No. 3429115). Available from ProQuest Dissertations and Theses Global. Retrieved from http://search.proquest.com.proxy.library.vcu.edu/docview/760081777?accountid=14780.

Segal, E. (1994). *Mothering a child with attention-deficit hyperactivity disorder: Learned mothering* (Order No. 9612115). Available from ProQuest Dissertations and Theses Global. Retrieved from http://search.proquest.com.proxy.library.vcu.edu/docview/304166370?accountid=14780.

Segal, E. S. (2001). Learned mothering: Raising a child with ADHD. *Child and Adolescent Social Work Journal, 18*(4), 263–271.

Segal, R. (1998). The construction of family occupations: A study of families with children who have attention deficit/hyperactivity disorder. *Canadian Journal of Occupational Therapy/Revue Canadienne D'Ergothérapie*, 65(5), 286–292.

Segal, R. (2000) Adaptive strategies of mothers with children with attention deficit hyperactivity disorder: Enfolding and unfolding occupations. *American Journal of Occupational Therapy*, 54(3), 300–306. doi:10.5014/ajot.54.3.300.

Segal, R., and Frank, G. (1998). The extraordinary construction of ordinary experience: Scheduling daily life in families with children with attention deficit hyperactivity disorder. *Scandinavian Journal of Occupational Therapy*, 5(3), 141–147.

Sikirica, V., Flood, E., Dietrich, C., Quintero, N., Harpin, J., Hodgkins, V., et al. (2015). Unmet needs associated with attention-deficit/hyperactivity disorder in eight European countries as reported by caregivers and adolescents: Results from qualitative research. *The Patient – Patient-Centered Outcomes Research*, 8(3), 269–281.

Singh, I. (2000). *A crutch, a tool: How mothers and fathers of boys with ADHD experience and understand the work of ritalin* (Order No. 9961219). Available from ProQuest Dissertations and Theses Global. Retrieved from http://search.proquest.com.proxy.library.vcu.edu/docview/304624673?accountid=14780.

Singh. I. (2003). Boys will be boys: Fathers' perspectives on ADHD symptoms, diagnosis, and drug treatment. *Harvard Review of Psychiatry, 11*(6), 308–316.

Singh, I. (2004). Doing their jobs: Mothering with Ritalin in a culture of mother-blame. *Social Science and Medicine*, 59(6), 1193–1205.

Singh, I. (2005). Will the "real boy" please behave: Dosing dilemmas for parents of boys with ADHD. *The American Journal of Bioethics*, 5(3), 34–47.

Smith, A. K. (2011). *Factors and symptoms contributing to parent stress in raising an ADHD child* (Order No. 3518283). Available from ProQuest Dissertations and Theses Global. Retrieved from http://search.proquest.com/docview/1033568055?accountid=14780.

Squire, M. D. (1993). *The impact of attention-deficit hyperactivity disorder in children on family members and family functioning* (Order No. 9400829). Available from ProQuest Dissertations and Theses Global. Retrieved from http://search.proquest.com/docview/9400829?accountid=14780.

Sullivan, M. D. (2008). *Coping strategies of single mothers of children with Attention Deficit/Hyperactivity Disorder (ADHD)* (Order No. MR34994). Available from ProQuest Dissertations and Theses Global. Retrieved from http://search.proquest.com/docview/304851012?accountid=14780.

Taylor, M., Houghton, S., and Durkin, K. (2008). Getting children with attention deficit hyperactivity disorder to school on time: Mothers' perspectives. *Journal of Family Issues*, 29(7), 918–943.

Taylor, M., O'Donoghue, T., and Houghton, S. (2006). To medicate or not to medicate? The decision-making process of Western Australian parents following their child's diagnosis with an attention deficit hyperactivity disorder. *International Journal of Disability, Development and Education*, 53(1), 111–128.

Villegas, T. V. (2007). *Experiences and challenges of parents who have children diagnosed with attention deficit/hyperactivity disorder* (Order No. 3274071). Available from ProQuest Dissertations and Theses Global. Retrieved from http://search.proquest.com.proxy.library.vcu.edu/docview/304722540?accountid=14780.

Wallace, N. (2005). The perceptions of mothers of sons with ADHD. *Australian and New Zealand Journal of Family Therapy*, 26(4), 193–199.

Wilcox, C. E., Washburn, R., and Patel, V. (2007). Seeking help for attention deficit hyperactivity disorder in developing countries: A study of parental explanatory models in Goa, India. *Social Science and Medicine*, 64(8), 1600–1610.

Wilder, J., Koro-Ljungberg, M., and Bussing, R. (2009). ADHD, motherhood, and intersectionality: An exploratory study. *Race, Gender and Class*, 16(3/4), 59–81.

Williams, M. A. (2009). *Exploration of effect of diagnosis of high school girls with attention deficit disorder on their mothers and the mother-daughter relationship* (Order No. 3440918). Available from ProQuest Dissertations and Theses Global. Retrieved from http://search.proquest.com.proxy.library.vcu.edu/docview/849715080?accountid=14780.

Williams, N. J., Harries, M., and Williams, A. M. (2014). Gaining control: A new perspective on the parenting of children with AD/HD. *Qualitative Research in Psychology*, *11*(3), 277–297. doi:10.1080/14780887.2014.902524.

Williams. C. (2008). *Parental explanatory models of children's attention deficit hyperactivity disorder* (Order No. 3398567). Available from ProQuest Dissertations and Theses Global. Retrieved from http://search.proquest.com.proxy.library.vcu.edu/docview/250292152?accountid=14780.

Wong, H., and Goh, E. (2014). Dynamics of ADHD in familial contexts: Perspectives from children and parents and implications for practitioners. *Social Work in Health Care*, 53(7), 601–616.

Yuen, A. (2008). *Cross-cultural effects in children diagnosed with attention-deficit hyperactivity disorder on parental and caregiver stress* (Order No. 3325344). Available from ProQuest Dissertations and Theses Global. Retrieved from http://search.proquest.com/docview/304382486?accountid=14780.

4 The lived experience of parents of children with autism spectrum disorders

Autism spectrum disorder (ASD) encompasses what used to include in DSM-IV (APA, 2000) autistic disorder, Asperger's disorder, childhood disintegrative disorder, and pervasive developmental disorder not otherwise specified (PDD-NOS) (APA, 2013). ASD is a neurological-developmental disorder with an onset during the first three years of life. The child with ASD demonstrates serious impairments in social interaction and communication, as well as odd repetitive behaviors and restricted interests (APA, 2013). Current US statistics indicate that one in 68 children are diagnosed with an autistic spectrum disorder (Centers for Disease Control, 2014).

A systematic review of the quantitative studies indicates that parents of children with autism spectrum disorders have higher rates of psychiatric disorders than parents of typically-developing children (Yirmiya and Shaked, 2005). This may be due to the stress and burden of parenting such a child (Lambrechts et al., 2012), but may also be because of genetic risk (Pozo, Sarriá, and Brioso, 2014).

Although some quantitative study has focused on these parents, the purpose of this study was to understand their lived experience from a synthesis of the qualitative research. Meta-synthesis is a recent methodology designed to systematically review and integrate results of primary qualitative studies that have been conducted on a similar topic using qualitative methods (Finfgeld, 2003; Sandelowski and Barruso, 2006). Although meta-synthesis is not without controversy (see Finlayson and Dixon, 2008; Jones, 2004), this methodology is a valuable way to build knowledge in a particular area of study, which may then be developed into policy and practice. Therefore, the purpose of this chapter is to conduct a meta-synthesis, embedded within a systematic review, of the lived experience of parents with a child on the autism spectrum. Sandelowski and Barruso (2006) have suggested that synthesis be done on studies conducted within a certain geographic area because policies and services delivered to these families will differ based on the country involved. For this reason, we limited the meta-synthesis to primary studies conducted in the United States.

Themes

After applying criteria, a total of 14 studies published between 2001 and 2012 with a total of 263 participants were included. A majority of the participants were mothers, though fathers and some non-biological parents were included as well. Caucasians and African-Americans were the most represented ethnicities in this sample. A majority of participants also had an income of at least $30,000 annually, lived in two-parent household, and were at least 30 years old. The participants were recruited most often using convenience, snowball, or purposive sampling methods and were frequently identified through online autism networks or through agencies serving children diagnosed with autism and their families. See Table 4.1 for more detail on studies.

A total of six major themes were identified in the results: (1) emotional stress and strain; (2) adaptation; (3) impact on the family; (4) services; (5) stigmatization; and (6) appreciating the little things (see Table 4.2).

Emotional stress and strain

Caring for a child with ASD is an emotionally taxing experience and parents reported intense negative emotions. From the point of diagnosis parents spoke about denial, grief, and disappointment. There was some initial denial with some parents, not wanting to believe their children had an autism spectrum-disorder, and husbands were often described as maintaining this denial for a longer period than mothers (e.g., Schwartz, 2001).

Then, once the diagnosis was accepted, parents described feeling intense grief. One parent expressed her reaction to the diagnosis as: "I fell into a deep grief.... I was lost, blaming myself or figuring out who to blame. I was angry" (Lutz et al., 2012, p. 209). Another parent stated: "When the doctor told me, I had the same feeling as when my grandmother died" (Hutton and Caron, 2005, p. 184), and in Schwartz (2001), a mother described it as getting a diagnosis of cancer. Another parent stated: "It was almost like a grieving period.... There's a part that you've lost; the part, a part of a dream of that everybody has about their children growing up, going to college, getting married and all that..." (Ewart, 2002, p. 59).

Feelings of disappointment were also common. One parent said: "I guess the biggest part is just trying to accept the reality and try to let go of your hopes and dreams" (Lutz et al., 2012, p. 211). Another parent described a similar sense of disappointment, of not being able to take pleasure in things "that I thought I was going to take pleasure in like making friends and stuff with school and stuff with girls" (Schwartz, 2001, p. 129). Parents felt they were not going to experience the normal joys of watching their child grow up and felt let down by the limited possibilities for their children.

Once time went on, parents spoke about "worry about what is going to happen to him when I am not around" (Schwartz, 2001, p. 128). Another parent stated: "I worry about his future and if something would happen to me, what would happen to him" (Kalash, 2009, p. 63). The main concern for parents was whether or not their child would be supported once the parents were no longer able to do this. They worried whether their child would be able to live a productive and fulfilling life without their continuous help.

Another subtheme was the stress and strain of taking care of children with autism. One mother described how exhausted she was at having "to take it all on" (Lutz et al., 2012, p. 209). Parents described extensive planning and accommodating, having to assist with daily living activities even when the child was older, and having to invest a lot of time and money into finding services. One parent described her experience as "very stressful all around" stating that "emotionally, it is the single most challenging event in my life" (Phelps et al., 2009, p. 29). Another parent talked about the difficulties in the following way: "Now, I feel like having child S is having five normal kids. I did not know it was going to be this hard. I try not to cry all the time because it hurts me a lot" (Lendenmann, 2010, p. 64). Yet another parent described isolation and frustration: "But it's hard to make friends you really can't you can't, you're just kind of stuck in the house with your kids. It's kinda hard.... So, it's just very frustrating. Very confining, very lonely actually" (Ewart, 2002, p. 67).

Adaptation

Another theme that emerged was parents speaking of the need to adapt and accommodate to the needs of the child with ASD. Adaptation for families included extra planning for any task, learning how to recognize and avoid children's triggers, and adjusting schedules. Parents talked about having to be hypervigilant and, constantly monitoring the environment and the child's behavior; having to take extra time and precautions to complete tasks like grocery shopping and haircuts. One parent in Ewart (2002) captured this need: "I think when you have a kid with autism, it's like you go from one little crisis to the next" (p. 74). Another parent summed up her thoughts on adaptation as: "You have to rearrange your life ... there is no more spontaneous ... everything is planned" (Lutz et al., 2012, p. 211).

One participant talked about the adaptation in terms of "the whole family had autism, not just the child" (Lutz et al., 2012, p. 210). Thus, the family has to learn to cope and adapt. Some families made life-changing decisions. One named frequently was for the mother to give up her work outside the home (Ewart, 2002; Kalash, 2009; Kent, 2011; Lendenmann, 2010; Ryan and Cole, 2009, Schwartz, 2001):

> ...either because of the number of appointments they had to go to for their children, because they felt that their children needed to have them at home, because they had to support their children in school or because they could not organize appropriate childcare.
>
> (Ryan and Cole, 2009)

As one mother described: "I just gave up work because it was just so tense and I knew Simon would have more acute problems settling into school" (Ryan and Cole, 2009, p. 47).

Impact on the family

As mentioned, autism affects the family as a whole and the parents as a couple. Participants described the difficulty of balancing the needs of the family – and the marital relationship – with the needs of the child with ASD. Husbands and wives sometimes had different ideas on how to parent children (Hunt-Jackson, 2007; Schwartz, 2001). Family activities and vacations often had to be curtailed (Ewart, 2002; Kent, 2011; Lendenmann, 2010).

However, strengths also developed in the family. Some people's marriages (Kent, 2011; Kuhaneck et al., 2010) and families became stronger from withstanding struggles (Lendenmann, 2010). Aside from helping share the logistical and financial burdens, spouses were often named as the most important support system. One mother talked about her husband as being a "safe person that I can say or share anything and know that he is not going to judge me or look differently at me" (Martinez, 2009, p. 62).

As well as the impact on the family and the couple, parents spoke of their concerns about their typically-developing children. Parents described feeling guilty about giving so much more time and attention to the child with autism and feeling like they were neglecting their other children (Ewart, 2002; Kent, 2011; Lendenmann, 2010; Kuhaneck et al., 2010). Many parents expressed feeling "torn between" their child with autism and their other children.

One parent described that her daughter had told her: "We don't give her enough attention, that it is always her brother. I often feel torn between the two of them and trying to give them enough time each" (Kalash, 2009, p. 61). Another parent described a similar situation: "My daughter will say that I love my son (with autism) more than her and that I spend more time with him" (Hutton and Caron, 2005, p. 186). Yet another said: "Our son has a hard time and often feels hurt. He has told us that he feels sad because he thinks we love his brother more than him which hurts us" (Hutton and Caron, 2005, p. 187). Participants further talked about the burden being placed on siblings both to care for their sibling with autism and to tolerate their sometimes embarrassing behaviors. According to many parents, their relationships with their other children are characterized by guilt, hurt, and confusion.

Services

Most studies described parents' use of different services for their child, including the types of services and interventions used, as well as the availability of services and overall satisfaction with services received. Parents described an array of different interventions and services. Support groups were used by some parents, who found them helpful (Ryan and Cole, 2009; Schwartz, 2001).

While some parents really appreciated the services they received, many others described frustration at various points in the diagnosis. Their first frustrating experience often related to the process of diagnosis. Parents concerns about their inability to manage their children and their children's behavioral signs were brushed off and dismissed by pediatricians and even specialists so that diagnosis was delayed (e.g., Martinez, 2009; Schwartz, 2001).

Once a diagnosis was made, one of the major sources of frustration was the difficulty in obtaining services, as expressed by one parent:

> My child was put on a waiting list for being assigned to a case manager. I was told that in the meantime, I should do the case management and coordination of services, which was appalling since I was already so stressed.
>
> (Hutton and Caron, 2005, p. 185)

In Ewart (2002), parents described feeling overwhelmed and lost when faced with the array of different interventions and no one route to access them. Some parents even described relocating to cities where there were more resources and services offered (Kent, 2011; Lendenmann, 2010). Specific to respite services, which parents desperately needed, Larson (2010) reported that mothers did not often use them because of the children's emotional reactions to being with another person, the amount of planning required, and the fact that respite workers couldn't handle their children's needs.

A second frustration that parents described was the lack of direction and support from service providers. One parent talked about the process as hopeless: "From the diagnosis we were not given any real direction ... such as what to pursue and when ... they made it sound pretty hopeless" (Kalash, 2009, p. 56). Parents talked about having to try on their own to educate themselves about the services available and having to make repeated efforts in order to get their child enrolled in them. Another parent talked about the doctors' lack of support for the family members, saying that "Professionals in the medical field lack the patience and understanding of dealing with persons with autism" (Phelps et al., 2009, p. 31). This lack of support was described mostly in the medical setting, but also with regard to the school system as well, with parents talking about "lots of phone calls and they wouldn't return my phone calls for a long time" (Schwartz, 2001, p. 134). Both Kuhaneck et al. (2010) and Ewart (2002) talked about a "continuous fight" to get school services and that it was incumbent upon the parents to learn the processes and structures within the school system.

The final frustration was the overwhelming time commitment required by parents in order for their children to participate in the necessary services. Parents complained about having "too many doctors' offices to go to" (Martinez, 2009, p. 46). In addition to the medical appointments, parents talked about how all the services together really required an extraordinary amount of their time. As one participant noted:

> There has been just an enormous amount of paperwork and hours ... of therapy each week ... which is stressful on our family because it disrupts home schedules and meal times. Our time and our home is not our own because we are always going to meetings or having people in our home.
>
> (Hutton and Caron, 2005, p. 185)

The parents recognized the need for their children to receive services, but there was also a significant amount of frustration and exhaustion surrounding this aspect of caring for their child with autism. This theme was present in a majority of the studies, suggesting that it is a common experience amongst parents caring for children with autism spectrum disorders.

Stigmatization

Another theme was that of stigmatization. Parents often described negative interactions in public where people misjudged them as bad parents who had no control over their children (e.g., Schwartz, 2001). Parents described that people would interfere, thinking they were being too physical with their children, when parents were only trying to restrain dangerous or out-of-control behaviors. The children were also judged with people often referring to them as "spoiled brats." Parents talked about getting "the look" that captured the disgust and pity so often expressed by the public (Hunt-Jackson, 2007, p. 57; Kalash, 2009, p. 65). They described how both embarrassing and annoying it would be to receive "the look."

Many parents believed that part of the reason they were judged so harshly was that autism is "invisible" in that the child does not look disabled; therefore, people have a hard time believing that the negative behaviors are due to a disorder. One parent stated: "If there was something that could show that he was different instead of just being bad, it would be easier – but he appears normal so therefore he should be normal" (Neely-Barnes et al., 2011, p. 213). Another parent expressed a similar notion saying that "Just because a child looks normal doesn't mean they are normal" (Kalash, 2009, p. 66).

Parents often struggled with whether or not to bring the child into public because of the potential for negative interactions. One parent commented: "I just try to get my son to a place where nobody can look at him" (Lutz et al., 2012, p. 209), while other parents took exactly the opposite stance stating that "I'm not going to shut my son in a room" (Neely-Barnes et al., 2011, p. 216). Parents described feeling like not only did they have to pick their battles with their children, but also with people in the general public.

In Ryan and Cole (2009), parents used some of the reactions from the public and used them as opportunities to advocate about autism. As one participant explained:

> I want him to feel part of society. I want people to see him doing things and think he has got a right to be there, because at the moment some

> people … don't think that a disabled child has the right to everything that other children have.
>
> (p. 50)

Appreciating the little things

Despite the negativity and struggle that surround raising a child with ASD, the parents also describe many positive consequences as well. Ten of the 14 studies discussed the concept of appreciating the little things as learning how to recognize their child's strengths and accomplishments. One parent described this phenomenon as: "I've learned to see the positive in things that people normally wouldn't see … making lemonade out of a lemon" (Lutz et al., 2012, p. 210). One father talks about a moment when his son returned a wave and a blown kiss: "I was just blown away … I was so elated" (Hunt-Jackson, 2007, p. 55). When asked what the experience of parenting an autistic child has been like, some parents expressed that "It has been an honor to be given a child like this – to parent a child like this" (Hutton and Caron, 2005, p. 186) and that "He has been a joy and a sweetheart. I wouldn't change anything" (Hutton and Caron, 2005, p. 186). Others described the joy of parenting their child or positive attributes of ASD: "The joy is when he is happy there is not a happier kid in the world, and that makes me so happy" (Kuhaneck et al., 2010, p. 346); "My son is a joyful child. I think that when you have delayed cognitive development, you don't develop the uglier aspects of the human personality. I don't think he has it in him to feel jealousy or rage" (Lendenmann, 2010, p. 70). Overall, parents talk about appreciating their children's differences because they make them unique and that they have helped to strengthen the parents and family as well. Some are even thankful for the experience with statements from parents, such as: "I feel I was given this job because maybe God thinks I can handle it" (Lendenmann, 2010, p. 67); "I am blessed to have a kid like him because I am very religious and God gave me child because I can take care of him" (Lendenmann, 2010, p. 68); and

> I realize that I had all kinds of interesting experiences and had learned so much that I never would have learned about otherwise and having a child with a disability has really enriched my life and really kind of broadened my horizons. So I consider it a blessing.
>
> (Kent, 2011, p. 99)

Discussion

This study provides an in-depth, qualitative overview of parent experiences with regard to raising children with autism spectrum disorders. Struggles involved the emotional strain involved with learning of a child's diagnosis of an autism spectrum disorder and managing the care of these children. Siblings were often affected negatively by the amount of time parents had to lavish on their child with a disability. Accessing services was a frustrating experience, and services and programs were woefully lacking.

However, strengths were also named. Although the family as a whole and the spousal relationship suffered strain, partners were still together, and, in some cases, drew closer as a result of the experience. Similarly, a quantitative study from the National Survey of Children's Health involving 77,911 parent interviews found that, after controlling for relevant covariates, results revealed that parents with children with ASD are not at increased risk for separation or divorce (Freedman et al., 2012). However, they do tend to have fewer subsequent children, according to a study of California birth records (Hoffmann et al., 2014). The reasons may include fear of having another child with an ASD, the enormous stress of rearing children with ASD, and concern about already neglecting other typically-developing children in the home.

Adaptation to the needs of the child was named as a necessity, and families demonstrated much flexibility in being able to change their family system in this way. An impressive strength as well was that parents were able to "appreciate the little things" and take pleasure and satisfaction in small accomplishments and triumphs.

As a result of the findings, several important practice implications can be identified. First, practitioners can share the themes and quotes from this study as a way to normalize parents' experiences and as a venue for them to speak of their own experiences. Difficulties can be validated and strengths can be affirmed and bolstered.

One notable theme of concern was the finding that services were difficult to locate and access and providers were neither consistently knowledgeable nor helpful. There were no positive remarks made about social service or medical providers, which can be taken as an indictment of current services in the US. Practitioners who work in this field, therefore, should strive to advocate for necessary programs and be familiar with the programs and services that exist in their communities so that appropriate information, guidance, and referrals can be provided to families.

The results of this study also indicate the great deal of emotional strain placed on these parents. Practitioners can act as a support system for these parents and help parents identify and strengthen their supports through counseling and referrals to additional services, such as support groups, recognizing that these parents have limited time.

Third, practitioners can address the negative impact on the siblings of the child with ASD through counseling and service referrals. Family counseling may help the parents and the siblings learn new ways to interact and bond with each other. In addition, services such as qualified respite can be recommended as well so that parents can spend time with typically-developing children.

Some limitations of this study involve the current controversies of qualitative research and, more specifically, meta-synthesis (Finlayson and Dixon, 2008). Criticisms of metasynthesis include its heavy reliance on secondary interpretation of experiences, which is likely to differ according to the researcher, and its synthesizing of studies that may be different in their orientation, methodological features, analysis, and quality.

Other limitations particular to this meta-synthesis was the fact that the majority of the participants were Caucasian; therefore, increasing the representation of minorities in samples is important. While there were males included in many of the studies, the participants' perspectives were mainly reflected by the females. Therefore, more emphasis should be placed obtaining the male perspective. A final limitation is that given the voluntary nature of participation in research, it is likely that subjects might have been higher-functioning, had more resources and supports, and been more articulate than parents who did not have the time or resources to make arrangements to be interviewed. Therefore, the results provided may not generalize to all parents of children with ASD. Despite these limitations, the synthesis of this literature aids in our understanding of the lived experience of parents with a child diagnosed with ASD.

Table 4.1 Data extraction of studies of parents of children with autism

Author and purpose	*Design*	*Sample*	*Findings*
Ewart (2002) To capture parents' experiences of having a child with ASD.	Phenomenological method of analysis.	$N = 8$ parents (5 mothers, 3 fathers); ages 32–45 years. Children ages 4–8 years with a diagnosis for at least 1 year prior to interview. Majority white. All married.	*Stages* 1 Getting the diagnosis. 2 Reactions to diagnosis. 3 Interventions, schooling, and changes in family roles. 4 Reactions to changes. 5 Recognized parents' increased knowledge, coping, and acceptance. 6 Future hopes and concerns.
Hunt-Jackson (2007) To explore how fathers view themselves as parents of children with Autistic Spectrum Disorders (ASD) by drawing out stories about their involvement with their children.	One-on-one in-depth interviews.	$N = 14$ fathers. Snowball sampling. Age range of children 9–23 years. Age range of parents 35–51 years. All Caucasian.	1 Diagnosis. 2 Acceptance. 3 Future issues. 4 Behavior. 5 Education. 6 Challenges. 7 Feelings. 8 Fixing the problem.
Hutton and Caron (2005) To find out what the impact of having a child with autism has on the family.	Semi-structured phone interviews.	$N = 21$. Convenience sampling from Autism Society mailing list.	1 Recognition. 2 Intervention services. 3 Family coping ability.

continued

Table 4.1 Continued

Author and purpose	*Design*	*Sample*	*Findings*
Kalash (2009) To understand the experiences and perceptions parents of a child with an autism spectrum disorder have had.	Phenomenological interview.	*N* = 12. Convenience sampling (support groups); snowball (asking those interviewed to recommend others). 4 geographic locations in a midwestern US state. 8 mothers, 4 fathers.	1 Early signs and diagnostic struggles. 2 Lack of guidance from medical professionals. 3 Limited daycare options and financial stressors. 4 Torn between. 5 Concerns for the future. 6 Judgment of others. 7 Parent perceptions of vaccinations.
Kent (2011) To look at the experiences and perceptions of parents of children with ASD and impact on the family.	Individual semi-structured interviews.	*N* = 8 (7 mothers, 1 father). Each had a child with ASD and at least one typically developing child. Ages 28–49. Children ages 5–13 (5 boys, 2 girls). 5 white; 1 white and Hispanic; 1 Hispanic/ Mexican American; 1 black and Japanese. Wide variety of education backgrounds and socioeconomic status . Convenience sampling via fliers at agencies for children with ASD, website advertisements, and snowball sampling.	1 Impact on parent and non-ASD child relationship. 2 Impact on parents. 3 Impact on marital relationship. 4 Impact on siblings and sibling relationship. 5 Broader impact on family.

Kuhaneck et al. (2010) To explore mothers' perceptions of effective coping strategies for their parenting stressors.	Individual semi-structured interviews.	$N = 11$ parents (all mothers). Ages 40–46 years. Children ages 6–11 years. Parent ethnicities: 9 white, 2 African American. Employment: 1 full-time, 6 part-time, 4 not employed. 9 married, 1 divorced, 1 widowed. All living in an affluent, suburban community in northeastern US. Convenience sampling; recruited through Autism Spectrum Support Group (ASSG).	Coping strategies included: 1 "me time"; 2 planning; 3 knowledge is power; 4 sharing the load; 5 lifting the restraints of labels; 6 recognizing the joys.
Larson (2010) To find out why caregivers of children with autism are often found to be more stressed by their caregiving than caregivers of other children with disabilities.	Individual semi-structured interviews.	$N = 9$ parents (all mothers). Children ages 3–14 years (all boys). Varied ethnicities. Wide income range ($16,000–$250,000). Convenience sampling.	1 Functions of vigilance: • facilitating performance in daily routines; • assisting social negotiations. 2 Monitoring safety and sensory triggers in the environment.

continued

Table 4.1 Continued

Author and purpose	*Design*	*Sample*	*Findings*
Lendenmann (2010) To explore the lived experience of parenting a preschool aged child with ASD and moderate mental retardation (MR).	Individual interviews.	N = 16 parents (13 mothers, 3 fathers). Convenience sampling from a major children's hospital in the mid-Atlantic region of the US. Ages 26–48 years. Children ages 3–5 years (11 males, 4 females). 8 white, 3 Hispanic, 3 Asian, 2 African American. All fathers employed, 1 mother employed. 14 married, 1 separated, 1 single.	*Four themes of parenting an autistic child* 1 Total life change. 2 Limited personal time. 3 Concurrent growth. 4 Hope.
Lutz et al. (2012) To explore the experiences of families of individuals with autism as perceived by the mother.	Face-to-face and telephone interviews	N = 16. Convenience sampling recruited by word of mouth and through AutismLink, an email listserve. 14 Caucasian, 2 African American. Ages between 30 and 50 years.	1 Grief and anger. 2 Seeking answers. 3 Dis-ease and relationship strain. 4 Support, socialization, and spirituality. 5 Guilt and doubt. 6 Appreciating and defining life and multiple roles. 7 Disappointment and sacrifice. 8 Adaptation.

Martinez (2009) To explore the experiences, perspectives, influences and challenges of selected mothers with children with autism spectrum disorders.	Semi-structured interviews.	$N = 13$. Purposive sampling. All mothers. 8 Caucasian, 2 African American, 1 Asian American, 2 Hispanic. 3 Protestants, 5 Catholics, 2 Lutheran, 1 Unity, 1 Christian, 1 other. 1 married, 1 single, 1 divorced/separated. 1 high school diploma, 3 associate degrees, 7 Bachelor's degrees, 2 Master's degrees. Income level: $100,000–$149,000 (1); $99,000–$75,000 (8); $74,000–$35,000 (3); $34,000–below (1). 4 employed, 8 unemployed, 1 in-between jobs.	1 Mother's experiences and perspectives during early detection and diagnosis. 2 Changes in lifestyle. 3 Avoidance of public places. 4 Difficulty in social relationships. 5 Allowance for more medical appointments and specialists' visits. 6 Mothers' perspectives on recovery or healing from autism. 7 Feelings of denial, sadness, uncertainty and grief. 8 Acceptance of the diagnosis and maternal empowerment: tenacity for the present and hope for the future. 9 Creating positive experiences for child. 10 Determination in obtaining information, resources, and services for the children: the quest for researching the diagnosis. 11 Recapturing one's sense of being and maturity. 12 Knowledge sharing. 13 Identification of mothers' social supports.

continued

Table 4.1 Continued

Author and purpose	*Design*	*Sample*	*Findings*
Neely-Barnes et al. (2011) To examine experiences of parents through their conceptualizations of autism and the theme of parental blame.	Focus groups.	N = 11. Participants: mothers = 9, fathers = 2. Purposive sampling. Demographics: 7 in first focus group, 4 in second focus group; 2 foster parents, 9 biological parents; 4 African American, 5 white, 1 Asian American, 1 Latina. Mean age = 42.8 years. 4 high-school education, 3 some college, 1 college degree, 3 graduate degrees.	1 Constructions of the parent and the child with autism by outsiders: • autism is invisible; • the shopping experience; • extended family; • people who understand. 2 Parents' responses to the public construction: • confrontation; • presence in the community; • picking your battles/choosing to ignore. 3 Parents' constructions of themselves and the child with autism: • the child's strengths; • extraordinary family; • overcoming/living/coping with autism. *Subthemes – influence of demographics* 1 Difference between mothers and fathers. 2 Role of race/ethnicity. 3 Differences between biological and foster parents.
Phelps et al. (2009) To explore the biopsychosocial-spiritual, systemic, and ecological implications of having a child with autism on family's lives and overall functioning.	Written narratives.	N = 80. Participants: anonymous; convenience sampling (Autism Society of North Carolina). Demographics: unknown.	1 Psychological implications. 2 Familial implications. 3 Social implications. 4 Services. 5 Spiritual benefits. 6 Economic challenges. 7 Focus on future.

Ryan and Cole (2009) Broader study: To explore the experiences of living with ASD from the parents' perspective; this analysis of that data: to understand the roles of advocacy and activism in the life of parents of children with ASD.	Individual semi-structured interviews.	$N = 36$ parents (all mothers). Convenience and snowball sampling via support groups, newsletters, online communities, special schools, and parent coordinators. Wide range of ages, ethnicities, marital status, and income but not specified. 17 full-time caregivers, 9 worked full-time, 10 worked part-time.	1 A different kind of mothering. 2 Individual approaches. 3 Individual activism. 4 Collectivism. 5 Social model mothers.
Schwartz (2001) To better understand what families of autistic children experience in adapting to and coping with their autistic child, and how it has influenced their lives.	Semi-structured individual interviews.	$N = 7$. Snowball sampling (identified by members of agencies serving families with autistic children). All parents were married. Combined income between $80,000 and $130,000. 6 Caucasian, 1 other.	1 Support: a friends; b husband; c community: • stigma and public judgment; d extended family; e counseling. 2 Emotional issues. 3 Coping before diagnosis. 4 Coping after diagnosis. 5 Child's developmental level. 6 Services.

Table 4.2 Final themes from studies of parents of children with autism

	Emotional stress and strain	*Adaptation*	*Stigmatization*	*Appreciating the little things*	*Impact on siblings*	*Future concerns*	*Services*
Total number of studies	14	8	6	5	4	6	6
Ewart (2002)	x	x	x	x	x		x
Hunt-Jackson (2007)	x	x	x	x	x	x	x
Hutton and Caron (2005)	x	x		x	x		x
Kalash (2009)	x		x		x	x	x
Kent (2011)	x	x		x	x		
Kuhaneck et al. (2010)	x	x		x	x		
Larson (2010)	x	x			x		
Lendenmann (2010)	x	x		x	x		
Lutz et al. (2012)	x	x	x	x	x	x	
Martinez (2009)	x	x	x			x	x
Neely-Barnes et al. (2011)	x	x	x				
Phelps et al. (2009)	x	x		x		x	x
Ryan and Cole (2009)	x	x		x			x
Schwartz (2001)	x	x	x	x		x	x

References

* Denotes an article used in the meta-synthesis.

APA (American Psychiatric Association). (2000). *Diagnostic and statistical manual of mental disorders* (Text revision). Washington, D.C.: Author.

APA (American Psychiatric Association). (2013). *Diagnostic and statistical manual of mental disorders* 5. Washington, D.C.: Author.

Centers for Disease Control. (March 28, 2014). Prevalence of Autism Spectrum Disorder Among Children Aged 8 Years – Autism and Developmental Disabilities Monitoring Network, 11 Sites, United States, 2010. *Morbidity and Mortality Weekly Report (MMWR)*. Retrieved from www.cdc.gov/mmwr/preview/mmwrhtml/ss6302a1.htm?s_cid=ss6302a1_w.

*Ewart, K. H. (2002). *Parents' experience of having a child with autism* (Doctoral dissertation). Available from ProQuest Dissertations and Theses Global (Order No. 3062724).

Finfgeld, D. L. (2003). Metasynthesis: The state of the art – so far. *Qualitative Health Research*, *13*(7), 893–904.

Finlayson, K. W., and Dixon, A. (2008). Qualitative meta-synthesis: A guide for the novice. *Nurse Researcher*, *15*(2), 59–71.

Freedman, B., Kalb, L., Zablotsky, B., and Stuart, E. (2012). Relationship status among parents of children with autism spectrum disorders: A population-based study. *Journal of Autism and Developmental Disorders*, *42*, 539–548.

Hodge, D., Hoffman, C., and Sweeney, D. (2011). Increased psychopathology in parents of children with autism: Genetic liability or burden of caregiving. *Journal of Developmental and Physical Disabilities*, *23*, 227–239.

Hoffmann, T., Windham, G., Anderson, M., Croen, L., Grether, J., and Risch, N. (2014). Evidence of reproductive stoppage in families with autism spectrum disorder: A large, population-based cohort study. *JAMA Psychiatry*, *71*(8): 943–951.

*Hunt-Jackson, J. (2007). *Finding fathers' voices: Exploring life experiences of fathers of children with Autistic Spectrum Disorders*. Available from ProQuest Dissertations and Theses Global (UMI No. 3261989).

*Hutton, A. M., & Caron, S. L. (2005). Experiences of families with children with autism in rural New England. *Focus on Autism and Other Developmental Disabilities*, *20*(3), 180–189.

Jones, M. (2004). Application of systematic review methods to qualitative research: Practical issues. *Journal of Advanced Nursing*, *48*(3), 271–278.

*Kalash, L. A. (2009). *Perspectives of parents who have a child diagnosed with an autism spectrum disorder* (University of North Dakota) (Order No. 3406196). Available from ProQuest Dissertations and Theses Global. Retrieved from http://search.proquest.com/docview/276068082?accountid=14780.

*Kent, M. C. (2011). *Autism spectrum disorders and the family: A qualitative study*. (Doctoral dissertation). Available from ProQuest Dissertations and Theses Global (Order No. 3459692).

*Kuhaneck, H. M., Burroughs, T., Wright, J., Lemanczyk, T., and Darragh, A. R. (2010). A qualitative study of coping in mothers of children with an autism spectrum disorder. *Physical and Occupational Therapy in Pediatrics*, *30*(4), 340–350. doi: 10.3109/01942638.2010.481662.

Lambrechts, G., Van Leeuwen, K., Boonen, H., Maes, B., and Noens, I. (2011). Parenting behaviour among parents of children with autism spectrum disorder. *Research in Autism Spectrum Disorders*, *5*, 1143–1152.

*Larson, E. (2010). Ever vigilant: Maternal support of participation in daily life for boys with autism. *Physical and Occupational Therapy in Pediatrics*, *30*(1), 16–27. doi:10.3109/13668250.2012.736614.

*Lendenmann, M. M. (2010). *The lived experience of parenting a preschool age, moderately mentally retarded autistic child* (Doctoral dissertation). Available from ProQuest Dissertations and Theses Global (Order No. 3391263).

*Lutz, H. R., Patterson, B. J., and Klien, J. (2012). Coping with autism: A journey toward adaptation. *Journal of Pediatric Nursing*, *27*(3), 206–213. doi: 10.1016/j.pedn.2011.03.013.

*Martinez, V. R. (2009). *The ecology of experiences and supports of mothers with children with autism spectrum disorder during the children's early years* (Michigan State University) (Order No. 3396072). Available from ProQuest Dissertations and Theses Global. Retrieved from http://search.proquest.com/docview/304951373?accountid=14780.

Meade, M. O., and Richardson, W. S. (1997). Selecting and appraising studies for a systematic review. *Annals of Internal Medicine*, *127*, 531–537.

*Neely-Barnes, S. L., Hall, H. R., Roberts, R. J., and Graff, J. C. (2011). Parenting a child with an Autism Spectrum Disorder: Public perceptions and parental conceptualizations. *Journal of Family Social Work*, *14*(3), 208–225. doi: 10.1080/10522158.2011.571539.

Noblit, G. W., and Hare, R. D. (1988). *Meta-ethnography: Synthesizing qualitative studies*. Newbury Park, CA: Sage.

*Phelps, K., Hodgson, S., McCammon, S., and Lamson, A. (2009). Caring for an individual with Autism Disorder: A qualitative analysis. *Journal of Intellectual and Developmental Disability*, *34*(1), 27–35.

Pozo, P., Sarriá, E., and Brioso, A. (2014). Family quality of life and psychological well-being in parents of children with autism spectrum disorders: A double ABCX model. *Journal of Intellectual Disability Research*, *58*(5), 442–458. doi:10.1111/jir.12042.

*Ryan, S., and Cole, K. (2009). From advocate to activist? Mapping the experiences of mothers of children on the autism spectrum. *Journal of Applied Research in Intellectual Disabilities*, *22*(1), 43–53. doi:10.1111/j.1468–3148.2008.00438.x.

*Schwartz, M. (2001). *Understanding the well-being of the primary care-takers of Autistic children*. Available from ProQuest Dissertations and Theses Global (UMI No. 3323874).

Ruiz-Robledillo, N., De Andrés-García, S., Pérez-Blasco, J., González-Bono, E., and Moya-Albiol, L. (2014). Highly resilient coping entails better perceived health, high social support and low morning cortisol levels in parents of children with autism spectrum disorder. *Research in Developmental Disabilities*, *35*, 686–695.

Yirmiya, N., and Shaked, M. (2005). Psychiatric disorders in parents of children with autism: A meta-analysis. *Journal of Child Psychology and Psychiatry*, *46*, 69–83.

5 The lived experience of parents of youths with intellectual disability

Intellectual disability (ID) is a complex neurodevelopmental disorder that takes into account both a person's cognitive capacities and the quality of his or her interactions with the environment. The diagnosis was once based primarily on tests of one's intelligence quotient, but this has changed in the United States, with less emphasis on measured cognitive functioning in the fifth edition of the Diagnostic and Statistical Manual (APA, 2013). A meta-analysis of 52 studies worldwide revealed that the prevalence rate of intellectual disabilities was 10.37 per 1,000 people (Maulik et al., 2011).

Parents of this sizeable population of people afflicted with intellectual disabilities have been subject to research. This literature has emphasized both the problems and the strengths involved with parenting a child with such a disability. Depression has been a focus of studies, according to Glidden's (2012) review, and depression is common, at least in response to initial diagnosis. Over time, as parents adjust to the child and revise their expectations, the depression seems to dissipate. However, depression and negative reactions may persist if behavioral problems are present in the child.

In another literature review, Hauser-Cram et al. (2001) found that results in studies are mixed as to whether parental well-being in parents of children with disabilities compared to those without is compromised. Results of studies seem to agree that parents with economic support (Olsson and Hwang, 2008; Resch et al., 2012; Trute et al., 2007), social support (Hauser-Cram et al., 2001; Resch et al., 2012; Trute et al., 2007) and coping styles that include problem-focused coping (i.e., active, planful approaches to stress) (Hauser-Cram et al., 2001; Resch et al., 2012), low appraisals of threat (Resch et al., 2012), and positive perception and meaning toward the disability (Trute et al., 2007, 2010). The more recent studies indicate that it is not the presence of a child with ID by itself that predicts parental well-being or the child's functional impairment or severity of the disability (Resch et al., 2012; Trute et al., 2007). In a Swedish study, the majority of mothers of children with ID (68 percent) possessed high well-being (Olsson and Hwang, 2008). Additionally, a survey conducted with 2,044 parents of down's syndrome children indicated that the vast majority reported positive experiences: 97 percent were proud of them; 79 percent felt their outlook on life was more positive because of them (Skotko et al., 2011); 5 percent felt embarrassed by them; and 4 percent regretted having them.

These quantitative studies on parents of children with ID often combine types of disability (for example, autism-spectrum or physical disabilities were included). A focus only on intellectual disabilities is needed as this may pose unique parenting challenges. Additionally, qualitative research is ideal for uncovering more nuanced expressions of parents' experiences and to gain more depth of understanding into their perceptions and daily challenges. At this point, qualitative studies have accumulated in sufficient numbers to justify the use of meta-synthesis, a methodology designed to systematically review and integrate results of primary qualitative studies that have been conducted on a similar topic (Finfgeld, 2003; Sandelowski and Barroso, 2006). Although meta-synthesis is not without controversy (see Finlayson and Dixon, 2008; Jones, 2004), it is a valuable way to build knowledge in a particular area of study so that practice and policy implications may be developed from qualitative research.

Only one meta-synthesis appears to have been conducted in the field of intellectual disabilities. Griffith and Hastings (2014) located 17 published studies that involved the experience of caregivers of children (both youth and adults) that had intellectual disabilities accompanied by behavioral challenges, and especially the supportive services that were used. Themes were the following: (1) caregivers experienced love for their children and this dominated narratives; (2) caregivers gave up their own identity, at least in part, to become the carers of their children; (3) crisis management when challenging behavior became dangerous; (4) the support caregivers sought were not specifically for the behavior problems but were more general in nature; (5) caregivers had to battle professionals and support services and generally found accessing services a difficult and overwhelming process.

The purpose of the current meta-synthesis is to examine more broadly the experience of parents of children with intellectual disabilities, residing in Western countries, that were elementary-school-aged children and adolescents and that lived in the home. Two meta-syntheses were produced out of the search: one involved the lived experience of parents of children and adolescents; the other centered solely on parental perceptions of the transition process from high school. Although these topic areas both involved youth, the focus of some studies on the transition process itself seemed to warrant gathering these studies and synthesizing them into their own meta-synthesis.

Themes of parents with children and adolescents with intellectual disability

The inclusion criteria for parents of children and adolescents produced a total of eight studies. The majority of the participants were Caucasian married couples. Most of the studies were conducted in the US, but the UK and Australia were also represented. The majority of studies were presented in peer-reviewed journal articles but there were also dissertations. Further detail on primary studies is elaborated in Table 5.1.

Certain themes emerged across studies and these included: (1) negative experiences with the medical system; (2) grief reactions at the time of diagnosis; (3) normalization; (4) stigma; (5) fears for the future; (6) impact on the family – both positive and negative; (7) religious and spiritual support (see Table 5.2).

Negative experiences with the medical system

A common theme involved negative experiences with doctors and other medical providers. A lack of warmth, understanding, sensitivity, and support characterized parental interactions from time of the diagnosis on. Some doctors relayed negative and hopeless attitudes and made dire predictions (Glenn, 1987). As one mother stated: "Well, I think the obstetricians seemed to be very poorly informed. One didn't say anything at all. The other one came in and cried and told me that I should think about institutionalizing the child" (Glenn, 1987, p. 82). Another participant described:

> [The pediatrician] came right in after I delivered him. It was Christmas morning and she said I have a Down's syndrome child and he has a hole in the heart and he has an inverted testicle and he has a double hernia and I should take him home and that he wouldn't live six months. Very cold, very heartless attitude. I think they did not know how to act ... everything was just thrown at me.
>
> (Glenn, 1987, p. 82)

In Pillay et al. (2012), a mother reported how the doctor delivered the initial diagnosis. "The Doctor had very bad bedside manners.... I felt like he was blaming me for the birth of my child. He kept saying, 'So you didn't have a test did you? You didn't have a test did you?' " (Pillay et al., 2012, p. 1503).

Heer et al. (2012) were scathing of professionals. They said that they couldn't get a diagnosis, they blamed medical professionals for why their children had an intellectual disability, they were unhappy with the services provided, especially by South Asian providers, and felt like providers blamed them for their children's condition (e.g., "marrying relations").

Lin *et al.* (2010) also discussed the way medical providers diminished the personhood of ID. As one participant in that study said: "Another doctor had said 'Oh they probably won't do anything about his ears because he's got Downs Syndrome,' and I felt that was ... but it was not medical profession, it's not been people" (p. 37).

A father's statement embodies the sentiments of a number of the parents regarding what they experienced or sensed in their contacts with physicians:

> Well, I think the problem with some pediatricians was the attitude about having handicapped children. They made it quite obvious that while they

> were going to do the professional thing, there wasn't any extra that they would give a normal child. We discovered that a lot of doctors didn't want to touch handicapped children that it was almost like a reflection on themselves. They only wanted to deal on perfect models.
>
> (Glenn, 1987, p. 108)

One mother discussed the condescending attitudes of doctors:

> Medical professionals are very condescending to parents, especially moms. You are the parent, you're with the child 24 hours a day. Just because he doesn't do what you tell the doctor he's been doing in the five minutes you're there, doesn't mean you don't know what you are talking about. They pass if off as mom just overreacting or panicking. Or they say well kids like these, that happens to them, don't worry.
>
> (Brown, 1993, p. 89)

Over time, parents stated that they took on an advocacy role, believing that they knew their child better than the doctors did, and pushed for services their children needed and deserved (Glenn, 1987; Prussing et al., 2004).

Grief reactions at the time of diagnosis

Even though it had been years since diagnosis, parents described having strong emotional reactions – shock, devastation, grief, and depression – to learning of their child's diagnosis (Brown, 1993; Glenn, 1987; Pillay et al., 2012). Brown (1993) commented on the level of detail in the stories about the initial diagnosis and their reactions. In Pillay et al. (2012), another mother stated: "Just dreadful grief. Extreme distress … it's a whole different pathway. So tremendous grief when she was first born for my normal baby that I didn't have" (p. 1503).

Normalization

Rejecting ideas of suffering and hardship, many families seem to turn instead to definitions of family life as similar to those of typically-developing children (Lalvani, 2008). Many parents strove to make their families as normal and as ordinary as possible (Glenn, 1987; Povee et al., 2012; Todd and Jones, 2005). Note that the term "normalization" (Hayes and Batey, 2013) refers to making conditions normal for the person with ID rather than making the person "normal."

However, Todd and Jones (2005), in particular, discussed that this strategy became more difficult as the child grew into adolescence. Siblings would leave home, and school was ending for the child with ID with other roles uncertain, so more responsibility fell on parents.

Stigma

Mothers expressed anger and sadness at the stigma in society of how children and families with Downs are viewed (Glenn, 1987; Povee et al., 2012). When family and friends found out about the diagnosis prenatally, some pressured mothers to abort. After the child was born, family and friends referring to mothers as "saints," which gave the implicit message that having a child with Down syndrome was largely undesirable (Brown, 1993; Povee et al., 2012). One mother stated:

> People are often patronizing. I don't really appreciate that. They will say things like, "Oh, you must be a saint and this and that." I'm not a saint, do you think my child isn't human, that I should have put him in an institution or killed him?
>
> (Brown, 1993, p. 85)

Even more distressing to parents "was the lack of value society placed on their child" (Brown, 1993, p. 85):

> A big issue is what's M's place in the world? Just what role do people really see for a child like this in society? It comes down to society just wanting to take care of him forever. I see that was a way to separate him from people. All these systems designed to help the handicapped, what is the purpose – just to be caretakers for them. I think they should try to really find some role for them.
>
> (Brown, 1993, pp. 85–86)

Fears for the future

One of parents' current stressors was fear of the future, present in almost all studies (Glenn, 1987; Heer et al., 2012; Pillay et al., 2012; Todd and Jones, 2005). They were worried about what would happen to the child in terms of income, employment, and housing, as parents aged or died and could no longer be responsible. They did not want to burden siblings, and wondered about how much governmental support would be available (Glenn, 1987).

Impact on the family

Positive impact

Mothers reported may positive impacts from having a child with ID. They had grown as individuals in terms of compassion and acceptance, were more patient, and had their priorities straight (Povee et al., 2012). As well as an individual impact, mothers stated that there was a positive result on the family from the presence of the child with the intellectual disability pulling everyone together (Glenn 1987; Pillay et al., 2012; Povee et al., 2012).

Some mothers also said that it had improved their relationships with their husbands, bringing them closer than perhaps they would have been. One mother in Glenn (1987) said:

> I'd say our big coping thing would be that we have depended on each other. With (husband) and I, we lean on each other so much that we find that we really don't need to lean on other people that much.
>
> (p. 119)

Parents also claimed there was a positive impact on siblings from having to live with a child with a disability, with such children being more responsible and understanding (Glenn, 1987; Pillay et al., 2012).

Negative impact

Perhaps more common than a positive impact on the family was an expressed negative impact. Most often parental concerns revolved around the effect on siblings in terms of their receiving less attention, having a restricted social life, and assuming caretaker duties (Povee et al., 2012). As one mother stated: "My son has helped to bring her up.... Less time for him to build up own friendships" (Povee et al., 2012, p. 969). Indeed, as children grew older, parents became worried about siblings leaving the home because then they would have to assume even more care (Todd and Jones, 2005). In Glenn (1987), some parents decried the loss of a "normal sibling relationship" that typically developing siblings missed out on. Additionally, siblings, as part of the family, experienced curtailment of family activities and holidays because of socially inappropriate behaviors (stubborness, aggression, tantrums), the child's need for routine and anxiety in new and unfamiliar surroundings and situations, and safety issues (children wandering away) (Povee et al., 2012). As one parent said: "It is very hard to go places as Dylan tends to run off and not listen. We are always worried he may get lost" (p. 969). The low functional ability of the child with Down syndrome was another factor commonly identified as having a negative impact on the family. The care demands of the child with Down syndrome, including transportation, dressing, feeding and toileting, were described as being stressful and exhausting, a financial burden and limiting the time that could be spent with other family members (Povee et al., 2012, p. 969).

Some of the negative impact of having a child with an intellectual disability was the resultant strain on the marriage (Pillay et al., 2012). Lack of time as a couple, differences in parenting strategies, and financial stress, were reasons given for marital strain (Povee et al., 2012). Financial stress was related to "[t]he cost of special education, medical and therapy appointments, childcare and entertainment for the child with Down syndrome was described by parents/carers as having a major impact on the family's finances" (Povee et al., 2012, p. 969).

Spirituality and religion

Another, smaller theme, revolved around the role of religious and spirituality beliefs for coping (Pillay et al., 2012). Spiritual beliefs provided comfort and strength (Prussing et al., 2004). A mother in Glenn's (1987) study noted: "It has made it possible to stay sane and hopeful and appreciate him as he is" (p. 119), and a father said: "When we have a problem, we do a lot of praying. It doesn't change anything, but it gives you a peace of mind. You have a special child and with God's help you're going to do it" (p. 119). Spiritual beliefs also facilitated acceptance of the situation. For example, in Heer et al.'s (2012) study of a South Asian sample living in the UK, participants believed "it's God's choice."

Attendance at religious institutions could also be helpful for some women in terms of not only the spiritual benefits, but also more tangible benefits involving inclusion in church-related activities and a social network (Prussing et al., 2004). That depended a great degree on how supportive the institution and its members were of their child (Prussing et al., 2004). "People at the church have always just accepted J. and worked around him and that's been helpful," a father stated (Glenn, 1987, p. 118).

Findings of meta-synthesis on parents of adolescents going through the transition process

This meta-synthesis on parents' perspectives of their adolescent children going through the transition process and leaving school involved eight studies in total. Studies were published mainly in the US but also the UK and Australia. The findings coalesced around the following themes: (1) the meaning of the transition process; (2) lack of resources and access to services; (4) transition planning; (5) the need for parental advocacy; and (6) parents' experience of negative emotions. See Table 5.3 for details on methodology of studies and Table 5.4 for themes.

Meaning of the transition process

The meaning of the transition process was seen by parents or caregivers of adolescents with intellectual disabilities as an opportunity for the adolescents to assume similar roles to peers without intellectual disabilities (Hanley-Maxwell, Whitney-Thomas, and Pogoloff, 1995). A sense of normality was given to roles such as holding on to more permanent employment, being able to live independently, and having the ability to make decisions for oneself. One mother of an individual with intellectual disabilities stated:

> Well we would love her to leave home and have a place on her own, maybe sharing with somebody, and have some carers looking after … that would be the ideal situation.… I hope she will continue working and yeah, ideally I would like her to be more involved with work and not…
>
> (Dyke et al., 2013, p. 155)

In Hanley Maxwell et al. (1995), parents had specific visions in terms of employment, housing arrangements, and social life that they wanted for their child.

Lack of access to services and resources

The dominant theme for this meta-synthesis, the lack of access to services and resources, was expressed by participants in all studies. The lack of available services after putting the transition plan in place was a "charade," as one participant described it. Long waiting lists, fragmentation of services, and bureaucracy and inflexibility were detailed. One mother reported: "In the last 12 months, I was most affected by the failure of my application for accommodation support funding on behalf of my disabled son.... I experienced the most heartrending sorrow of all the past 21 years" (Rapanaro et al., 2008, p. 37). Another mother in Raghaven *et al.* (2013) said:

> I asked for respite care a year ago and nothing ... and I'm very dissatisfied with the reaction that I got from the social worker. I'm at the edge of saying I can't cope with it anymore, I want him to go into respite or a group home. But it shouldn't had to get to this point, I'm so angry about it.
>
> (p. 940)

Problems with service providers was a subtheme to general lack of services and inability to access them. Unprofessionalism and lack of training were described. A parent in Rapanaro et al. (2008) detailed an incident:

> When going to ... enrol him in a course, I was treated as if I was disabled or intellectually impaired ... they would not let me assist him in making decisions and as a result would not enrol him in a life skills class. I went home feeling desperate, discouraged and depressed.
>
> (p. 38)

Schools were seen mostly as a high-support environment (Dyke et al., 2013; Gillan and Coughlan, 2010; Sagen and Ytterhus, 2015), and parents lamented the lack of services and supports that could never come close to matching up. As one father said in Hanley-Maxwell et al. (1995): "It's absurd to think of these kids leaving school and finding a substitute for school" (p. 10), and another said: "It's just like in the community, when you get into the adult program nobody knows you're there" (p. 10). A parent in Dyke et al. (2013) was concerned about loss of progress that had been made in the school system:

> The people at the adult program ... none of them have any real training ... but ... what frustrates me the most is ... it is all a waste of time because as soon as you get to adult services none of it is used ... so they lose all of these skills.
>
> (p. 153)

The only positive mentioned about service providers was that their children had relationships with staff that they did not have with people in their social network; people with ID were dependent on paid staff for friendship and companionship.

Need for parental advocacy

Advocacy was another important theme that arose from the primary studies. The success of the transition was often dependent upon how much advocacy was done by the adolescent's parent. The caregivers at times aligned themselves with professionals, such as social workers, adult service workers, and special education school teachers to aid with their advocacy and offer insight (Gillan and Coughlan, 2010). This advocacy was done to acquire services to help fill unmet needs (Dyke et al., 2013). An individual with Down syndrome reported: "Yeah I had lots of support like I've got a mother that really, like wrote so many letters to the Ministers, to every Minister you can imagine, to Canberra, to all the local ones here…" (Dyke et al., 2013, p. 154). In Rapanaro et al.'s study (2008), parents wrote in the following statements:

> I have become more resourceful and will not take "no" for an answer anymore. [I] try more avenues, speak to more people.… My daughter is a normal teenager with problems and I'm not shy about getting us the help we need.…

Stress and negative emotions in parents

The transition process for adolescents with intellectual disabilities was *extremely stressful for their parents*. This theme was present in most studies, either implicitly or explicitly. Many parents reported feelings of anxiety with the uncertainty and loss that the transition represented. As one person expressed it:

> I was really scared … it was a really emotional time and because you are leaving this environment that you've been a part of for 15 years.… I think I was struggling more to think how am I going to cope not having this network of people because I've known them for so long.
>
> (Dyke et al., 2013, p. 155)

Another parent experienced stress as a result of being unable to access enough support so she could continue employment: "My son is leaving school at the end of this year and trying to get enough money from post-school options and enough [support] hours [to enable me] to continue working is so stressful" (Rapanaro et al., 2008). In the same study, Rapanaro et al. (2008) listed a series of statements written by parents demonstrating how painful the process was for them:

> "I cried on and off for weeks thinking about the way we were treated."

> "… constant clock watching and worry about the same thing happening again."

> "I resent his hold over my personal life and the fact that it still feels like the responsibility for a small child, but he is 18 and bigger and stronger…"

> "… feelings of guilt, sorrow, useless mother, irresponsible…"

> "I often feel very frustrated and stressed."

> "I am sometimes resentful of how much responsibility he creates and that it will always be the same…"

> "[a] sense of helplessness, of my life never being likely to improve. [A] sense of annoyance and frustration with myself for feeling like this…"

> "I worry about him … sometimes I feel I can't help [him] … I feel I failed as a mum…"

> "My overwhelming feeling is sadness, that [she] cannot have the life of any normal twenty year old."

Some of the painful feelings were about the transition process but some of them were about the fact that the child would not have a "normal lifestyle" and that the demands of caregiving would continue, unadulterated.

Discussion

These meta-syntheses of the qualitative research offer insight into the experience of parents with children diagnosed with an intellectual disability. Like the quantitative literature, there is discussion of both the hardships of raising such a child – the grief reactions at learning of the diagnosis, caregiving demands having a negative impact on the family, especially siblings, and fear for the child's future – and the positive experience – growing as individuals, closeness among family members.

We compared the results of the meta-synthesis on parent perspectives of children and adolescents to the meta-synthesis conducted on caregiver experiences with children's intellectual disability accompanied by behavioral challenges (Griffith and Hastings, 2014). Griffith and Hastings located more studies than ours (17 versus 8) given the differing inclusion criteria and age restrictions. Some of the themes found overlapped with ours whereas others were entirely different. We agree that love and caring underlaid the tone of caregivers' descriptions of their children, but it did not rise up as a theme. Identity concerns also did not emerge as a theme, although participants in both studies spoke about the high demand of caregiving. Crisis management was not a topic in this meta-synthesis but recall that one of the criteria of Griffith and Hastings (2014) was the presence of challenging behavior. In both meta-syntheses, there was an emergent theme of negative experiences with formal services. In Griffith and Hastings (2014), caregivers described the overwhelming nature of having to seek out services, and struggle through bureaucratic challenges to obtain them, with little help from professionals. In our meta-synthesis, the nature of the relationship was also negative, but it revolved around the medical system specifically. Doctors were characterized as uniformly insensitive and harsh and unable to see the personhood of the child with ID. These negative interactions occurred at the birth of the child and continued on as the child developed.

In the second meta-synthesis, parents seemed much more stressed at this stage, and a strengths-based theme did not emerge. Parents were upset and frustrated, among other negative emotions, about the lack of planning for transition, and the difficulty of accessing services, and, in general, a lack of services. They decried the loss of the school system and all the supports available when having to face the adult system that was fragmented, full of gaps, long waiting lists, and bureaucracy. At this level, staff were much less well trained than school personnel had been. Although parents had a vision of where they wanted their child to be, they were frustrated, sad, and scared about what they faced with their child's transition into adulthood. They attributed any successes to their own efforts at advocacy, at times coupled with that of a social worker or teacher who was particularly supportive.

The US Individuals with Disabilities Education Act in 1990 required that special education services in schools provide services and instruction that enabled students with intellectual (and other disabilities) to "transition" after high school to postsecondary education, independent living and work roles (Wehmeyer and Webb, 2012). Wehmeyer and Webb (2012) review evidence from quantitative studies, including the National Longitudinal Transition Study of Special Education Students, that in terms of adult outcomes – employment, income, postsecondary education, and living independently – youth with disabilities fared poorly. However, there were noticeable improvements between the first and second National Longitudinal Transition Studies.

Despite these improvements, the participants talked with one voice about the hardships of transition planning and then having their child actually obtain those needed resources and supports in the community that had been put in the plan. The Division on Career Development and Transition developed a comprehensive definition with guidelines about transitioning from school to postschool settings (Halpern, 1994, as cited in Wehmeyer and Webb, 2012). The suggestion that it should begin at age 14 as a minimum, that students should have as much responsibility as possible in the process, and involve families in the planning stage. Families were involved, but often felt "in the dark" and left out of the process. Despite these recommendations, the participants in this study did not experience transition in line with these guidelines.

Implications

Given the negative interactions with medical doctors, particularly at the time of diagnosis, it seems incumbent that social workers and other social service professionals are involved with families from the initial point of diagnosis. Such providers can educate medical doctors on how to make sensitive disclosures and referrals for follow-up services. Alternatively, social workers/social service practitioners could be involved in the delivery of news in a way that is unbiased, non-blaming, and supportive of a range of reactions, including grief, shock, and anger. Povee et al. (2012) described the necessity of this process to find a level of acceptance. As one parent said: "It's more like a puzzle, or maybe a mosaic. It's never really finished. It just takes time and its bit-by-bit – the emotions. I guess its finding contentment in where she's at and also seeing the beauty in her" (Pillay et al., 2012, p. 1504). The medical system is a dominant system for intellectual disability, particularly because of the medical comorbidities involved. Therefore, it is imperative that interactions with doctors are improved for the quality of life experienced by parents and their children with ID.

Another implication for social service providers is to recognize and validate the burden associated with care demands, as well as the behavioral and health challenges that youth with ID often manage. Reducing these burdens, whenever possible, by facilitating referrals to a work-force of competent care workers who can provide respite and assistance is critical. Although participants didn't generally mention attendance at support groups as helpful (an exception was Glenn, 1987), it seems that social workers and other social service providers are poised well to assist with the potential impact on siblings, creating support for them, and providing concrete services so that parents can pay more attention to siblings.

The picture from the perspectives of parents in the qualitative studies of the transition process is a grim portrayal of what this is like for parents. Although they had high hopes for their children assuming adult roles in the community, they struggled to obtain the services their children needed. Services were often unavailable and when they were, hard to locate and to access. Clearly needed are supports in the environment; these supports would have to be coordinated and streamlined and parents would need essential information to navigate the service system (Stewart et al., 2008).

Key elements of successful transitioning have been identified to include the following (Wehmeyer and Webb, 2012, p. 6): assessment of strengths, needs, preferences, and interests; development of a set of transition activities/services that is included in the IEP and then implemented; coordination among key school and adult service agency personnel; and family involvement.

Summary

This chapter described through two meta-syntheses, parents' experience raising youth with IDD. One meta-synthesis was of parents' experiences with children, and the other involved parenting adolescents. The second focused more specifically on the transition process of children moving from the school system to the community. Challenges occurred at each of these stages with parents of adolescents particularly concerned about the transition process.

Table 5.1 Data extraction of studies of parents of children with intellectual disabilities

Author and purpose	*Design*	*Data analysis*	*Sample*	*Findings*
Brown (2003) To explore the usefulness of family stress and coping theory in understanding family response to having a child with mental retardation. Insight into families' perceptions of events and the meanings they attributed to having a child with intellectual disabilities	Combination of in-depth interviews with mothers and fathers.	Interview data was coded for coping strategies and challenges/issues.	$N = 46$. Families recruited from five special education districts in southeastern Michigan. Child with mental retardation must be between the ages of 1 and 12 years and child had to be placed in either the Educable Mentally Impaired or Trianable Mentally Impaired program. Median age of mothers: 36 years, fathers: 52 years. Race: 96% white, 4% black/Hispanic. Child's gender: 52.2% female, 47.8% male. All two-parent families.	Difficulty with transition from early intervention program to regular school. Multiple roles. Distress due to stereotyping and labeling of the child (stigma).

continued

Table 5.1 Continued

Author and purpose	*Design*	*Data analysis*	*Sample*	*Findings*
Glenn (1987) To explore parental perceptions of raising a child with an intellectual disability and the meaning of the child to the family.	In-depth interviews.	The coding categories were developed from the topics in the interview schedule; these categories were called "topical" categories and represent the first level of analysis the investigator identified and explored relationships and themes within and among the topical coding categories.	N = 49 parents of children who were diagnosed as moderate intellectual disability. 25 two-parent families, 5 single-parent families. Child's mean age = 11.3 years, 90% white, most had Down syndrome. Parents were contacted through two agencies serving handicapped children. Both agencies provide services to children based on contractual agreements with local public school districts. The agencies are located in a large metropolitan area in the midwestern US and educate students between ages of 3 and 21.	Parental descriptions of the initial period of learning of their child's handicap were characterized by considerable emotion, as well as detailed recollections. Parents believed in the importance of their child being dealt with in as normal a manner as possible. A major concern was the uncertainty of the future for their child. Generally, felt support at church, but some felt that church was not sensitive to ID. Grandparents were noted by half (N = 15) of the families as a source of support. Parents experienced educational system as major resource. Both positive and negative impact on siblings and positive impact on family. Support groups or associations for parents of mentally retarded children were also noted as source of support (attended by about half of sample).

Heer et al. (2012) "To explore the cultural context of care-giving amongst South Asian communities caring for a child with intellectual disabilities in the United Kingdom" (p. 179).	2 focus groups; 1 of Muslims and 1 of Sikhs.	Interpretative phenomenological analysis.	*N* = 9 parents (5 mothers, 4 fathers). 4 Sikhs, 5 Muslims, recruited from existing carers' support groups in the UK. All participants biological parents of children with intellectual disabilities and caring for them at home; all children born in the UK; all Sikh parents born in India, all Muslim parents born in Pakistan.	1 Making sense of the disability: • "God's choice": using religious beliefs to make sense of disability; • making sense of disability in relation to behavior problems; • believed children had problems with expression, not with understanding; • struggle getting a diagnosis: belief by parents that medical negligence was to blame for child's disability. 2 Feeling let down by services: • anger at unresponsive doctors; • feeling blamed by service providers; • difficult interactions with Asian service providers. 3 Looking to the future: • concerns for future well-being; • wanting help vs. giving up.
Lin et al. (2010) To understand the formal support needs and experiences of mothers of adolescents with intellectual disabilities	Semi-structured interviews at 3 6-month intervals in time.	Constant comparative analysis.	*N* = 7 mothers. Recruited from 2 caregiver organizations in Edinburgh. Mean age of children = 13.86 years.	Dissatisfaction with medical providers, seen as having a lack of sympathy and emotion, diminishment of personhood of ID. Social workers were seen as more favorable, especially in the area of arranging respite care, although still mixed reviews. Liked support of disability living allowance, but they had to fight to get it even though they were supposed to be eligible. School was also passive, and parents had to be vocal about getting the services that they are mandated to provide.

continued

Table 5.1 Continued

Author and purpose	*Design*	*Data analysis*	*Sample*	*Findings*
Pillay et al. (2012) To understand the experiences of mothers who have a child with Down syndrome and the possible role of spirituality and religion in the adjustment.	In-depth interviews.	Open-coding method described by Glaser & Strauss (1967).	$N = 8$ mothers of children with Down syndrome between ages of 7 and 12 years. Purposive sample recruited through *Down Syndrome NOW study*, a population-based database of families of children with Down syndrome living in Western Australia. All were either married or living with a partner.	Stress and difficulty when first getting diagnosis (postnatal). Frustration and heartbreak in seeing child struggle and fail to do things that normally developing children can do. Mothers preferred mainstreamed public schools because of their greater need for accountability. Support from other mothers in the organization Down Syndrome WA. Maternal stress was related to child behavioral problems, comorbid health conditions, stigma, "work-life balance, schooling, future planning and financial" strain (p. 1504). Fear about the future – how could the child be independent? Important to accepting the diagnosis was a working through of emotions and finding the beauty in the child. Frustration and heartbreak in seeing child struggle and fail to meet normal developmental milestones.

				Stress was related to comorbid health or behavioral conditions, financial strain, stigma. Personal coping style of optimism was found helpful. Felt like they had grown as people. Spiritual beliefs. Support from husbands and family (mothers' parents especially) – emotional and physical support – childcare, cooking, and cleaning. Despite support, sometimes felt strain with husbands because child is taking attention A change in life plans meant reductions in friendships and socializing.
Povee et al. (2012) "To explore the factors that predict functioning in families with a child with Down syndrome" (p. 961).	Write-in responses to four questions.	Thematic analysis using method by Braun & Clarke (2006).	$N = 224$ caregivers of children identified through the Down Syndrome NOW study. Most were low income. Average child age: 13 years.	Family provided emotional support and respite care. Normality: no difference from normal families. Family activities and vacations were curtailed. Some parents: child had positive impact on family life but, more commonly, child had negative impact, most often for impact on siblings and marital strain.

continued

Table 5.1 Continued

Author and purpose	*Design*	*Data analysis*	*Sample*	*Findings*
Prussing et al. (2004) To explore parents' perceptions of the extent and quality of communication about complementary/alternative medicine (CAM) with pediatricians, and to obtain parents' recommendations for improvement.	Qualitative semistructured parent interviews.	Data was tape-recorded and analyzed with assistance from qualitative data analysis software. Comprehensive content analysis of the interview data, identifying and coding themes with the assistance of qualitative data analysis software. Additionally, narrative analysis was conducted.	$N = 30$. All were parents of children with Down Syndrome under age of 18 years. A convenience sample, as all were recruited with assistance of Down Syndrome Association of San Diego. The sample was culturally and linguistically diverse, but all participants were fluent in English.	Parents described how they advocated with their pediatricians about biomedical concerns, but commonly avoided discussing nonbiomedical concerns, such as CAM. Many parents expressed that they expected pediatricians to initiate conversations about CAM. Among families who used CAM therapies ($N = 26$), most parents (67%) described communicating none or only some of this use to their pediatricians. Parents emphasized their identities as healthcare coordinators for their children, and linked their advocacy to tensions and frustration in their interactions with pediatricians. Parents most frequently ($N = 19$) related an absence of communication to pediatricians' lack of knowledge about CAM and lack of time during visits.

Todd and Jones (2005) Looking at the future and seeing the past: the challenge of the middle years of parenting a child with intellectual disabilities.	Conversational interviews.	In-depth interviews with mothers of children with intellectual disabilities.	$N = 30$. Location: Wales, UK. Mother's age: average age: 48 years; age range: 34–56 years. Child's age: 11–19. Sample size was opportunistically selected from various places: • social services; • parental support groups; • participants of previous groups who had worked with other researchers.	• Mothers of children with intellectual disabilities saw themselves as having a normal and ordinary life like any other mother. • Parents reported needing the same amount of assistance with care of their adult children with ID but receiving less help with caring duties. • Parents reported that their resources in care for their adult children with ID diminished significantly.

Table 5.2 Themes from studies of parents of children with intellectual disabilities

Author	*Initial reactions to diagnosis*	*Normalization*	*Fear for future*	*Stigma*	*Impact on family*	*Religion and spirituality*	*Negative interactions with medical system*
Brown (2003)				Distress due to stereotyping and labeling of child.			Negative interactions with medical professionals. Had to advocate for child.
Glenn (1987)	Parental descriptions of initial period of learning of their child's handicap were characterized by considerable emotion, as well as detailed recollection of their feelings and reactions at that time.	Parents believed in importance of their child being dealt with in as normal a manner as possible.	Uncertainty about future for their child when parents were no longer able to be responsible.		*Positive* Both positive and negative impact on siblings. Brought spouses closer together. The child was not only valued as an individual, but seen as enriching to the life of the family. *Negative* Both positive and negative impact on siblings.	Almost half of families saw involvement in their church as resource, but some did not find churches receptive to ID.	Insensitive reactions of medical providers, parents turned to advocacy role to get their children's health needs met.

Heer et al. (2012)			Fear for the future.			"God's choice" – explanation for ID.	Dismissal by medical professionals; feeling blamed by medical professionals; looking for a diagnosis; blame Asian providers more than white providers; blame disability on medical negligence.
Lin et al. (2010)							Dissatisfaction with medical providers, seen as having lack of sympathy and emotion, diminishment of personhood of ID.
Pillay et al. (2012)	Stress and difficulty when first getting diagnosis (postnatal).		Fear about the future – how could the child be independent and hold job?	Maternal stress was related to, among other factors, stigma.	*Positive* Felt like they had grown as people. Felt that it had strengthened family relationships and pulled everyone together. But siblings had also developed positive characteristics as result of being sibling to disabled child.	Spirituality and religion.	Dissatisfaction with way medical providers gave diagnosis.

continued

Table 5.2 Continued

Author	*Initial reactions to diagnosis*	*Normalization*	*Fear for future*	*Stigma*	*Impact on family*	*Religion and spirituality*	*Negative interactions with medical system*
					Support from husbands and family (mothers' parents especially) – emotional and physical support – child care, cooking, and cleaning. *Negative* Felt guilty that attention was being taken away from siblings. Sometimes felt strain with husbands.		
Povee et al. (2012)		Normality: no difference from normal families.		Support: family – emotional support and respite care.	*Positive* Some parents: child had positive impact on family life, shaping life philosophy and helping people become better.		

		Negative Financial costs. Family activities and vacations were curtailed. More common among parents: that child had negative impact, most often for effect on siblings. Marital strain.		
Prussing et al. (2004)			Spirituality and religious beliefs and institutions helped to facilitate and shape acceptance.	Parents had to advocate with doctors but this was uncomfortable because most doctors did not want to be challenged. Discussion of complementary medicines avoided as doctors believed to be unsupportive.
Todd and Jones (2005)	Parents reported other stressors were thoughts about future, and death for themselves and their adult children with ID.			

Table 5.3 Data extraction of studies of parents of adolescents with intellectual disabilities undergoing transition

Author and purpose	*Design*	*Data analysis*	*Sample*	*Findings*
Bhaumik et al. (2011) To explore carers' perceptions of transition process, identify unmet needs, and offer ideas for addressing these unmet needs.	Face-to-face, semi-structured interviews.	Grounded theory approach.	*N* = 24 parents of teenagers aged 16–19 years diagnosed with intellectual disabilities (ID) living in city of Leicester and counties of Leicestershire and Rutland. Purposive sampling. Ethnicity: 92.4% Caucasian or South Asian. ID level: profound (17); severe (52); moderate (10). Type of accommodation: 83.5% living with family; 10.1% living in residential/foster care.	Services did not take into account those who could not communicate needs directly or who lived at home. Services needed to have more flexibility and less bureaucracy.
Cooney (2002) To explore perspectives on transition of youth with disabilities: voices of young adults, parents, and professionals.	Study completed in two phases: 1 first year of study followed 4 young adults with severe disabilities and their families; 2 second year of study included use of purposive sampling to select second group of 5 participants.	Qualitative content analysis.	*N* = 9 young adults with severe disability during their last year of high school in the US. Purposing sampling was used in this study. 5 male, 4 female. 3 from small-sized urban community and 6 from surrounding rural towns. 6 attended community-based life skills classroom, 2 in rural high school, and 1 in local urban central high school. 8 parents were interviewed. 7 teachers and 8 adult agency professionals were interviewed.	• Findings are not representative of larger population, but are important indicators of prevailing patterns that exist during transition periods. • Young adults are able to articulate aspirations for future and pursuit of independence. • Parents' goals for children included achieving fulfillment through use of skills, contributing to the greater community, and keeping children safe from harm. • Professionals formally planned and implemented transition for the young adults.

				• Perspectives on the young adults, viable options, and coping strategies to deal with insufficient transition plans.
Dyke et al. (2013) To identify life trajectory of young adults with Rett syndrome and Down syndrome after they transition from high school into adulthood.	Semi-interviews were administered to mothers of young adults with intellectual disabilities over the phone ranging from 15 to 70 minutes. Questions were comprised of information from literature reviews, ICF framework, and authors' knowledgeable on intellectual disabilities.	Content analysis.	$N = 18$. Purposive sampling method. Participants chosen from databases at Telethon Institute for Child Health Research in Perth, Western Australia. 11 mothers with daughters with Rett Syndrome, 7 mothers with either sons (3) or daughters (4) with Down Syndrome. Been out of school for 0 to 5 years. Range between ages of 19 to 33 years. 15 females, 3 males.	Adult roles assumed during day: • transition to day placement program, business service, open employment, vocational or educational placement; • success of transition dependent on level of parent's advocacy. Living a "good" life: • under half ($N = 8$) reported that outcome/good life they hoped for their child was not achieved; mainly connected to option of living independently with support and more permanent employment. Family impact: • anxiety for mother associated with leaving safety of school; timing of transition/loss of other informal supports; concerns about mother being able to continue work; transportation.

continued

Table 5.3 Continued

Author and purpose	*Design*	*Data analysis*	*Sample*	*Findings*
Gillan and Coughlan (2010) To highlight lack of information given to parents living in southern Ireland with children who have a mild intellectual disability that are transitioning from special education to post-school services. It also focuses on the different factors and psychological impacts that can occur to the family when a young adult with ID is transitioning to post-school services.	Semi-structured interviews were conducted with parents who had a child suffering from a mild intellectual disability.	Grounded theory.	*N* = 12: 4 married couples, 4 single mothers. Purposive sampling was used in this study. Parent/caregiver participant's ages ranged from 42 to 65 years. Children participants' ages ranged from 19 to 24 years. All had a mild intellectual disability. All participants were recruited through organizations working with families who live within one of the following counties: Cork, Kerry, Waterford, Wexford, Carlow, Tipperary, and Kilkenny (all located in southern Ireland). Children of parents participating in this study were attending either supported employment program or vocational training program provided by National Learning Network.	Post-school transition process in southern Ireland was viewed by parents as uncertain and stressful, especially when dealing with bureaucratic aspect of process. Results also showed many gaps between policy and transitional planning and post-school services for young adults with an intellectual disability and their families, which pose as obstacles and affect success of transition process from school-based services to post-school services.

Hanley-Maxwell et al. (1995) To examine issues relating to transition from school to adulthood for individuals with disabilities.	In-depth interviews.	Coding, memo-writing and domain analysis.	15 participants (parents of students who graduated from a medium-sized midwestern US city school district's program for individuals with cognitive disabilities). Purposive sampling was used in this study. 8 female, 7 male. 1 American Indian, 2 African American, 12 Caucasian.	Parents of students who are involved in transition process have specific vision for what they want for their child. Many of the parents reported that specific teachers throughout their children's educational careers had big influence on their child's ability to transition well.
Raghavan et al. (2013) Small et al. (2013) "To explore the family carers' views and experiences on transition from school to college or to adult life with special reference to ethnicity" (p. 936).	Interviewed twice.	Content analysis (not described).	*N* = 43 families. Recruited from social services, respite care homes, carer groups and organizations, and schools in West Yorkshire, UK. Convenience sample. Children aged from 14 to 22. White 37%, South Asian 60%.	1 Transition. 2 Formal support. 3 Family involvement, expectations, and coping. 4 Culture, language, and acculturation. 5 Religion. 6 Ethnicity and socioeconomic status.

continued

Table 5.3 Continued

Author and purpose	*Design*	*Data analysis*	*Sample*	*Findings*
Rapanaro et al. (2007) Perceived benefits and negative impact of challenges encountered in caring for young adults with intellectual disabilities in transition to adulthood.	Questionnaire that was completed by primary parental carer. Questionnaire asked that carer recall stressful events encountered while caring for their child. Experiences were categorized as: a unpleasant or upsetting feelings; b feelings of being unable to do things to level that they would have liked or expected; and c negative and positive outcomes associated with chronic demands of caring for child transitioning to adulthood.	Qualitative content analysis.	*N* = 119. Parents of young adults with intellectual disabilities aged 16–21 years. Purposive sampling was used in this study. Parents were identified by Western Australia's Disability Services Commission. 90% female. 77.8% metropolitan area. Mean age of parents: 48.05 years.	• Parents identified transition into adulthood as stressful. • Parents attributed difficulty of transition to lack of access to post-school services for their children, problematic interactions with service providers, issues relating to their children's independence or dependence, sexuality and behavioral problems, and children's vulnerability and well-being. • Despite difficulties experienced, 64.7% of parents reported perceived benefits or positive outcomes. • Nearly half of parents in study reported experiencing both negative and positive outcomes simultaneously.

Sagen and Ytterhus (2015) To examine “how the self-determination of pupils with intellectual disabilities is practised in secondary school in Norway” and to discuss “possible challenges connected to this practice” (p. 344).	Qualitative interviews and observation of school activities.	Hermeneutic design.	$N = 55$, with primary focus on 10 pupils ages 13-16 (6 boys, 4 girls); remainder of sample ($n = 45$) were parents and guardians, employees of the schools, and counselors at local educational and psychological counseling services. Participants selected through purposive sampling from schools in different midsize cities in Norway; children were selected on basis of mild to moderate intellectual disability diagnosis and with spoken language abilities.	• Widely varying degrees of self-determination for pupils in regards to their IEP plan and their learning activities: some had little influence over what they did, some had almost total control. • Content of IEP plans and what pupils actually did were often not correlated. • About half of pupils were able to decide when they wanted to work with mainstream class. • Pupils with high degree of self determination often suffered from not having education experiences that were structured and goal-oriented-allowed to do whatever they wanted. • Some teachers used self determination for pupils to increase learning outcomes by utilizing dialogue-based teaching and motivation.

continued

Table 5.3 Continued

Author and purpose	*Design*	*Data analysis*	*Sample*	*Findings*

				• Teachers' lack of focus on self determination to increase pupils' learning outcomes a result of lack of expectation for pupils' educational progress:
				  • apparent in how they prioritized subjects and what skills they believed the pupils were learning in those subjects;
				  • most pupils spent more time doing activities of daily living and physical education than academic activities.
				• Concern from parents that children did not have enough opportunity to develop academic abilities.

Table 5.4 Themes from studies of parents of adolescents with intellectual disabilities undergoing transition

	Meaning of the transition	*Services*	*Transition planning*	*Parental advocacy*	*Parental stress*
Bhaumik et al. (2011)		Services didn't take into account those who could not communicate needs directly or who lived at home. Services needed to have more flexibility and less bureaucracy.			
Cooney (2002)		Program options did not allow for full use of children's potential. Adult system was unfamiliar, and it was difficult to learn the in's and out's.	Parents found it awkward at school team meetings when planning occurred. Limited information was provided.		
Dyke et al. (2013)	Had a vision of their children's future which was holding "normal" adult roles.	Loss of supports and services that were provided in the educational system.	Limited information given about options.	Parents needed to push for services.	

continued

Table 5.4 Continued

	Meaning of the transition	*Services*	*Transition planning*	*Parental advocacy*	*Parental stress*
Gillian and Coughlin (2010)		Inflexible and unresponsive services: lack of information about available options; waiting lists for available services; lack of person-centered practices in vocational training service; lack of coordination between child and adult services; problematic interactions with staff in adult services; vocational training staff "not listening" to parents; lack of facility to be involved in adult services; difficulty experienced in terms of assisting their children to obtain and sustain jobs in the open labor market.	Lack of parent involvement in decisions and planning; lack of facility with transition planning.	Parents' experience was partly characterized by "fighting" or "battling" for the child to get services.	Stress, worry, and frustration.
Hanley-Maxwell et al. (1995)	Parents had specific visions for what they wanted for their child.	Did not want to leave school system since all the services that had been provided were no longer there. Felt like there were no options, only waiting lists.	Parents felt like they were not being listened to. Specific teachers throughout their children's educational careers had large influence on their child's ability to transition well. Wanted longer time to transition from school to work.		Fear for child being out of the home, and uncertainty and vulnerability involved.

Raghavan et al. (2013) Small et al. (2013)	Expectation in South Asian culture that person with ID would get married at some point.	Lack of respite care.	A plan was not put into place in the school.		
Rapanaro et al. (2007)		Difficulties accessing services and dissatisfaction with service provision/actions of service staff. Difficulty gaining and maintaining access to post-school services for their child.		Had to develop advocacy skills	Parents experienced a range of painful feelings with transition process.
Sagen and Ytterhus (2015)				Most advocacy done by parents.	

References

APA (American Psychiatric Association). (2013). *Diagnostic and statistical manual of mental disorders* (5th edn.). Arlington, VA: Author.

Field, M., and Jette, A. (2007). *Institute of Medicine (U.S.) Committee on Disability in America: The future of disability in America.* Washington, D.C.: National Academies Press (US).

Finfgeld, D. L. (2003). Metasynthesis: The state of the art – so far. *Qualitative Health Research, 13*(7), 893–904.

Finlayson, K. W., and Dixon, A. (2008). Qualitative meta-synthesis: A guide for the novice. *Nurse Researcher, 15*(2), 59–71.

Glidden, L. (2012). Family well-being and children with intellectual disability. In J. Burack, R. Hodapp, G. Iarocci, and E. Zigler (Eds.) *The Oxford handbook of intellectual disability and development* (pp. 303–317). New York: Oxford University Press.

Griffith, G. M., and Hastings, R. P. (2014). "He's hard work, but he's worth it." The experience of caregivers of individuals with intellectual disabilities and challenging behaviour: A meta-synthesis of qualitative research. *Journal of Applied Research in Intellectual Disabilities, 27*(5), 401–419. doi:10.1111/jar.12073.

Hauser-Cram, P., Warfield, M. E., Shonkoff, J. P., and Krauss, M. W. (2001). Children with disabilities: A longitudinal study of child development and parent well-being. *Monographs of the Society for Research in Child Development*, 66(3), i–viii, 1.

Hayes, C., and Batey, G. (2013). Understanding intellectual disability in healthcare practice. *British Journal of Nursing, 22*(7), 384–386.

Jones, M. (2004). Application of systematic review methods to qualitative research: Practical issues. *Journal of Advanced Nursing, 48*(3), 271–278.

Maulik, P. K., Mascarenhas, M. N., Mathers, C. D., Dua, T., and Saxena, S. (2011). Prevalence of intellectual disability: A meta-analysis of population-based studies. *Research in developmental disabilities, 32*(2), 419–436.

Olsson, M., and Hwang, C. (2008). Socioeconomic and psychological variables as risk and protective factors for parental well-being in families of children with intellectual disabilities. *Journal of Intellectual Disability Research, 52*, 1102–1113.

Resch, J. A., Benz, M. R., and Elliott, T. R. (2012). Evaluating a dynamic process model of wellbeing for parents of children with disabilities: A multi-method analysis. *Rehabilitation Psychology, 57*(1), 61–72.

Skotko, B. G., Levine, S. P., and Goldstein, R. (2011). Having a son or daughter with down syndrome: Perspectives from mothers and fathers. *American Journal of Medical Genetics. Part A, 155A*(10), 2335–2347.

Stewart, D., Freeman, M., Law, M., Healy, H., Burke-Gaffney, J., Forhan, M., Young, N., and Guenther, S. (2008). In M. Blouin, and J. Stone (Eds.), Transition to adulthood for youth with disabilities: Evidence from the literature. *International Encyclopedia of Rehabilitation.* Retrieved from http://cirrie.buffalo.edu/encyclopedia/en/article/110.

Trute, B., Hiebert-Murphy, D., and Levine, K. (2007). Parental appraisal of the family impact of childhood developmental disability: Times of sadness and times of joy. *Journal of Intellectual and Developmental Disability, 32*(1), 1–9.

Trute, B., Benzies, K. M., Worthington, C., Reddon, J., and Moore, M. (2010). Accentuate the positive to mitigate the negative: Mother psychological coping resources and family adjustment in childhood disability. *Journal of Intellectual and Developmental Disability, 35*(1), 36–43.

Wehmeyer, M., and Webb, K. (2012). An introduction to adolescent transition education. In M. Wehmeyer, and K. Webb (Eds.), *Handbook of adolescent transition education for youth with disabilities*. New York: Routledge.

Studies included in parents of children with intellectual disabilities

Brown, R. L. (1993). *Sense of coherence, perceptions and coping: Family adaptation to a child with mental retardation* (Order No. 9409642). Available from ProQuest Dissertations and Theses Global. Retrieved from http://search.proquest.com/docview/304062177?accountid=14780.

Glenn, M. W. (1987). *Mental retardation: A parental perspective* (Order No. 8808145). Available from ProQuest Dissertations and Theses Global. Retrieved from http://search.proquest.com/docview/303635475?accountid=14780.

Heer, K., Larkin, M., Burchess, I., and Rose, J. (2012). The cultural context of care-giving: Qualitative accounts from South Asian parents who care for a child with intellectual disabilities in the UK. *Advances in Mental Health and Intellectual Disabilities*, 6(4), 179–191.

Lalvani, P. (2008). Mothers of children with Down Syndrome: Constructing the socio-cultural meaning of disability. *Intellectual and Developmental Disabilities*, 46(6), 436–445.

Lin, M., Macmillan, M., and Brown, N. (2010). The formal support experiences of mothers of adolescents with intellectual disabilities in Edinburgh, UK: A longitudinal qualitative design. *Journal of Nursing Research*, 18(1), 34–43.

Pillay, D., Girdler, S., Collins, M., and Leonard, H. (2012). "It's not what you were expecting, but it's still a beautiful journey": The experience of mothers of children with Down syndrome. *Disability and Rehabilitation*, 34(18), 1501–1510.

Povee, K., Roberts, L., Bourke, J., and Leonard, H. (2012). Family functioning in families with a child with Down Syndrome: A mixed methods approach. *Journal of Intellectual Disability Research*, 56(10), 961–973.

Prussing, E., Sobo, E. J., Walker, E., Dennis, K., and Kurtin, P. S. (2004). Communicating with pediatricians about complementary/alternative medicine: Perspectives from parents of children with down syndrome. *Ambulatory Pediatrics*, 4(6), 488–494.

Todd, S., and Jones, S. (2005). Looking at the future and seeing the past: The challenge of the middle years of parenting a child with intellectual disabilities. *Journal of Intellectual Disability Research*, 49(6), 389–404.

Studies included in parents of adolescents with intellectual disabilities undergoing transition

*Bhaumik, S., Watson, J., Barrett, M., Raju, B., Burton, T., and Forte, J. (2011). Transition for teenagers with intellectual disability: Carers' perspectives. *Journal of Policy and Practice in Intellectual Disabilities*, 8(1), 53–61.

*Cooney, B. F. (2002). Exploring perspectives on transition of youth with disabilities: Voices of young adults, parents, and professionals. *Mental Retardation*, 40(6), 425.

*Dyke, P., Bourke, J., Llewellyn, G., and Leonard, H. (2013). The experiences of mothers of young adults with an intellectual disability transitioning from secondary school to adult life. *Journal of Intellectual and Developmental Disability*, 38(2), 149–162.

*Gillan, D., and Coughlan, B. (2010). Transition from special education into post school services for young adults with intellectual disability: Irish parents' experience. *Journal of Policy and Practice in Intellectual Disabilities*, *7*, 196–203.

*Hanley-Maxwell, C., Whitney-Thomas, J., and Pogoloff, S. M. (1995). The second shock: A qualitative study of parents' perspectives and needs during their child's transition from school to adult life. *Journal – Association of Persons With Severe Handicaps*, *20*(1), 3.

*Raghavan, R., Pawson, N., and Small, N. (2013). Family carers' perspectives on post-school transition of young people with intellectual disabilities with special reference to ethnicity. *Journal of Intellectual Disability Research*, *57*(10), 936–946. doi: 10.1111/j.1365–2788.2012.01588.x.

*Rapanaro, C., Bartu, A., and Lee, A. H. (2008). Perceived benefits and negative impact of challenges encountered in caring for young adults with intellectual disabilities in the transition to adulthood. *Journal of Applied Research in Intellectual Disabilities*, *21*(1), 34–47.

Sagen, L. M., and Ytterhus, B. (2015). Self-determination of pupils with intellectual disabilities in Norwegian secondary school. *European Journal of Special Needs Education*, *29*(3), 3444–3357. doi:http://dx.doi.org.proxy.library.vcu.edu/10.1080/08856257.2014.909174

*Small, N., Raghavan, R., and Pawson, N. (2013). An ecological approach to seeking and utilising the views of young people with intellectual disabilities in transition planning. *Journal of Intellectual Disabilities*, *17*(4), 282–300. doi: 10.1177/1744629513500779.

Part II

Disorders in adults

6 The lived experience of people with bipolar disorder

Bipolar disorder is a disorder of mood instability in which, over time, a person experiences one or more *manic episodes* that are usually accompanied by one or more *major depressive episodes* (APA, 2013). There are two types of bipolar disorder. Bipolar I disorder is characterized by one or more manic episodes accompanied by recurrent major depressive episodes. Bipolar II disorder is characterized by one or more major depressive episodes accompanied by at least one hypomanic episode. The National Comorbidity Study reported a lifetime prevalence of nearly 4 percent for bipolar disorder (Kessler et al., 2005). Bipolar disorder has been considered the most expensive behavioral healthcare diagnosis, costing more than twice as much as depression (CDC, 2014; Laxman et al., 2008; Peele et al., 2003). The economic burden includes a 39.1 percent greater inpatient hospitalization compared to 4.5 percent for other behavioral health diagnoses, resulting in high out-of-pocket, deductible, and medication related costs for both insured and uninsured individuals (CDC, 2014).

For individuals diagnosed with bipolar disorder, behaviors resulting from manic and depressive episodes can have negative and lasting consequences. A significant burden of bipolar disorder is suicide-related as it is estimated that between 25 and 60 percent of bipolar individuals will attempt suicide once in their lives, and between 4 and 19 percent will complete the act (Angst, 2004; Novick et al., 2010). Bipolar disorder has a significant negative effect on quality of life in the areas of education, work, financial functioning, social support, and intimate relationships (IsHak et al., 2012; Michalak et al., 2006). The person's mood swings and erratic behavior may be a source of ongoing turmoil in family, peer, and professional relationships, testing the limits of those relationships until others are exhausted. Fewer than half of bipolar adults report having a job, and those who do experience problems in the areas of employment continuity, job loss, managing the illness, stigma, and interpersonal problems in the workplace (Michalak et al., 2007; Sanchez-Moreno et al., 2009). Long-term studies of persons with BD report that 19–23 percent of their months feature moderate impairment and 7–9 percent feature severe impairment (Treuer and Tohen, 2010).

One meta-synthesis on bipolar disorder has previously been published (Russell and Moss, 2013). However, it was not part of a comprehensive systematic review and only dealt with the experience of symptoms and diagnosis. Nine studies were located in that study, which were mostly conducted in Western countries (Australia, the UK, and the US), and nine themes were identified: (1) struggles with identity; (2) loss of control; (3) disruption, uncertainty and instability; (4) negative impact of symptoms across life and the experience of loss; (5) negative view of the self; (6) positive or desirable aspects of mania; (7) struggling with the meaning of diagnosis; (8) stigma; and (9) acceptance and hope.

Methodology

The methodological process for meta-synthesis has been described in Chapter 2. Our comprehensive search yielded 41 studies on bipolar disorder. From this larger pool, the decision was made to narrow the scope of the meta-synthesis to just one geographic area (Sandelowski and Barroso, 2006) – the United States – since the highest proportion of studies were conducted there.

A total of 12 studies conducted between 1995 and 2014 were included in our final synthesis, representing 234 participants. Both published refereed articles and dissertations were represented. A majority of participants were women and identified as Caucasian or European-American. For more detail, see Table 6.1. Four themes were identified in our results: (1) experience of the diagnosis; (2) negative impact on relationships with others; (3) internal coping strategies; and (4) external coping strategies (see Table 6.2).

Themes

Experience of diagnosis

Receiving a diagnosis of bipolar disorder is fraught with emotion and involves a process of coming to terms with new information to reach an adjusted view of the self. Many participants described the process of diagnosis as frustrating and lengthy, occurring years after symptoms began (e.g., Freedberg, 2011). For some, the delay was a function of incorrect diagnosis or not feeling "heard" within the medical field. One woman stated: "It basically took me five years and eight doctors to get an accurate diagnosis … ridiculous" (Driscoll, 2004, p. 70). A few studies suggested that denial is often present and accompanied by anger and despair over one's acceptance of the disorder (Pollack, 1995; Pollack and Aponte, 2001). As one participant indicated: "I chose to ignore it for a long time.… I knew there was something wrong but, at the same time, I didn't want to get diagnosed" (Chapman, 2002, p. 83).

All participants expressed that they had experienced strong emotions upon receiving the bipolar diagnosis. However, depending on their self-awareness and self-motivation, those emotions ran the gamut from negative to positive. A participant in Pollack's (1995) study referenced the denial he had seen in others with bipolar disorder: "You're still going to have the ones that are going to throw them [bipolar-related informational pamphlets] out, because they don't want your lousy information" (p. 126). Some participants experienced shock and distress, believing the diagnosis implied they were somehow "different" from other, normal people. One study participant recalled thinking her diagnosis meant she was "nuts. Manic. A manic depressive is somebody's who's institutionalized … out of control … somebody that has to be locked up" (Goldberg, 2007, p. 138).

But diagnosis can also bring relief and greater understanding. One person shared: "I was so happy to have somebody assess me and evaluate me and give a name to how I felt" (Driscoll, 2004, p. 71). Another described the diagnosis as putting a "piece into the puzzle" (Freedberg, 2011, p. 53), because it finally helped give her behavior a framework for self-understanding. People who had always felt they were different found solace in the diagnosis' explanation. They judged their past behaviors less harshly and began to question the validity of their negative self-views (e.g., Chapman, 2002).

Several studies described coming to terms with a bipolar diagnosis as a process or journey. Participants indicated that they went through adjustment phases similar to Elisabeth Kubler-Ross's stages of grief, including denial, anger, and despair (Pollack and Aponte, 2001). One person recalled going through "several phases of denial" (Goldberg, 2007, p. 134). Another reported: "So there is just a lot of grieving, grieving is a really good word for it because you grieve for the life you thought you would have" (Driscoll, 2004, pp. 74–75). Additionally, Chapman (2002) described a process of moving through different diagnosis-related stages, including ignoring and denying diagnostic information, protecting the pre-diagnosis identity, using diagnostic information to restructure identity, and, eventually, getting on with life.

Several study participants had come to see positive aspects of having bipolar disorder: "I think it is kind of a positive illness to have. I truly believe that in many ways it has made me more insightful" (Driscoll, 2004, p. 78). Individuals mentioned gaining compassion, a richer life, a deeper sense of spirituality, and a desire to help others from their experiences with the disorder (Chapman, 2002). Many participants expressed optimism about the effects of intervention on their mood, functional level, and stress level (Sajatovic et al., 2011). In Sajatovic et al.'s 2009 study, participants shared their hopes that the medications would "reduce symptoms and balance mood" (p. 364). Others expressed short-term hopes for managing their lives: "I think my future's looking up. My goal is not to be in the hospital.… I have a good job, I have a good manager, I have my own little house … I want to stay positive" (Freedberg, 2011, p. 97).

Negative impact on relationships with others

Relationships were often negatively affected by a bipolar diagnosis and its related symptoms because of the person's social withdrawal, which was described as a way to protect others and to avoid being a burden (Chapman, 2002; Doherty and MacGeorge, 2013; Driscoll, 2004; Goldberg, 2007). As one participant said: "You end up just going off by yourself to protect them [family] and myself and letting it just pass" (Driscoll, 2004, p. 63). In addition to withdrawing for other people's protection, participants often noticed strong reactions to their diagnoses, including fear and anxiety among partners, friends, and family members (Freedberg, 2011; Sajatovic et al., 2009). As a result, people with bipolar disorder report having fewer close friends, mainly due to fear about disclosing their condition (Driscoll, 2004; Freedberg, 2011). One young woman shared: "I prefer not to [have friends] actually because I just kind of get screwed over" (Freedberg, 2011).

People with bipolar disorder often must renegotiate their relationships. One woman described "being-in-relationship in a new way," focusing on only the relationships that nurture her (Driscoll, 2004, p. 78). Another woman mentioned having to decrease the time she spent with some friends because they "didn't know how to act" after her diagnosis (Chapman, 2002, p. 120).

Coping strategies

People with bipolar disorder used a variety of coping strategies; some internal and some external, to help them manage the condition.

Internal strategies

Internal coping strategies included vigilance over one's mood and other self-care practices. Goldberg (2007) and Driscoll (2004) determined that participants practice forms of constant self-monitoring of their feelings in order to control the disorder. This vigilance helps them catch early warning signs of mania or depression: "Yes, it's on my mind constantly. What are my motives?... I'm always doing a check. Am I being too happy?... Am I ... you know, overreacting?" (Goldberg, 2007, p. 194). Many people with bipolar disorder stressed the importance of self-care with a variety of practices including regular routines, good nutrition, journaling, mood charting (Kemp, 2010); listening to music, meditating, painting, reading, practicing their faith, and napping (Chapman, 2002; Freedberg, 2011); exercising (Driscoll, 2004; Kemp, 2010); learning to communicate needs and maintaining healthy boundaries (Driscoll, 2004); and remembering the past in order to stay on track with recovery (Kemp, 2010).

External strategies

Support from friends, family, and practitioners represented the primary external coping strategy. According to Pollack (1995), "the existence of a support system that encourages positive efforts toward self-management" represents a significant factor "that influence[s] a person's ability to select useful self-management strategies" (p. 127). For one participant (Kemp, 2010), "family [mom, spouse, cousin] and support group" helped her observe her moods and "kind of know if I'm becoming a little bit manic or if I am getting depressed" (p. 54). Another (Driscoll, 2004, p. 77) recommended:

> always have a safety net of people who know you, I mean counseling people and doctors who have met you when you're well and then when it hits the fan you can go back and they see right off that this isn't the high functioning girl I know.

Doherty and MacGeorge's (2013) study highlighted the importance of the emotional, everyday, and illness-management support offered by family and friends. One participant recognized that his mother "really emphasized that she and the rest of my family love me unconditionally.... I have this idea that, like, nobody cares about me.... So I think that that's something that's helpful to keep hearing that" (p. 366). Another shared an example of her friend's support:

> If she starts to notice I'm not slowing down but not as interested in my job or she, for some reason she can tell before I can that I've been off my medication for a while. So she'll be like, "You know you need to be on your meds."
>
> (p. 368)

Discussion

The present meta-synthesis developed several themes that cut across the qualitative research, although it offered more personal, nuanced understandings of the experience of living with a diagnosis of bipolar disorder. The dominant theme emerging from the data was the challenge of accepting the diagnosis. It often involved a process of struggle to determine if the diagnosis fit and learning more about the disorder as the person went along, with ambivalence being a key characteristic. On one hand, having a diagnosis explained the problems and symptoms the participants faced and reduced some of their self-blame, but at the same time, acceptance of such a serious diagnosis was a struggle for what it implied about the future. Participants realized that having a bipolar diagnosis was considered a life-long condition. They had to consider whether their goals for the future were realistic given their current capacities. Some were hopeful and retained their goals.

This theme, the struggle to accept the diagnosis, seemed to encapsulate the following themes delineated by Russell and Moss (2013): struggles with identity; loss of control; disruption, uncertainty, and instability; negative impact of symptoms across life and the experience of loss; negative view of self; struggling with the meaning of diagnosis; and acceptance and hope. Even though there was only slight overlap between these two meta-syntheses (three studies), the present study lends credence to the process of accepting the diagnosis as a difficult challenge that involves many aspects of the self and life situation, and might involve a stage process.

In comparison to Russell and Moss (2013) and their focus on diagnosis and symptoms, the current study dealt with broad aspects of bipolar disorder. Another theme to emerge was the ambivalence participants felt about medication use.

The quantitative literature has established that non-adherence to medication is high (Clatworthy et al., 2007; Crowe et al., 2011). A systematic review indicated that 20–60 percent of clients are intentionally non-adherent during their course of medication therapy (Busby and Sajatovic, 2010). Another systematic review studying the reasons for this behavior included poor insight about the disorder and doubts about the ongoing need for medication; concurrent substance use; and concerns about current or future adverse effects (LeClerc et al., 2013). Additionally, barriers to care and the fact that medication does not produce a sufficient response are other explanations for non-adherence (Bowden et al., 2012; Crowe et al., 2011). The likelihood that persons with bipolar disorder will eventually experience a relapse – 90 percent of persons who have a manic episode develop future episodes (Treuer and Tohen, 2010) – means they should be informed that one of the most common reasons for relapse is the discontinuation of an effective medication regimen.

Despite their ambivalence in other areas, participants in this review were adamant about their need to be aware of warning signs and other triggers that may herald a developing mood episode. They also talked about making lifestyle changes, including having a routine schedule and getting proper diet and exercise, to help maintain their mood. Social workers could emphasize the development of self-management techniques, taking a strengths-based approach with people to help them find what is helpful in terms of self-care and bolstering their efforts to avoid mood swings. Interventions – psychoeducation (Lucksted et al., 2012; Prasko et al., 2013; Schulte et al. (2012), family-focused, cognitive-behavioral (Castle et al., 2009; Reinares et al., 2014), and interpersonal therapies – have been designed and subjected to testing, showing effectiveness in addressing the kinds of concerns that were prominent in this study, by increasing client awareness and understanding of the disorder, as well as the importance of medication compliance, stable social and sleep rhythms, avoidance of heavy substance use, and relapse prevention planning for ongoing stability (Popovic et al., 2013).

The theme that coalesced around negative impacts on relationships confirms the importance of clinical discussions that address the burden on relationships experienced by persons with bipolar disorder. The chronicity of the disorder negatively affects family life, which is characterized by less cohesion and organization, greater conflict, lower rates of intact family, and higher rates of maternal and paternal tension (Koutra et al., 2013). These features, in turn, increase the risk for the client member's relapse (Sullivan et al., 2012). In one large longitudinal study, 89, 52, and 61 percent of caregivers, respectively, reported moderate or high burden in relation to client problem behaviors, role dysfunction, and disruption in household routines (Perlick et al., 2007).

What also emerged in our review, however, was that not only relations and friends feel burden; the person with the disorder at times also withdraws from relationships in order to protect others from the interpersonal impact of the mood swings. Apparently, some people with bipolar disorder actively try to protect their relationships when they think they might act in ways that are detrimental (Chapman, 2002; Doherty and MacGeorge, 2013; Driscoll, 2004; Goldberg, 2007).

The desired goal of participants in this study of developing positive social support, and the opportunity to engage in previous activities of social life, is well supported in the quantitative literature. Deficient social support is associated with more mood symptoms and interruptions to circadian rhythms (Eidelman et al., 2012). Persons who are able to maintain a work, social, and family life experience fewer symptoms and are able to develop and maintain a higher quality functioning (Gutierrez-Rojas et al., 2011). Miklowitz and colleagues have formulated and tested a specific intervention for families in which one member has bipolar disorder, called Family Focused Treatment (FFT) (Miklowitz and Taylor, 2006). The components of FFT include family education, communication skills development, and problem solving. A systematic review indicated that this model is effective in reducing relapse rates for persons with bipolar disorder (Reinares et al., 2014).

Limitations

While this study makes a contribution to the knowledge of the experiences of people with bipolar disorder, it has several limitations. The study encapsulates only the experiences of participants within the United States since its aim was not to provide consideration of varying cultural contexts. Another limitation is the controversial application of qualitative meta-synthesis itself (Finlayson and Dixon, 2008). Interpreting individuals' experiences with a secondary lens gives concern to issues of varying possible interpretations and the quality of analysis. The functioning levels of participants could also be a limitation in that, in attempting to solicit responses, only high functioning individuals were considered. The majority of participants in the studies were women and thus the biological component of gender may also have skewed results. For example, Kriegshauser et al. (2010) reported that women with bipolar disorder had a better quality of social relationships and lower levels of self-medicating through substance abuse than men. Despite these limitations, this study adds to the current knowledge base of the lived experiences of persons diagnosed with bipolar disorder.

Table 6.1 Data extraction of studies of people with bipolar disorder

Author and purpose	*Design*	*Sample*	*Findings*
Chapman (2002) To explore sources of challenges to identity and how participants dealt with those challenges.	Semi-structured, open-ended interviews. Analysis used grounded theory methodology. Sampling: purposive (participants were referred by clinicians).	$N = 12$. BD-I 50%, BD-II 50%. Ethnicity: all Caucasian or mixed-Caucasian. Median age 40 years, age range 22–62 years. Males 25%, females 75%. Married 60%, single 40%.	*Several themes surrounding the concept of identity* 1 Challenges to identity: a symptoms as challenges; b timing of symptoms has different implications. 2 Protecting identity: a discounting information; b strategies for protecting identity; c denial, reinterpreting information, ignoring information, preventing others from seeing symptoms, self-medicating. 3 Restructuring identity; deciding whether to use information: a using information to restructure identity; b self-monitoring; c dealing with issues of control; d reevaluating views of the past. 4 Getting on with life: a self-monitoring, integrated identity, negotiating relationships, finding positives, spirituality, helping others.

Doherty and MacGeorge (2013) To explore those types of behaviors from support networks which young adults with BD perceive as helpful in coping with the disorder.	Semi-structured interviews. Ethnographic evaluation. Sampling: Purposive at first (contacted clinicians), then convenience (posted flyers on campus and in community).	*N* = 30. Age range was 18–30. Mean age = 23 years, median age = 24 years. 24 women, 6 men. All had a BD diagnosis. No information on ethnicity provided.	Eleven types of helpful behavior were identified: 1 emotional support (especially helpful in depressive states): a conversational; b reappraisal of situation; c esteem/encouragement; d expressions of love. 2 Everyday support tangible: a activities (helpful in depressive states). 3 Illness-management support: a advice (some identified this as important before mania) and information; b treatment support (anything that helped treatment adherence); c vigilance support (checking in, monitoring moods) (some identified this as important before mania); d educational support (support provider wants to learn more about BD); e maintenance support (help with managing day-to-day life/everyday tasks).
Driscoll (2004) To explore phenomenon of experience of women living with bipolar II disorder. Provided a voice for women, as the qualitative literature was silent during the time of dissertation.	Colaizzi's (1978) phenomenological method is used to investigate (qualitative). Sampling: purposive (referred by therapists).	11 women were interviewed, all diagnosed with bipolar II disorder. Age range 30–61 years. All Caucasian. 8 married, 3 divorced.	Four themes emerged: 1 Melancholy to mayhem at flick of a switch. 2 Dwelling in the maze: the journey toward diagnosis to treatment. 3 Emerging in steadiness; regaining control. 4 Cultivation of a new self. The study resulted in increased understanding and awareness of a woman's experience of living with bipolar II disorder. Results will help with education, practice, and research in women's healthcare.

continued

Table 6.1 Continued

Author and purpose	*Design*	*Sample*	*Findings*
Freedberg (2011) To gain a better understanding of the lived experiences of adults diagnosed with bipolar and how they use cognitively, affectively, and spiritually oriented strategies to cope with life stressors and circumstances.	Qualitative phenomenological method used to analyze interview transcripts. Sampling: convenience (recruited through a classified advertisement).	8 English speaking adults age 18 years or older and diagnosed with bipolar disorder at least one year or longer. Mean age = 31.4 years, median age = 31 years. 7 females, 1 male. 6 Caucasian, 1 African American, 1 other.	Four themes emerged: 1 Diagnosis brings understanding accompanied by irrevocable change. 2 Finding effective treatment is an interminable process. 3 Bipolar disorder is the third partner in every relationship. 4 Caring for oneself is as important as receiving formal treatment. A wide variety of coping strategies were reported, placing importance on assessment and nurturance of client self-care strategies by mental health professionals.
Goldberg (2007) To examine impact of American society's construction of bipolar disorder on individuals diagnosed with it.	Open-ended interviews using narrative research theory. Autoethnography. Sampling: snowball (recruited classmates who then suggested other participants).	*N* = 6. 1 male, 5 females. Aged 39–55 years. All with BD diagnosis. All identified as European Americans.	How bipolar clients make meaning of their diagnosis in light of societal values: 1 Meaning making: a interactive process between individual and societal experience; b self-labeling; c choose from society's labels; d labels were negative post-diagnosis; e later they grew to encompass divergent experiences but the definition became almost too broad.

			2 Identity – conflicting selves: a hard to feel "selfsameness"; b difference between unmedicated and medicated self was the most difficult; c societal explanations of BD make identity tasks hard; d participants preferred explanations involving personal responsibility over biochemical explanations; e participants both reflected and impacted societal understanding of BD.
Kang (2013) To explore inner experience of persons living with bipolar disorder, as it remains largely unknown despite diagnostic criteria.	Hurlburt (1990,1993, 2011) Descriptive Experience Sampling (DES) Method: qualitative. Sampling: convenience (recruited from database of neuropsychology research participants).	4 individuals diagnosed with bipolar disorder. 2 male, 2 female. 1 Multi-cultural, 1 African American, 2 Caucasian. Mean age 39.25 years.	All 4 individuals had clear and prevalent experiences of sensory awareness, difficulty apprehending and conveying their inner experiences, and a deficit or lack of coherence in the experience of feelings.
Kemp (2010) To give voice to individuals diagnosed with bipolar disorder who adhere to their medication regime, through eyes of provider also living with the disorder.	Qualitative; autoethnographic. Sampling: convenience (support group) and snowball.	5 individuals living with bipolar disorder and adhering to medications including researcher's own experience. Age range 26–68 years, mean age = 51 years. 3 males, 2 females. 3 Caucasian, 2 Hispanic.	Four themes emerged: 1 Feeling fear. 2 Feeling challenged. 3 Feeling balanced. 4 Feelings toward providers. Results provide illumination of why sample participants adhere to medications, challenges they faced, their coping strategies to manage the disorder, and desired communications to providers.

continued

Table 6.1 Continued

Author and purpose	*Design*	*Sample*	*Findings*
Kriegshauser et al. (2010) To examine gender differences related to adherence to treatment for BD.	SEMI (semi-structured/ in-depth interview. Sampling: purposive (referred by clinicians).	*N* = 90, pooled data from 3 studies. Referred by clinicians or volunteered at BD treatment centers (academic medical center mood disorders clinic, community mental health clinic, private hospital or state hospital). Mean age was 36.5 years. 46 male, 44 female. 66 Euro-Americans, 14 African Americans, 10 identified as other.	No gender difference in experience of stigma, self-medicating through drug abuse, or value of lessened irritability and impulsivity because of medications. Women experienced more fear of weight gain because of medications, had higher quality social relationships, and had lower rates of self-medicating through alcohol abuse.
Pollack (1995) To examine how people with BD strive to go on despite their illness.	In-depth, semi-structured interviews. Grounded theory methodology. Sampling: convenience (all participants were in the hospital).	*N* = 33. Participants were hospitalized average of 23 days for treatment of bipolar disorder. 17 Euro Americans, 11 African American, 4 Hispanic, 1 Pakistani. Ages ranged from 20 to 57 years with average of 35 years. 20 women, 13 men.	For people striving to achieve stability, normalcy, and control in face of the disorder, the processes of information seeking and self-management are continuous. Denial of the disorder represented a major barrier to coping. Information seeking; realization of need for (acceptance is a key) information, critical juncture in treatment (medication stabilization, motivation to go on), self-management.

Pollack and Aponte (2001) To explore perceptions of illness of people in public hospital setting for treatment of BD.	Structured interviews. Sampling: Convenience (all participants were in the hospital and were referred by their physicians).	$N = 15$. Participants were between ages of 18 and 70 years and were hospitalized in a university managed, state and country funded facility. Voluntary and involuntary. 5 African Americans, 5 Hispanics, 5 Euro-Americans. Male = 7, female = 8	Three major themes: 1 Coming to terms with diagnosis: lengthy process full of phases of denial, anger, hopelessness and acceptance. Seen as injury to self-identity. 2 Importance of personal metaphors: bipolar disorder as a gift, caused by stress, being patient until Jesus comes. 3 Dealing with medical model: focused on medication. Dissatisfaction with quality of their lives, feeling disconnected from others and not being able to fulfill their life dreams.
Sajatovic et al. (2009) To evaluate attitudes and perceptions of medication treatment along with hopes/ expectations for treatment.	Semi-structured interviews/ ethnographic evaluation combined with quantitative assessment (scales). Sampling: purposive and convenience (all participants were receiving outpatient care or hospitalized).	$N = 90$, pooled data from 3 studies. Referred by clinicians or volunteered at BD treatment centers (academic medical center mood disorders clinic, a community mental health clinic, a private hospital or a state hospital. Mean age 36.5 years. 46 participants male, 44 female. 66 Euro-Americans, 14 African Americans, 10 identified as other.	42% believed medication stabilized or balanced mood; 19% believed they decreased anxiety/ depression symptoms; 10% believed they improved sleep. Perceptions tended to focus on achieving euthymic mood and decreasing depressive symptoms. Fears of long-term side effects could be barrier. Media feeds fears.

continued

Table 6.1 Continued

Author and purpose	*Design*	*Sample*	*Findings*
Sajatovic et al. (2011) To evaluate “factors related to adherence among 20 poorly adherent community mental health clinic patients with bipolar disorder” (p. 280).	Mixed method, with qualitative interview. Sampling: convenience (all participants were receiving outpatient care at a community MH clinic).	$N = 20$. 14 female. Age range 18–59 years, with mean of 37 years. 14 African Americans, 4 European Americans, 1 Native American, 1 Asian participants. Diagnosis of BP-I or BP-II for at least 2 years and had treatment of antipsychotic or mood stabilizer. They were identified as non-adherent.	These poorly adherent clients identified the following reasons for non-compliance with medication treatment: 1 Forgetting. 2 Side effects. 3 Belief that the meds are not needed. 4 Disorganized home settings. 5 Poor social networks.

Table 6.2 Themes from primary studies of people with bipolar disorder

Author	*Experience of diagnosis*	*Coping strategies*	*Relationships with others*	*Barriers to recovery*
Chapman (2002)	Resistance to diagnosis: • ignoring • reinterpreting the information. Does it "fit"? • denial as a way to protect identity. Stages of acceptance/ adjustment to diagnosis.	*Internal* Gaining compassion. Developing self awareness. Developing a richer life. Deeper spirituality. Helping others. Self-care. Self-monitoring. Finding the positive aspects of BD. *External* Negotiating relationships.	Social isolation results from symptoms/moods and others' reactions to those. Renegotiating relationships with friends who don't know how to handle the diagnosis.	*Internal* Denial that there's anything wrong. I'm feeling ok., so there's nothing wrong. Depressive symptoms prevent action. Self-medicating with substances. Alternative explanations for behavior. Lacking information/ framework to deal with the diagnosis. *External* Negative experiences with the medical model.
Doherty and MacGeorge (2013)		*External* Importance of support from: • family; • friends; • intimate partners. Emotional, everyday, and illness management support. Different types of support needed at different times (during depression, before/ during mania).	Relationships with close supports can facilitate recovery and treatment adherence. Not wanting to burden others with symptoms and moods.	

continued

Table 6.2 Continued

Author	*Experience of diagnosis*	*Coping strategies*	*Relationships with others*	*Barriers to recovery*
Driscoll (2004)	Dwelling in the maze: it can take many years to get an accurate diagnosis from the medical model. Feeling unseen/unheard. Some experienced relief at diagnosis. Some experienced shame. Stages of acceptance (anger, grief, acceptance). Worries about costs of healthcare, medication side effects, heredity in children, stigma.	*Internal* Finding positive aspects of BD. Greater insights/authenticity. Constant self monitoring. Some framed process as a journey. *External* Exercise. Importance of having a "safety net" of people who can help monitor mood/ symptoms.	Developed and maintained healthier boundaries with people. Importance of having a "safety net" of people who can help monitor mood/symptoms. Desire to protect family and friends from mood/symptoms. Fears about disclosure of diagnosis.	Costs of healthcare. Medical model: • medication trials; • feeling unseen/unheard.
Freedberg (2011)	Diagnosis can take many years. Often accompanies hospitalization, which was reported as a negative experience. There can be relief in the diagnosis: • it gives meaning to past experiences/behaviors. Medication trials can be difficult. Finding effective treatment is an interminable process.	*Internal* Self-care is as important as formal, medical treatment. Hopes for future were short-term. Self-awareness, self monitoring: • journaling; • music; • time alone. *External* Therapy is effective if fully engaged in it. Exercise for stress relief .	Partners can react with fear, anxiety, and/or support. It's hard to maintain friendships. Fear of disclosure. Stigma.	*Internal* Cognitive effects of BD. *External* Medication trials are difficult. Finding effective treatment is an interminable process. Reports of mixed relationships with medical personnel. Costs of care. Difficulty connecting with providers.

Goldberg (2007)	Negative self-labels after diagnosis: • "Crazy"; • "Nuts." Several phases of denial.	*Internal* Vigilant self-monitoring of moods.	Social isolation resulted from diagnosis.	*Internal* Negative self-labels. *External* Societal constructions of, and labels for, BD. Medical model. Lack of information on BD. Difference between unmedicated and medicated self difficult to reconcile.
Kang (2013)				*Internal* Cognitive deficits caused by BD may affect ability to apprehend inner experience and manage BD.
Kemp (2010)	Embarrassment and stigma over their BD. Feeling fear: • suicidal depression; • re-hospitalization. Cut off from family. Dependence on facility for all needs: • no free choice; • relapse (to pre-medication functioning). Lack of control. Loss of contact with reality.	Feeling balanced (how to achieve success in managing BD): • daily maintenance. Gaining self control: • routines, nutrition, exercise. Stabilization efforts: • support from family and support groups; • journaling/mood charting; • reminder notes to take meds; • remember the past (how I don't want to be).	Support from family and support groups. Family observation of mood, so they can observe if I'm becoming manic or depressed.	*Internal* Feeling challenged. Feeling fear. Feelings toward providers (advice they would give providers). Embarrassment. *External* Providers listening to verbal and nonverbal communication. Medication issues: • cost, dosages, combinations of meds. Stigma.

continued

Table 6.2 Continued

Author	*Experience of diagnosis*	*Coping strategies*	*Relationships with others*	*Barriers to recovery*
Kriegshauser et al. (2010)	Men and women had equal experiences of stigma. Lessened irritability/impulsivity due to meds.	Self-medicating through drug abuse (negative coping strategy). Valuing of lessened irritability/impulsivity due to meds.	Women had better quality social relationships.	*Internal* Self-medicating through drug abuse. *External* Stigma.
Pollack (1995)	Information-seeking process. Critical juncture in treatment: • occurs once information has been obtained; • ability to analyze (cognitive effects of BD); • requires will, stability, energy, access to resources.	Self-management: • advanced activity; • requires information, motivation, ability to apply knowledge, support system.	Information seeking from support system. Not telling others when suicidal. Poor living arrangement: • support system can encourage positive efforts toward self-management.	*Internal* Barriers to this phase. Self management, med non-compliance, poor living arrangements, low tolerance, not telling others when suicidal, denial, stubbornness. Success and failure. Denial, lack of acceptance of the need for help.
Pollack and Aponte (2001)	Coming to terms with diagnosis: • phases: denial, anger, hopelessness, acceptance (similar to Kubler-Ross); • these led to non-adherence. Diagnosis an injury to identity.	Wanted practitioners to incorporate their strengths and other aspects of identity into treatment. Art, poetry, and religion. Importance of personal metaphors: • subjective ways to make sense of BD (meaning making).	Disconnected with others. Telling their stories is important.	*Internal* Quality of life. Disconnected with others. Not able to fulfill dreams. Not incorporated other self-care activities. *External* Dealing with medical model. Dissatisfaction with medical model.

	Importance of personal metaphors: • subjective ways to make sense of BD (meaning making). Integrating the illness as part of self.	Integrating the illness as part of self, telling their stories is important, causes of BD (no one is to blame), timeline (this is for life), control (meds can control).		
Sajatovic et al. (2009)	Fear of medication side effects. Hope/expectations include mood stabilization, elimination of symptoms, being "normal" and "cured." Reduce symptoms and balance mood.	Mood stabilization, elimination of symptoms.	Interaction with family and friends. Friends' and family members' reactions. Limited support network.	*Internal* Fears expressed by client, relating to family, friends, media, worries. *External* Relationships with media, friends, family (reactions).
Sajatovic et al. (2011)	Not wanting to take meds for the rest of life. Optimism about effects of treatments on their mood, function, and stress levels.		Limited support network; specifically: • one-third described home as tense, unpleasant, disorganized; • one-third had inadequate social contact; • one-third didn't feel there were people to talk to about BD; • one-third had people in their lives who discouraged taking meds.	*Internal* Medication non-compliance. Forgetting. Not wanting to take meds for rest of life. *External* Side effects of medication. Judgment.

References

* Denotes an article used in the meta-synthesis.

Abraham, K. M., Miller, C. J., Birgenheir, D. G., Lai, Z., and Kilbourne, A. M. (2014). Self-efficacy and quality of life among people with bipolar disorder. *The Journal of Nervous and Mental Disease*, *202*(8), 583. doi:10.1097/NMD.0000000000000165.

Aguirre, R. T. P., and Bolton, K. W. (2014). Qualitative interpretive meta-synthesis in social work research: Uncharted territory. *Journal of Social Work*, *14*(3), 279–294. doi:10.1177/1468017313476797.

Andreasen, N. C., and Black, D. W. (2006). *Introductory Textbook of Psychiatry* (4th edn.). Washington, D.C.: American Psychiatric Publishing.

Angst, J. (2004). Bipolar disorder: A seriously underestimated health burden. *European Archives of Psychiatry and Clinical Neuroscience*, *254*, 59–60. Retrieved from http://search.library.vcu.edu/primo_library/libweb/action/dlSearch.do?institution=VCU&vid=VCU&search_scope=all_scope&dym=true&query=any,contains,%22Bipolar%20Disorder%3A%20a%20seriously%20underestimated%20health%20burden%22.

APA (American Psychiatric Association). (2013). *Diagnostic and statistical manual of mental disorders* (5th edn.). Arlington, VA: Author.

Aydemir, O., and Akkaya, C. (2011). Association of social anxiety with stigmatisation and low self-esteem in remitted bipolar patients. *Acta Neuropsychiatrica*, *23*(5), 224–228. doi:10.1111/j.1601–5215.2011.00565.x.

Bauer, M., McBride, L., Shea, N., Gavin, C., Holden, F., and Kendall, S. (1997). Impact of an easy-access VA clinic-based program for patients with bipolar disorder. *Psychiatric Services*, 48: 491–496. Retrieved from http://search.library.vcu.edu/primo_library/libweb/action/display.do?frbrVersion=3&tabs=viewOnlineTab&ct=display&fn=search&doc=TN_medline9090732&indx=1&recIds=TN_medline9090732&recIdxs=0&elementId=0&renderMode=poppedOut&displayMode=full&frbrVersion=3&dscnt=0&frbg=&scp.scps=scope%3A%28VCU_CONTENTDM%29%2Cscope%3A%28VCU%29%2Cscope%3A%28VCU_ALMA%29%2Cprimo_central_multiple_fe&tab=all&dstmp=1414611686609&srt=rank&mode=Basic&&dum=true&tb=t&vl(freeText0)=Impact%20of%20Easy%20access%20VA%20clinicbased&vid=VCU.

Blairy, S., Linotte, S., Souery, D., Papadimitriou, G. N., Dikeos, D., Lerer, B., and Mendlewicz, J. (2004). Social adjustment and self-esteem of bipolar patients: A multicentric study. *Journal of Affective Disorders*, *79*(1–3), 97–103. doi:http://dx.doi.org.proxy.library.vcu.edu/10.1016/S0165-0327(02)00347-6.

Bowden, C. L., Perlis, R. H., Thase, M. E., Ketter, T. A., Ostacher, M. M., Calabrese, J. R., et al. (2012). Aims and results of the NIMH systematic treatment enhancement program for bipolar disorder (STEP-BD). *CNS Neuroscience and Therapeutics*, *18*(3), 243–249. doi:10.1111/j.1755-5949.2011.00257.x.

Busby, K. K., and Sajatovic, M. (2010). Patient, treatment, and systems-level factors in bipolar disorder nonadherence: A summary of the literature. *CNS Neuroscience and Therapeutics*, *16*, 308–315.

Castle, D. J., Berk., L., Lauder, S., Berk, M., and Murray, G. (2009). Psychosocial interventions for bipolar disorder. *Acta Neuropsychiatrica*, *21*, 275–284.

CDC (Centers for Disease Control and Prevention). (2014). *Burden of mental illness*. Retrieved from www.cdc.gov/mentalhealth/basics/burden.htm.

Cerit, C., Filizer, A., Tural, Ü., and Tufan, A. E. (2012). Stigma: A core factor on predicting functionality in bipolar disorder. *Comprehensive Psychiatry*, *53*(5), 484–489. doi:10.1016/j.comppsych.2011.08.010.

*Chapman, J. R. (2002). *Bipolar disorder: Responding to challenges to identity* (Order No. 3099430). Available from ProQuest Dissertations and Theses Global. Retrieved from http://search.proquest.com/docview/305470796?accountid=14780.

Clatworthy, J., Bowskill, R., Rank, T., Parham, R., and Horne, R. (2007). Adherence to medication in bipolar disorder: A qualitative study exploring the role of patients' beliefs about the condition and its treatment. *Bipolar Disorders*, 9(6), 656–664. doi:10.1111/j.1399-5618.2007.00434.x.

Col, S. E., Caykoylu, A., Karakas Ugurlu, G., and Ugurlu, M. (2014). Factors affecting treatment compliance in patients with bipolar I disorder during prophylaxis: A study from Turkey. *General Hospital Psychiatry*, 36(2), 208–213. doi:10.1016/j.genhosppsych.2013.11.006.

Crowe, M., Wilson, L., and Inder, M. (2011). Patients' reports of the factors influencing medication adherence in bipolar disorder: An integrative review of the literature. *International Journal of Nursing Studies*, 48(7), 894–903. doi:10.1016/j.ijnurstu.2011.03.008.

Crowe, M., Whitehead, L., Wilson, L., Carlyle, D., O'Brien, A., Inder, M., and Joyce, P. (2010). Disorder-specific psychosocial interventions for bipolar disorder: A systematic review of the evidence for mental health nursing practice. *International Journal of Nursing Studies*, 47(7), 896–908. doi:http://dx.doi.org.proxy.library.vcu.edu/10.1016/j.ijnurstu.2010.02.012.

*Doherty, E. F., and MacGeorge, E. L. (2013). Perceptions of supportive behavior by young adults with bipolar disorder. *Qualitative Health Research*, 23(3), 361–374.

*Driscoll, J. W. (2004). *The experience of women living with bipolar II disorder* (University of Connecticut) (Order No. 3134781). Available from ProQuest Dissertations and Theses. Retrieved from http://search.proquest.com/docview/305207265?accountid=14780.

Edge, M. D., Miller, C. J., Muhtadie, L., Johnson, S. L., Carver, C. S., Marquinez, N., and Gotlib, I. H. (2013). People with bipolar I disorder report avoiding rewarding activities and dampening positive emotion. *Journal of Affective Disorders*, 146(3), 407–413. doi:10.1016/j.jad.2012.07.027.

Eidelman, P., Gershon, A., Kaplan, K., McGlinchey, E., and Harvey, A. G. (2012). Social support and social strain in inter-episode bipolar disorder. *Bipolar Disorders*, 14(6), 628–640. doi:10.1111/j.1399-5618.2012.01049.x.

Finlayson, K. W., and Dixon, A. (2008). Qualitative meta-synthesis: A guide for the novice. *Nurse Researcher*, 15(2), 59.

Frank, E. (2007). Interpersonal and social rhythm therapy: A means of improving depression and preventing relapse in bipolar disorder. *Journal of Clinical Psychology: In Session*, 63(5), 463–473.

*Freedberg, R. P. (2011). *Living with bipolar disorder: A qualitative investigation* (PhD). Available from ProQuest Dissertations and Theses Full Text (900443417).

Fulford, D., Peckham, A. D., Johnson, K., and Johnson, S. L. (2014). Emotion perception and quality of life in bipolar I disorder. *Journal of Affective Disorders*, 152–154, 491–497. doi:10.1016/j.jad.2013.08.034.

Geddes, J., and Miklowitz, D. (2013) Treatment of bipolar disorder. *Lancet*, 381, 1672–1682.

Gergen, K. J. (1985). The social constructionist movement in modern psychology. *American Psychologist*, 40(3), 266–275. doi:10.1037/0003–066X.40.3.266.

Gershon, A., Johnson, S. L., and Miller, I. (2013). Chronic stressors and trauma: Influences on the course of bipolar disorder. *Psychological Medicine*, 43, 2583–2592.

*Goldberg, S. G. (2007). *The social construction of bipolar disorder: The interrelationship between societal and individual meanings* (Order No. 3296060). Available from ProQuest Dissertations and Theses Global. Retrieved from http://search.proquest.com/docview/304705338?accountid=14780.

Goodwin, F., and Jamison, K. (1990). *Manic-depressive illness*. New York: Oxford University Press.

Gutierrez-Rojas, L., Jurado, D., and Gurpegui, M. (2011). Factors associated with work, social life, and family life disability in bipolar disorder patients. *Psychiatry Research, 186*, 254–260.

Hawke, L. D., Parikh, S. V., and Michalak, E. E. (2013). Stigma and bipolar disorder: A review of the literature. *Journal of Affective Disorders, 150*(2), 181–191. doi:http://dx.doi.org.proxy.library.vcu.edu/10.1016/j.jad.2013.05.030.

Hollon, S. D., and Ponniah, K. (2010). A review of empirically supported psychological therapies for mood disorders in adults. *Depression and Anxiety, 27*, 9891–9832.

Inder, M. L., Crowe, M. T., Moor, S., Luty, S. E., Carter, J. D., and Joyce, P. R. (2008). "I actually don't know who I am": The impact of bipolar disorder on the development of self. *Psychiatry, 71*(2), 123–133. doi:10.1521/psyc.2008.71.2.123.

IsHak, W. W., Brown, K., Aye, S. S., Kahloon, M., Mobaraki, S., and Hanna, R. (2012). Health-related quality of life in bipolar disorder. *Bipolar Disorders, 14*(1), 6–18. doi:10.1111/j.1399-5618.2011.00969.x.

*Kang, J. Y. (2013). *Examining the inner experience of four individuals with bipolar disorder using descriptive experience sampling* (University of Nevada, Las Vegas) (Order No. 1553241). Available from ProQuest Dissertations and Theses. Retrieved from http://search.proquest.com/docview/1513233292?accountid=14780.

*Kemp, B. S. (2010). *Living with bipolar disorder: We adhere to our medication* (MS). Available from ProQuest Dissertations and Theses Global (750063381).

Kessler, R., Chiu, W., Demler, O., Merikangas, K., and Walters, E. (2005). Prevalence, severity, and comorbidity of 12-month DSM-IV disorders in the National Comorbidity Survey Replication. *Archives of General Psychiatry*, 62, 617–627. Retrieved from http://search.library.vcu.edu/primo_library/libweb/action/display.do?frbrVersion=10&tabs=viewOnlineTab&ct=display&fn=search&doc=TN_medline15939839&indx=1&recIds=TN_medline15939839&recIdxs=0&elementId=0&renderMode=poppedOut&displayMode=full&frbrVersion=10&dscnt=0&frbg=&scp.scps=scope%3A%28VCU_CONTENTDM%29%2Cscope%3A%28VCU%29%2Cscope%3A%28VCU_ALMA%29%2Cprimo_central_multiple_fe&tab=all&dstmp=1414611953639&srt=rank&mode=Basic&&dum=true&tb=t&vl(freeText0)=Prevalence%2C%20severity%2C%20and%20comorbidity%20of%2012-month%20DSM-IV%20disorders%20in%20the%20National%20Comorbidity%20%09Survey%20Replication&vid=VCU.

Kilbourne, A., Goodrich, D., Lai, Z., Clogston, J., Waxmonsky, J., and Bauer, M. (2012). Life Goals Collaborative Care for patients with bipolar disorder and cardiovascular disease risk. *Psychiatric Services, 12*: 1234–1238. Retrieved from http://search.library.vcu.edu/primo_library/libweb/action/display.do?frbrVersion=3&tabs=viewOnlineTab&ct=display&fn=search&doc=TN_medline23203358&indx=1&recIds=TN_medline23203358&recIdxs=0&elementId=0&renderMode=poppedOut&displayMode=full&frbrVersion=3&dscnt=0&frbg=&scp.scps=scope%3A%28VCU_CONTENTDM%29%2Cscope%3A%28VCU%29%2Cscope%3A%28VCU_ALMA%29%2Cprimo_central_multiple_fe&tab=all&dstmp=1414612051642&srt=rank&mode=Basic&&dum=true&tb=t&vl(freeText0)=Life%20goals%20collaborative%20care%20for%20patients&vid=VCU.

Kilbourne, A., Goodrich, D., O'Donnell, A., and Miller, C. (2012) Integrating bipolar disorder management in primary care. *Current Psychiatry Reports, 14*: 687–695. Retrieved from http://search.library.vcu.edu/primo_library/libweb/action/display.do?frbrVersion=4&tabs=viewOnlineTab&ct=display&fn=search&doc=TN_springer_jour10.1007%2fs11920-012-0325-4&indx=2&recIds=TN_springer_jour10.1007%2fs11920-012-0325-4&recIdxs=1&elementId=1&renderMode=poppedOut&displayMode=full&frbrVersion=4&dscnt=0&frbg=&scp.scps=scope%3A%28VCU_CONTENTDM%29%2Cscope%3A%28VCU%29%2Cscope%3A%28VCU_ALMA%29%2Cprimo_central_multiple_fe&tab=all&dstmp=1414612153675&srt=rank&mode=Basic&&dum=true&tb=t&vl(freeText0)=Integrating%20bipolar%20care%20in%20a%20primary%20care%20setting&vid=VCU.

Koutra, K., Basta, M., Roumeliotaki, T., Stefanakis, A., Triliva, S., Lionis, S., and Vgontzas, C. (2013). Family functioning, expressed emotion, and family burden in relatives of first-episode and chronic patients with schizophrenia and bipolar disorder: Preliminary findings. *European Psychiatry, 28*(1), 1.

*Kriegshauser, K., Sajatovic, M., Jenkins, J. H., Cassidy, K. A., Muzina, D., Fattal, O., et al. (2010). Gender differences in subjective experience and treatment of bipolar disorder. *The Journal of Nervous and Mental Disease, 198*(5), 370.

Laxman, K., Lovibond, K., and Hassan, M. (2008). Impact of bipolar disorder in employed populations. *American Journal of Managed Care, 14*, 757–784. Retrieved from http://search.library.vcu.edu/primo_library/libweb/action/display.do?frbrVersion=2&tabs=viewOnlineTab&ct=display&fn=search&doc=TN_medline18999910&indx=1&recIds=TN_medline18999910&recIdxs=0&elementId=0&renderMode=poppedOut&displayMode=full&frbrVersion=2&dscnt=0&frbg=&scp.scps=scope%3A%28VCU_CONTENTDM%29%2Cscope%3A%28VCU%29%2Cscope%3A%28VCU_ALMA%29%2Cprimo_central_multiple_fe&tab=all&dstmp=1414612277220&srt=rank&mode=Basic&&dum=true&tb=t&vl(freeText0)=Impact%20of%20Bipolar%20disorder%20in%20employed%20populations&vid=VCU.

Leclerc, E., Mansur, R. B., and Brietzke, E. (2013). Determinants of adherence to treatment in bipolar disorder: A comprehensive review. *Journal of Affective Disorders, 149*, 247–252.

Lucksted, A., McFarlane, W., Downing, D., Dixon, L., and Adams, C. (2012). Recent developments in family psychoeducation as an evidence-based practice. *Journal of Marital and Family Therapy, 38*(1), 101–121.

McIntyre, R. S., Rosenbluth, M., Ramasubbu, R., Bond, D. J., Taylor, V. H., Beaulieu, S., et al. (2012). Managing medical and psychiatric comorbodity in individuals with major depressive disorder and bipolar disorder. *Annals of Clinical Psychiatry, 24*(2), 163–169.

Meade, M. O., and Richardson, W. S. (1997). Selecting and appraising studies for a systematic review. *Annals of Internal Medicine, 127*, 531–537.

Michalak, E. E., Yatham, L. N., Kolesar, S., and Lam, R. W. (2006). Bipolar disorder and quality of life: A patient-centered perspective. *Quality of Life Research: An International Journal of Quality of Life Aspects of Treatment, Care and Rehabilitation, 15*(1), 25–37. doi:10.1007/s11136–005–0376–7.

Michalak, E. E., Yatham, L. N., Maxwell, V., Hale, S., and Lam, R. W. (2007). The impact of bipolar disorder upon work functioning: A qualitative analysis. *Bipolar Disorders*, 9(1/2), 126–143. doi:10.1111/j.1399–5618.2007.00436.x.

Miklowitz, D. J., and Taylor, D. O. (2006). Family-focused treatment of the suicidal bipolar patient. *Bipolar Disorders*, 8, 640–651.

National Alliance on Mental Illness. (2014). What is bipolar disorder? Retrieved from: www.nami.org/Content/NavigationMenu/Mental_Illnesses/Bipolar1/Home_-_What_is_Bipolar_Disorder_.htm.

Novick, D. M., Swartz, H. A., and Frank, E. (2010). Suicide attempts in bipolar I and bipolar II disorder: A review and meta-analysis of the evidence. *Bipolar Disorders*, *12*(1), 1–9. doi:10.1111/j.1399–5618.2009.00786.x.

Peele, P., Xu, Y., and Kupfer, D. (2003). Insurance expenditures on bipolar disorder: Clinical and parity concerns. *American Journal of Psychiatry*, *160*, 1286–1290. Retrieved from http://search.library.vcu.edu/primo_library/libweb/action/display.do?frbrVersion=7&tabs=viewOnlineTab&ct=display&fn=search&doc=TN_medline12832243&indx=1&recIds=TN_medline12832243&recIdxs=0&elementId=0&renderMode=poppedOut&displayMode=full&frbrVersion=7&dscnt=0&frbg=&scp.scps=scope%3A%28VCU_CONTENTDM%29%2Cscope%3A%28VCU%29%2Cscope%3A%28VCU_ALMA%29%2Cprimo_central_multiple_fe&tab=all&dstmp=1414612350400&srt=rank&mode=Basic&&dum=true&tb=t&vl(freeText0)=Insurance%20expenditures%20on%20Bipolar%20Disorder&vid=VCU.

Perlick, D. A., Rosenheck, R. A., Miklowitz, D. J., Chessick, C., Wolff, N., Kaczynski, R., et al. (2007). Prevalence and correlates of burden among caregivers of patients with bipolar disorder enrolled in the Systematic Treatment Enhancement Program for bipolar disorder. *Bipolar Disorders*, 9, 262–273.

Perugi, G., Angset, J., Azorin, J.-M., Bowden, C., Vieta, E., and Young, A. H. (2013). The bipolar-borderline personality disorders connection in major depressive patients. *Acta Psychiatrica Scandinavica*, *128*, 376–383.

*Pollack, L. E. (1995). Striving for stability with bipolar disorder despite barriers. *Archives of Psychiatric Nursing*, 9(3), 122–129. doi:http://dx.doi.org.proxy.library.vcu.edu/10.1016/S0883-9417(95)80034-4.

*Pollack, L., and Aponte, M. (2001). Patients' perceptions of their bipolar illness in a public hospital setting. *Psychiatric Quarterly*, *72*(2), 167–179. doi:10.1023/A:1010371626859.

Popovic, D., Reinares, M., Scott, J., Nivoli, A., Murru, A., Pacchiarotti, I., et al. (2013). Polarity index of psychosocial interventions in maintenance treatment of bipolar disorder. *Psychotherapy and Psychosomatics*, *82*, 292–298.

Post, R. M., and Leverich, G. S. (2006). The role of psychosocial stress in the onset and progression of bipolar disorder and its comorbidities: The need for earlier and alternative modes of therapeutic intervention. *Development and Psychopathology*, *18*(4), 1181–1211. doi:10.1017/S0954579406060573.

Prasko, J., Latalova, K., Cerna, M., Grambal, A., Jelenova, D., Kamaradova, D., et al. (2013). Psychoeducation for patients with bipolar disorder. *European Psychiatry*, *28*(1), 1.

Provencher, M. D., Guimond, A. J., and Hawke, L. D. (2012). Comorbid anxiety in bipolar spectrum disorders: A neglected research and treatment issue? *Journal of Affective Disorders*, *137*, 161–164.

Reinares, M., Sanchez-Moreno, J., and Fountoulakis, K. N. (2014). Psychosocial interventions in bipolar disorder: What, for whom, and when. *Journal of Affective Disorders*, *156*, 46–55.

Russell, L., and Moss, D. (2013). A meta-study of qualitative research into the experience of 'symptoms' and 'having a diagnosis' for people who have been given a diagnosis of bipolar disorder. *Europe's Journal of Psychology*, 9(2), 385–405. doi:10.5964/ejop.v9i2.560.

Sajatovic, M., Davies, M., Bauer, M. S., McBride, L., Hays, R. W., Safavi, R., et al. (2005). Attitudes regarding the collaborative practice model and treatment adherence among individuals with bipolar disorder. *Comprehensive Psychiatry*, *46*(4), 272–277. doi:10.1016/j.comppsych.2004.10.007.

*Sajatovic, M., Jenkins, J. H., Cassidy, K. A., and Muzina, D. J. (2009). Medication treatment perceptions, concerns and expectations among depressed individuals with type I bipolar disorder. *Journal of Affective Disorders*, *115*(3), 360–366.

*Sajatovic, M., Levin, J., Fuentes-Casiano, E., Cassidy, K. A., Tatsuoka, C., and Jenkins, J. H. (2011). Illness experience and reasons for nonadherence among individuals with bipolar disorder who are poorly adherent with medication. *Comprehensive Psychiatry*, *52*(3), 280–287.

Sanchez-Moreno, J., Martinez-Aran, A., Tabarés-Seisdedos, R., Torrent, C., Vieta, E., and Ayuso-Mateos, J. (2009). Functioning and disability in bipolar disorder: An extensive review. *Psychotherapy and Psychosomatics*, *78*(5), 285–297. doi:10.1159/0002 28249.

Sandelowski, M., and Barroso, J. (2006). *Handbook of synthesizing qualitative research*. New York: Springer Publishing.

Schulte, P., Jabben, N., Postma, D., Knoppert, E., and Peetoom, T. (2012). Psychoeducation for bipolar disorder: A systematic review on efficacy and a proposal for a prototype. *European Psychiatry*, *27*(Supp).

Simon, G., Ludman, E., Unitzer, J., Bauer, M., Operskalski, B., and Rutter, C. (2004). Randomized trial of a population-based care program for people with bipolar disorder. *Psychological Medicine*. Retrieved from http://search.library.vcu.edu/primo_library/libweb/action/display.do?frbrVersion=6&tabs=viewOnlineTab&ct=display&fn=search&doc=TN_cambridgesgmS0033291704002624&indx=5&recIds=TN_cambridgesgmS0033291704002624&recIdxs=4&elementId=4&renderMode=poppedOut&displayMode=full&frbrVersion=6&dscnt=0&frbg=&scp.scps=scope%3A%28VCU_CONTENTDM%29%2Cscope%3A%28VCU%29%2Cscope%3A%28VCU_ALMA%29%2Cprimo_central_multiple_fe&tab=all&dstmp=1414612442994&srt=rank&mode=Basic&&dum=true&tb=t&vl(freeText0)=Randomized%20trial%20of%20population%20based&vid=VCU.

Steele, A., Maruyama, N., and Galynker, I. (2010). Psychiatric symptoms in caregivers of patients with bipolar disorder: A review. *Journal of Affective Disorders*, *121*, 10–21.

Sullivan, A. E., Judd, C. M., Axelson, D. A., and Milkowitz, D. J. (2012). Family functioning and the course of adolescent bipolar disorder. *Behavior Therapy*, *43*, 837–897.

Suto, M., Murray, G., Hale, S., Amari, E., and Michalak, E. E. (2010). What works for people with bipolar disorder? Tips from the experts. *Journal of Affective Disorders*, *124*(1/2), 76–84. doi:http://dx.doi.org.proxy.library.vcu.edu/10.1016/j.jad.2009.11.004.

Targum, S. D., Dibble, E. D., Davenport, Y. B., and Gershon, E. S. (1981). The family attitudes questionnaire: Patients' and spouses' views of bipolar Illness. *Archives of General Psychiatry*, *38*(5), 562–568. doi:10.1001/archpsyc.1980.01780300074009.

Treuer, T., and Tohen, M. (2010). Predicting the course and outcome of bipolar disorder: A review. *European Psychiatry*, *25*(6), 328–333. doi:10.1016/j.eurpsy.2009.11.012.

Van der Voort, T., Goossens, P., and Van der Bijl, J. (2007). Burden, coping and needs for support of caregivers for patients with a bipolar disorder: A systematic review. *Journal of Psychiatric and Mental Health Nursing*, *14*, 679–687. Retrieved from http://search.library.vcu.edu/primo_library/libweb/action/display.do?frbrVersion=12&tabs=viewOnlineTab&ct=display&fn=search&doc=TN_wj10.1111%2fj.1365-2850.2007.01158.x&indx=1&recIds=TN_wj10.1111%2fj.1365-2850.2007.01158.

x&recIdxs=0&elementId=0&renderMode=poppedOut&displayMode=full&frbrVersion=12&dscnt=0&frbg=&scp.scps=scope%3A%28VCU_CONTENTDM%29%2Cscope%3A%28VCU%29%2Cscope%3A%28VCU_ALMA%29%2Cprimo_central_multiple_fe&tab=all&dstmp=1414612511989&srt=rank&mode=Basic&&dum=true&tb=t&vl(freeText0)=Burden%2C%20coping%20and%20needs%20for%20support%20of%20caregivers%20for%20patients%20with%20a%20bipolar%20disorder%3A%20a%20systematic%20review%20&vid=VCU.

Van Rheenen, T. E., and Rossell, S. L. (2014). Objective and subjective psychosocial functioning in bipolar disorder: An investigation of the relative importance of neurocognition, social cognition and emotion regulation. *Journal of Affective Disorders*, *162*, 134–141. doi:10.1016/j.jad.2014.03.043.

Vázquez, G. H., Kapczinski, F., Magalhaes, P. V., Córdoba, R., Lopez Jaramillo, C., Rosa, A. R., et al. (2011). Stigma and functioning in patients with bipolar disorder. *Journal of Affective Disorders*, *130*(1), 323–327. doi:10.1016/j.jad.2010.10.012.

Victor, S. E., Johnson, S. L., and Gotlib, I. H. (2011). Quality of life and impulsivity in bipolar disorder. *Bipolar Disorders*, *13*(3), 303–309. doi:10.1111/j.1399-5618.2011.00919.x.

7 The lived experience of people with schizophrenia

Schizophrenia is a mental disorder characterized by abnormal patterns of thought and perception. It includes two types of symptoms (APA, 2013). *Positive* symptoms represent exaggerations of normal behavior, and include hallucinations, delusions, disorganized thought processes, and tendencies toward agitation. The *negative* symptoms of schizophrenia represent the diminution of what would be considered normal behavior, and include flat affect (the absence of expression), social withdrawal, non-communication, anhedonia (blandness), passivity, and ambivalence in decision making. Complete and permanent remission in schizophrenia is relatively uncommon (Van Os et al., 2008). A person with the disorder may experience a chronic course, with symptoms being more or less florid but never really disappearing, or one in which periods of psychosis are interspersed with periods of remission. Suicide is the leading cause of premature death in schizophrenia, as 20–40 percent of persons attempt suicide at some point in their lives and 5–10 percent succeed (Johnson et al., 2008). The average life span of persons with schizophrenia is approximately 10 years shorter than the national average in the United States due to lifestyle factors such as diet, physical health, and risks related to poverty (Heald, 2010).

The nature of schizophrenia has been a major research topic in the health sciences for more than a century, but most studies have focused on its causes and treatment. What has been studied less often is the personal experience of having schizophrenia. Qualitative studies have been illuminating in these regards, and the purpose of this meta-synthesis was to determine the themes that could be identified across those studies.

Themes

After applying the selection criteria, a total of 27 studies published between 1992 and 2013 were included in our meta-synthesis, with a total of 408 participants, all with diagnoses of schizophrenia or schizoaffective disorder. About one-third of the participants were women and two-thirds were men. Caucasians and African-Americans were the most represented ethnicities in this sample, although four studies focused on specific ethnic groups, including Thai, Indonesian, Chinese, and Korean populations. There was wide variation in the marital and parenting status of participants as well as age range, with most falling between 18 and 50 years. Some had college degrees but the majority had obtained a high school diploma or less. Participants were recruited most often using purposive and convenience sampling methods and were frequently identified through local mental health facilities. Most were receiving some kind of mental health services for their condition, in both inpatient and outpatient settings. (See Table 7.1.)

Four major themes were identified in the results: (1) experience of symptoms; (2) acceptance processes; (3) personal relationships; (4) treatment experiences; and (5) spiritual practices and faith.

Themes

Experience of symptoms

Within the rubric of "symptoms" are included the experience of hallucinations, disorientation, and the loss of a sense of self (see Table 7.2).

Hallucinations

The onset of hallucinations was described as gradual by some and immediate by others (Fernandes, 2009). In general the experience of hallucinations was described as frightening, confusing, and exhausting (Flanagan et al., 2012; Forchuk et al., 2003; Humberstone, 2002; Jarosinski, 2006; Yennari, 2011). Participants in Phripp's (1995) study reported that they heard voices in their heads but felt that the voices were separate from themselves. The voices were often associated with violence, negativity, and yelling (Forchuk et al., 2003; Humberstone, 2002; Walton, 2000). Participants in Suryani et al.'s (2013) study reported feeling the need to comply with orders given by the voices. One participant noted: "The voices seemed to command my brain.... In my mind I felt as if I was under their command" (p. 315). It was not uncommon for participants to hear the voices as coming from electronic media such as television or radio (Baier, 1995). Participants noted the importance of gaining some level of control or understanding of the voices as an important step in learning to cope with schizophrenia (Roe et al., 2004).

Disorientation

The disorientation felt with schizophrenia can be described as not knowing what is real or unreal (Anderson, 2011; Baier, 1995; Baker, 1996; Phripp, 1995; Roe et al., 2004; Sung and Puskar, 2006). Experiences of hallucinations, both visual and auditory, as well as delusions, leave individuals constantly questioning reality. In Phripp's (1995) study, participants commented that they felt time passed differently for them. Multiple studies noted that participants made use of reality testing (ways to evaluate one's sensory impressions) to distinguish symptoms from reality (Anderson, 2011; Roe et al., 2004).

Another aspect of schizophrenia that leads to disorientation stems from difficulties with concentrating and problems with memory (Evenson et al., 2008; Fernandes, 2009; Forchuk et al., 2003; Liu et al., 2012; Sung and Puskar, 2006). Participants described confusion and difficulty with remembering and tracking information (Fernandes, 2009). This makes the task of reality testing even more challenging. The combination of unpredictable symptoms, being out of touch with reality, and difficulty thinking and remembering work together to increase anxiety (Liu et al., 2012). As one participant noted: "For me, the future is unrealistic and unpredictable. The only thing I can do now is just to take care of my daily life" (Liu et al., 2012, p. 1711).

Loss of sense of self

In general, participants found that the symptoms of schizophrenia were so overwhelming that they experienced a lost "sense of self" (Phripp, 1995, p. 30), defined as a loss of self-control or personal agency (Baker, 1996; Phripp, 1995), and a loss of identity (Fernandes, 2009; Humberstone, 2002; Jarosinski, 2006; Phripp, 1995). Jarosinski described participants as wondering: "Are they who they are?" (2006, p. ix). Participants in Fernandes' (2009) study expressed feeling fragmented rather than whole. Jarosinski's (2006) participants reported on the difficulties of finding a sense of self separate from the hallucinations. This was consistent with Yennari's (2011) study, which found that participants struggled to find a sense of identity. A young man from one study explained it this way:

> There was nowhere I could go for – for a sense of privacy because I felt that everyone was understanding everything that I was thinking and it didn't matter where I was. And uh just the sense of being absolutely out of control and having absolutely no control in your life. No control for your thoughts, no control of your actions no control of anything. Just being completely manipulated by exterior forces. No sense of self.
>
> (Phripp, 1995, p. 144)

Process of acceptance

The theme of acceptance considers the progress that individuals make in living with and managing schizophrenia. In general, participants did not feel that "recovery" was an appropriate description of their reality (Phripp, 1995; Tooth et al., 2003). Due to the long-term nature of schizophrenia, recovery was seen as something that was never complete but an ongoing process better described as coping (Phripp, 1995). As one participant noted:

> I just don't think you can live through a psychosis and be – and be ah somehow immune to its effects even if you make a complete recovery. I don't think there's such a thing as a complete recovery from a psychosis.
>
> (Phripp, 1995, p. 153)

The subthemes considered in this section include feelings of pain and loss, regaining a sense of self, acceptance (as a continuum), and reengagement (see Table 7.1).

Pain and loss

As symptoms appeared and individuals first become aware of their diagnosis, their feelings of pain and loss could be overwhelming. Many study participants reported feeling like failures (Baker, 1996; Evenson et al., 2008; Sung and Puskar, 2006). There was a sense of shame at being diagnosed with schizophrenia and not being able to maintain control of their lives (Evenson et al., 2008; Fernandes, 2009; Sanseeha et al., 2009; Suryani et al., 2013). Feelings of shame were frequently connected with internalized stigma (Flanagan et al., 2012) and negative self-thoughts (Forchuk et al., 2003). Participants described feelings of low self-confidence and poor self-image (Liu et al., 2012; McCann and Clark, 2004).

These negative feelings were associated with a sense of loss. Participants expressed that they had lost the chance to have a normal life (Baker, 1996; Gould, DeSouza, and Rebeiro-Gruhl, 2005), lost relationships (Baker, 1996), and lost tangible resources such as jobs and homes (Humberstone, 2002). One participant stated this simply as: "I remember when I was normal" (Gould et al., 2005, p. 469). This, in turn, led to feelings of isolation, hopelessness, and depression (Fernandes, 2009; Forchuk et al., 2003; Liu et al., 2012; Ng et al., 2008; Sung and Puskar, 2006). For some, this led to thoughts of suicide: "I feel like a suicide. I feel like taking a knife and putting it right through my chest" (Baker, 1996, p. 27). As the symptoms they experienced were unpredictable and difficult to understand, participants were also filled with worry, anxiety, and fear for the future (Baker, 1996; Evenson et al., 2008; Fernandes, 2009). Confusing, overwhelming, and erratic symptoms left the individuals in these studies feeling shame, loss, and fear.

Regaining a sense of self

Participants reported regaining a sense of self as they began to feel some level of control over their symptoms (Eklund et al., 2012; Phripp, 1995; Roe et al., 2004). As one person described: "I feel like a human being again. I've got my emotions back. I've got my long-term memory. I've got my short-term memory. I'm just coping and doing fine" (Forchuk et al., 2003, p. 147). This control enabled them to feel safer and to move forward in other areas such as reengagement (Eklund et al., 2012). Participants noted that gaining this control was hard work and required determination (Fernandes, 2009; Tooth et al., 2003). The new sense of identity that formed tended to include the diagnosis of schizophrenia, which was incorporated and accepted as one part of the self (Baier, 1995; Phripp, 1995; Sung and Puskar, 2006). Some participants felt pride in their new sense of self and considered themselves to be survivors. One participant stated:

> You might notice that I'm very individual. I know that. I, myself, it's up to me, this person behind the face here. I know it's a bit fleshy, a bit funny, but that person that I am behind this face is responsible for all kinds of freedom.
>
> (Humberstone, 2002, p. 370)

Acceptance (as a continuum)

The participants in these studies fell along a continuum of acceptance. There were some who refused to accept their diagnosis or identify as mentally ill (Liu et al., 2012; Sung and Puskar, 2006). Others accepted the diagnosis and were able to incorporate it into their identity without being defined by it (Yennari, 2011).

Acceptance itself had many meanings beyond acceptance of the diagnosis. It also meant coming to terms with the long-term nature of the disorder (Baier, 1995), the many losses inherent in the diagnosis, and acknowledging the need for support (Gould et al., 2005). Psychosocial support and psychoeducation sometimes helped individuals gain a level of acceptance (Phripp, 1995; Tooth et al., 2003), which generally enabled them to cope better and to move on with their lives, as this participant described:

> But ah, so I think that I've come a long way in dealing with the schizophrenia so that I know it's not a healthy thing to have but it's not life threatening and it's not um, it doesn't have to control your life.
>
> (Phripp, 1995, p. 84)

Reengagement

Participants who were coping well with their schizophrenia showed signs of reengagement, most commonly involving social interactions (Baier, 1995; Phripp, 1995; Sung and Puskar, 2006; Tooth et al., 2003) but also in setting goals (Eklund et al., 2012; Jarosinski, 2006), such as having a job and living independently (Forchuk et al., 2003; Ng et al., 2008; Phillips, 2008). One participant, a young man, commented: "Yeah, I want to get out of the system.... I'd get me a job, my own apartment, and a car and maybe even get married.... I'm gonna walk out that door. I'm getting discharged soon" (Phillips, 2008, p. 60).

Personal relationships

Discussions of relationships with others dominated the narratives in 23 studies. Participants consistently expressed the belief that their ability to develop and maintain interpersonal relationships was profoundly affected by the disorder. Stigma and discrimination from others, as well as the necessity of support were also indicated. See Table 7.1.

Deterioration of existing relationships

The third subtheme involved the deterioration of relationships that had been established prior to the onset of psychosis. Individuals expressed that they had lost relationships, both by being rejected due to their symptoms and due to their own emotional disengagement and resentment (Baker, 1996; Evenson et al., 2008; McCann and Clark, 2004; Suryani et al., 2013; Yennari, 2011). The effect of the disorder on one father's relationship with his children is apparent in the following quote: "Well because you alienated them from your mind ... they're my children but they're not my children ... it's a horrible feeling" (Evenson et al., 2008, p. 634). Some expressed anger and resentment toward family members who they believed had betrayed them by participating in their involuntary hospitalizations (Baker, 1996; Phillips, 2008).

When relationships with friends and family members were maintained, they were often described as being limited or superficial (Baker 1996; Forchuk et al., 2003; Humberstone, 2002; Liu et al., 2012; Shepherd et al., 2012; Sung and Puskar, 2006). Participants often described feelings of loneliness and isolation as a result of this deterioration in relationships. One woman described this as an inherent feature of schizophrenia, noting: "That's the thing about schizophrenia, it leaves you alone emotionally and alone physically.... I got really lonely. People my own age left me alone ... the trouble with schizophrenia was loneliness" (Humberstone, 2002, p. 7).

Difficulty establishing new relationships

Difficulty relating to others, referenced in 13 studies, often prevented individuals from establishing relationships that mattered to them (Baker, 1996; Gee et al., 2003; McCann and Clark, 2004; Sung and Puskar, 2006). Difficulty connecting was related to paranoia, anxiety, fear regarding other people's motivations, and fear of being considered abnormal or psychotic (Baker, 1996; Liu et al., 2012; Suryani et al., 2013; Walton, 1992, 2000). As one woman noted: "You can't ever feel comfortable. I'm always nervous and tense with people" (Baker, 1996, p. 26). As a result, some individuals came to accept the idea of being alone, or limited their relationships to others with the diagnosis (Humberstone, 2002; Ng et al., 2008; Phillips, 2008). Some reported that they were eventually able to establish relationships with others, but only by utilizing a "false self" and hiding their true feelings and emotions (Fernandes, 2009; Yennari, 2011). As one man explained: "[Regarding relationships] suppose people go out with you and are willing to be your friends. You don't really tell them too much. You'd be afraid of how they might look at you after you tell them" (Ng et al., 2008, p. 125). Others reported that the sense of discomfort with others never truly disappeared, but eased somewhat as the individual made progress in recovery (Forchuk et al., 2003).

Stigma and discrimination

Individuals spoke of facing alienation and stigma from their families, friends, and their communities in 12 studies, based on both their diagnosis and actual symptoms (Gee et al., 2003; Humberstone, 2002; Jarosinki, 2006; Powell, 1998; Tooth et al., 2003; Yennari, 2011). Many expressed that this stigma led to feelings of shame, isolation, rejection, and distrust, and was a major contributor to voluntary isolation (Flanagan et al., 2012; Liu et al., 2012; Sanseeha et al., 2009). When discussing even brief encounters with the outside world, themes of paranoia often permeated the narrative:

> But I remember I used to walk around, and I'd know that these people were looking at me. I used to get really paranoid, and they were all dressed in black, and I thought ... that's why I used to freak out so much, because I used to think someone was after me.
>
> (Walton, 2000, p. 3)

Many discussed the ways in which discrimination led to major consequences, such as difficulty finding housing. As a result, participants often concealed their diagnosis (McCann and Clark, 2004; Walton, 1992, 2000). While some individuals expressed a sense of injustice regarding being treated or judged negatively, many expressed the belief that these experiences were an inevitable part of living with the diagnosis of schizophrenia (Walton, 1992, 2000).

Importance of social support in coping

The final subtheme was the importance of social support in coping with the illness (16 studies). Individuals described depending on others for basic survival, including necessities such as food, clothing, and housing (Baker, 1996; Walton, 1992, 2000). Positive relationships enabled them to cope with their illness and make progress in recovery (Baier, 1995; Evenson et al., 2008; Forchuk et al., 2003; Humberstone, 2002; Liu et al., 2012; Ng et al., 2008; Phillips, 2008; Sanseeha et al., 2009; Sung and Puskar, 2006; Tooth et al., 2003; Walton, 1992, 2000). One individual noted: "I believe that friends are very important. Don't have to keep talking about your illness. Just hanging out and interacting with friends is quite good" (Ng et al., 2008, p. 126). Many discussed the ways in which helping others suffering from schizophrenia was beneficial to their own recovery (Eklund et al., 2012; McCann and Clark, 2004; Phillips, 2008). In order to develop these relationships, many sought out support groups so they could maintain contact with other persons with schizophrenia and maintain awareness regarding their illness (Phripp, 1995).

Treatment

Participant views on treatment were discussed in 19 studies, with two subthemes emerging for contact with the mental health system and medication (see Table 7.1).

Contact with mental health system

This subtheme was present in 12 studies, falling into two categories: issues of control and negative contact with staff. Many individuals expressed concern that their illness had caused them to lose control over both their lives and their behaviors (Baker, 1996; Forchuk et al., 2003; Suryani et al., 2013). Many who were interviewed within an inpatient setting had fears related to being controlled by others, which had been exacerbated by non-voluntary hospitalizations and being forced to take medications (Baker, 1996; Forchuk et al., 2003; Humberstone, 2002; Liu et al., 2012; Phillips, 2008; Yennari, 2011). One man encapsulated this feeling of helplessness regarding treatment options by noting:

> I was put on various drugs. I don't know if I can remember them all.... Then I was told that I wasn't allowed to leave the hospital unless I agreed to six months of injections outside the hospital. I was never all right there.
> (Baker, 1996, p. 29)

Some reported they were not well informed about their illness by doctors and staff, and, as a result, felt subject to the will of seemingly arbitrary decisions related to policies and treatment methods (Ng et al., 2008). Many expressed frustration at not being consulted regarding treatment decisions (Baker, 1996; Forchuk et al., 2003; Liu et al., 2012; Phillips, 2008). This lack of knowledge regarding their illness, combined with a lack of agency and control over decisions related to their health, often resulted in fear, discomfort, and disempowerment (Powell, 1998; Walton, 1992, 2000).

The second category under encounters with the mental health system was negative contact with staff, discussed in 10 studies. Many individuals expressed the belief that providers did not fully appreciate what it was like to experience a mental illness, and, consequently, failed to understand the impact of treatment decisions on clients' lives (Forchuk et al., 2003; Liu et al., 2012; Walton, 1992, 2000). Some complained about staff members who were not well informed about schizophrenia and invalidated their psychotic experiences (Forchuk et al., 2003; Powell, 1998; Yennari, 2011). Others complained that staff members treated them like children (Forchuk et al., 2003), which, at times, resulted in a desire to fight the system. As one woman noted: "She [nurse] never really lets go, you know, she sort of always treats you like a patient or something like that and you just, you want to rebel, or that's how I felt" (Walton, 2000, p. 80). Many respondents believed that staff did not always know what was best for them, and some expressed doubt that providers even had their best interest in mind (Baker, 1996; Fernandes, 2009; Liu et al., 2012; Ng et al., 2008; Tooth et al., 2003; Walton, 1992, 2000). As a result, some avoided communication with staff: "I keep my mouth shut.... I want to keep it a short stay" (Forchuk et al., 2003, p. 148). Even when some trust was developed, many emphasized that their relationships with staff continued to be largely superficial: "I know what the doctors are thinking about. They just take me as a patient. I mean, they just want to treat me like a client" (Liu et al., 2012, p. 1712).

Medications

The subtheme of medication was present in 18 studies and divided into two categories of acceptance of medications (11 studies) and adverse effects (11 studies). While many were resistant to medications at first, a large number of respondents acknowledged their necessity (Baker, 1996; Humberstone, 2002; Liu et al., 2012; Sanseeha et al., 2009; Sung and Puskar, 2006; Walton, 1992, 2000). Some spoke of the beneficial aspects of medications in managing their symptoms, and even seemed to accept the idea of medication as a long-term solution (Evenson et al., 2008; Phillips, 2008). One man stated: "I'm hoping the medication keeps working for the rest of my life" (Forchuk et al., 2003, p. 146). Even for those who were unhappy with their medications, many expressed a willingness and desire to try new medications in hopes they would find something that would work (Forchuk et al., 2003). However, even when medications were accepted, many individuals expressed the belief that they would not be completely "recovered" from their illness until they were able to be free of them (Liu et al., 2012; Ng et al., 2008).

The second category under medications involved side effects. Individuals described a variety of concerning side effects including lack of energy, weight gain, concentration and memory problems, excessive sleeping, and impaired ability to show emotions (Baier, 1995; Evenson et al., 2008; Fernandes, 2009; Forchuk et al., 2003; Gee et al., 2003; McCann and Clark, 2004; Phripp, 1995; Sung and Puskar, 2006; Tooth et al., 2003). The effect on memory was often particularly troubling, as one man noted: "When I have those slips of memory, which are part of my illness, something major will get lost ... and when it relates to the kids, that makes it hard to be a dad" (Evenson et al., 2008, p. 635). Concern about over-medication was a frequent point of focus, as individuals were fearful that taking too many medications would negatively impact their ability to function normally (Forchuk et al., 2003). Opinions on the effectiveness of medications varied, as some described positive effects (symptom reduction), some described negative effects (anxiety, restlessness, etc.), and some noted no change as the result of taking medication (Forchuk et al., 2003). One man reported that when his side effects were at their worst, they were "sometimes worse than the actual illness" (Yennari, 2011, p. 102). When this was the case, side effects often resulted in noncompliance (Sung and Puskar, 2006; Yennari, 2011).

Faith/spirituality

Faith and spirituality were frequently listed as factors that helped the participants cope with schizophrenia. Humberstone (2002) noted that participants found hope and meaning in God, as well as feeling that God was the only thing more powerful than their psychosis. Liu et al. (2012) noted the use of traditional Chinese spiritual methods, and Sanseeha et al. (2009) described participants using Buddhist teachings, mindfulness, meditation, and prayer for coping. Roe et al. (2004) also noted the use of mindfulness for coping. Faith and spirituality in general were used to instill hope (Phillips, 2008) and as a means of support (Walton, 2000). One participant noted:

> Well, I go to church and pray and all that. It made me more confident that I'll go to heaven in a good way ... it gives me reassurance ... it makes me feel sure that I have a spot in heaven.
>
> (Phillips, 2008, p. 49)

See Table 7.1.

Discussion

A limitation of the meta-synthesis is the fact that many participants were interviewed in an inpatient setting and might differ in important ways from individuals without these conditions, so perspectives shared in this meta-synthesize might not generalize to all people with schizophrenia. Still, the comments provided by the participants in these studies are powerful and have many implications for professionals who wish to enhance the lives of persons with schizophrenia.

The strengths of this meta-synthesis are that it provides a rich, detailed portrait of individuals with schizophrenia and avoids reducing those persons to mere symptomology. The themes of the meta-synthesis illuminate a conceptualization of the illness from a purely clinical model to that of a human experience with sociocultural implications. Our meta-synthesis identified complex psychological themes such as issues of control and loss of sense of self that would not have emerged using a quantitative approach.

Also revealed in this meta-synthesis was the stigma people experience, which only worsens the pain and suffering involved in having a diagnosis of schizophrenia. For many people, coping with schizophrenia is made more difficult by the stigma, that is, other people's negative attitudes and behavior, they experience. This rejection can lead to their social marginalization and low quality of life. The effects of stigma were borne out in a 27-nation quantitative study that investigated the nature, direction, and severity of anticipated and experienced discrimination reported by people with schizophrenia (Thornicroft et al., 2009). Negative discrimination was experienced by 47 percent of study participants in making or keeping friends, by 43 percent from family members, by 29 percent in finding a job, by 29 percent in keeping a job, and by 27 percent when pursuing intimate relationships. Anticipated discrimination affected 64 percent of the respondents in applying for work, training, or education, and by 55 percent who were seeking close relationships. Almost three-quarters (72 percent) of respondents felt the need to conceal their diagnosis. A third of participants anticipated discrimination for job seeking and close personal relationships even when no discrimination was subsequently experienced.

One clinical issue that emerged from the meta-synthesis was the fact that persons with schizophrenia often have an incomplete understanding of their own illness, which heightens their feelings of fear and disorientation (Liu et al., 2012; Walton 2000). This supports the need for psychoeducation, focused on teaching people about symptoms and the skills for managing them, acceptance of the disorder, and education about medications. Findings in this study also support the inclusion of topics related to the process of acceptance and coping, the usefulness of faith and spirituality practices for some people, and the need for social support. Social workers need to promote realistic expectations of recovery to combat the viewpoint that recovered patients must be symptom-free and not take medication (Forchuk et al., 2003; Liu et al., 2012; Ng et al., 2008; Phripp, 1995). In a systematic review of 44 trials it was found that psychoeducation resulted in greater medication compliance and significantly decreased relapse or readmission rates for participants compared with standard care (Xia et al., 2011).

Participants in the meta-synthesis spoke about the need for social support, even though they tend to withdraw from others. Pracitioners should understand that a moderate amount of interaction with significant others is optimal (Harley et al., 2012). They respond favorably to attitudes of acceptance, reasonable expectations, opportunities to develop social and vocational skills, and a relatively small number, but broad range, of social supports. These may include family members, friends, neighbors, work peers, school peers, informal community relations, and perhaps members of shared religious groups and organizations (Gunnmo and Bergman, 2011).

Psychoeducation should also be available to the families and friends of person with schizophrenia. Family psychoeducation focuses on educating participants about the ill relative's schizophrenia, helping them develop social and resource supports in managing the disorder, and developing coping skills of their own (Griffiths, 2006). Pharoah et al. (2010) conducted a systematic review of the randomized studies done on family intervention in schizophrenia and concluded that while the interventions may reduce the risk of relapse and improve compliance with medications, differences with standard care are modest.

Psychotropic medication is, of course, a primary intervention modality for persons with schizophrenia, and there is approximately a 66 percent chance that a person will respond positively to an antipsychotic medication (Stahl, 2013). A systematic review of 65 controlled trials has affirmed that all of the antipsychotic drugs are effective in controlling the resurgence of symptoms in persons with schizophrenia, even though they tend to produce adverse effects of movement disorders, sedation, and weight gain (Leucht et al., 2012). They are comparable in effectiveness to each other but demonstrate variable adverse effects with regard to extrapyramidal symptoms, anticholinergic effects, weight gain, insomnia, headache, and increased heart rate (Komossa et al., 2011; Komossa, Rummel-Kluge, Hunter et al., 2010; Komossa, Rummel-Kluge, Schmid et al., 2010; Lobos et al., 2010). The findings of this meta-synthesis support the idea that many consumers have serious reservations about taking medications due to these adverse effects and should be encouraged to be open about their experiences so that appropriate medication regimen of medications can be determined.

While nursing and hospital staff are equipped to provide appropriate medical interventions, problems related to issues of trust and control suggest that poor therapeutic relationships can have a negative impact on recovery. Hewitt and Coffey (2005) conducted a meta-analysis of studies on the significance of the therapeutic relationship with persons who have schizophrenia and concluded that those who experience an empathic, positive, facilitative relationship have better outcomes. Professional development programs that aim to increase awareness of the relationship issues facing this population could help to combat their perceived stigma and prejudice.

Vocational rehabilitation is defined as work-related activity that provides clients with pay and the experience of participating in productive social activity. The goals of vocational programs may be full-time competitive employment, any paid or volunteer job, the development of job-related skills, and job satisfaction. These interventions are helpful to persons with schizophrenia who first achieve a level of cognitive stability (Tsang et al., 2010). One specific program known as Individual Placement and Support has been demonstrated effective in several systematic reviews (Bond and Drake, 2012).

Very much in keeping with the findings of this study, it is important to describe the recovery *philosophy* of mental illness (Walsh, 2013). Recovery in mental health refers to a person's journey toward wellness and emphasizes his or her primary role in achieving wellness. According to the Social Workers' Desk Reference, recovery is:

> A process of developing individual potential and realizing life goals while surmounting the trauma and difficulties presented by behavioral, emotional, or physical challenges. [It] involves a process of personal transformation in which the disorder becomes less central in a person's life as he or she achieves outcomes that increasingly bring personal meaning and life satisfaction.
>
> (Roberts, 2009, p. 1203)

That is, people with long-term disorders need not delay resuming a full life while waiting for their symptoms or illness to disappear.

Inherent in the recovery philosophy is the idea that mental illness does not take over the entirety of a person, but exerts varying degrees of impact on specific domains of functioning. Mental illness leaves many domains of functioning intact, so consumers retain areas of health and competence alongside their problem areas. Within this paradigm recovery refers to a person's right and ability to have a safe, dignified, and meaningful life in the community of his or her choice, despite continuing disability resulting from the illness (Beecher, 2009; Reindal, 2008). Professional approaches to recovery tend to focus on observable improvements in symptoms and social functioning, and on the role of professional intervention. Consumer models, however, tend to emphasize peer support, empowerment, and the primacy of personal experience, such as what was represented in the findings of the meta-synthesis. There is a stronger focus on life meaning within the context of a supposedly enduring disability. Recovery, then, involves consumers accepting and owning their disabilities, however they understand them, developing their own goals, and making their own decisions about the types of formal and informal services they wish to receive.

Table 7.1 Data extraction of studies of people with schizophrenia

Author and purpose	*Design*	*Data analysis*	*Sample*	*Findings*
Anderson (2011) To understand lived experience of schizophrenia in African American males.	Interpretive phenomenology. In-depth interviews, recorded and transcribed verbatim. One interview per participant of approximately 1 hour length. Field notes were also kept.	Thematic analysis post transcription of audio recordings.	$N = 5$. Purposive. Ages 21–57 years. All African American males diagnosed with schizophrenia and living independently. Recruited from outpatient psychiatric clinics.	Four themes emerged: 1 "They know that they are mentally ill." 2 "They make a special effort to test reality." 3 "They assert their autonomy." 4 "They experience reality differently, which they see as a gift" (p. x). Participants in this study did not talk of loss, but all were at a point of acceptance and viewed the disorder as only a part of themselves, not the whole.
Baier (1995) To understand how individuals with schizophrenia experience "insight and meaning" (p. 1).	Semi-structured interviews ranging from 10 to 75 minutes. Naturalistic inquiry. Contextual field notes were also used.	Content analysis of interviews, determination of themes, construction of framework for understanding insight. Interviews were recorded and transcribed, information was also added from recordings to field notes.	$N = 26$. Use of selective sampling and snowball sampling. Recruited from self-help support groups and community center serving those who are homeless and experiencing mental illness. 18 men, 8 women. Ages 27–68 years. Mean of 40 years. 22 Caucasian, 4 African Americans. Diagnosis of schizophrenia or schizoaffective.	Individuals with schizophrenia described insight as awareness that their positive symptoms were "distortions of reality" (p. 1). Insight was developed through use of medication, family support, and long term treatment. Problematic issues/symptoms reported included poor concentration, beliefs about electronic media, drug abuse, medication side effects. Finding meaning required: 1 understanding level of control with disorder; 2 viewing the disorder as one part of life; 3 acceptance of long-term nature and challenge. Acceptance included building new social relationships and making future plans.

				Components of meaning: stigma, loss, emotional reactions, triggers, impact, coping skills, and future/acceptance. Most felt disorder was caused and/or triggered by substance use and/or stress.
Baker (1996) To determine how self-care knowledge is acquired by individuals with schizophrenia, despite lack of instruments available to detect warning signs of decompensation.	One-on-one interviews guided by interpretative interactionism, a line of inquiry developed by Norman Denzin.	Husserlian phenomenonology; data analyzed by: 1 "bracketing", which refers to dissection of informants' narratives in order to isolate and list essential recurring elements; 2 construction, where brackets are reassembled into coherent whole by identifying how they occur within the experience; 3 contextualization, in which investigator relocates constructed processes in informants' biographies in order to determine how the specific experiences impacted the phenomenon.	$N = 15$, non-probabilistic, purposive sample. Recruited through three psychiatric institutions located in Moncton, New Brunswick, Canada. Respondents had to have been hospitalized at least once for schizophrenia. Acute psychotic symptoms must have been remitted and patients had to be able to be followed on outpatient basis. 10 Males, 5 Females. Ages: 1 – 18 years, 2 – 20–29 years, 6 – 30–39 years, 4 – 40–49 years, 1 – 50–59 years, 1 – 70 years. 11 single, 1 married, 3 divorced.	*Themes permeating the narrative* Pain, both in accompanying symptoms and resulting from symptoms: • Informants depict onset of schizophrenia as their introduction to life of persistent emotional discomfort. This pain often centered on being out of touch with reality and feeling "tormented" by their illness. Control: • Losing control – Informants felt that their life was unpredictable and uncontrollable; this could be major or minor from day to day. When symptoms were worst they found themselves disruptive and in danger. • Being controlled by others – Involuntary hospitalizations create fear. Have no control over their future and being dependent on others. Failure: • Letting oneself down – Felt disappointed that they were unable to become the person they wanted to be. Inability to meet goals.

continued

Table 7.1 Continued

Author and purpose	*Design*	*Data analysis*	*Sample*	*Findings*
			3 did not graduate high school, 2 graduated high school, 1 attended technical university, 2 attended university, 6 received a technical diploma, 1 received a university diploma. 9 unemployed, 2 employed part-time, 3 in a sheltered workshop, 1 retired.	• Letting others down – Their actions many times have resulted in others making it clear to them that they had failed in meeting expectations. Being "kicked out." Loss: • Losing a normal life – They have negative attitudes towards their illness and are sad that they have lost the chance to be normal. • Losing roles and relationships – Not being able to find jobs they liked, not being able to establish relationships that mattered to them. Synthesis: • People with schizophrenia are able to monitor illness by analyzing the elevations in intensity of their distress. These persons have sought help from mental health care system when symptoms have worsened. As problematic experiences with control, failure, and loss accumulate, a fear of relapsing allows individuals to begin to pay closer attention to symptoms and identify when they need help.

Eklund et al. (2012) To determine what brings meaning to lives of individuals with schizophrenia.	Semi-structured interviews.	Qualitative content analysis to determine categories. Interviews recorded and transcribed. Author consensus.	*N* = 10. 5 men, 5 women. Purposive sample from supported housing in Sweden. Age: 36–60 average age 51 years. None with occupation.	Five categories of meaning: 1 social – having social contacts, being part of a social context, and feeling accepted; 2 occupational – functional daily routine, hobbies, having a goal or "work"; 3 health – physical and mental; 4 memories; 5 positive feelings – feeling safe, feeling needed.
Evenson et al. (2008) To explore potential issues concerning fathers with psychosis (schizophrenia, schizoaffective, or other psychotic-type disorder).	Two-part interview including brief demographic questionnaire and semi-structured interview on fatherhood.	Interpretative phenomenological analysis (IPA), which attempts to gain insight into phenomena as experienced by a person by listening to their account and then making an interpretation.	*N* = 10, recruited from patients of community mental health teams in west and north London. Sample was both purposive and convenience, as participants were meaningfully selected but not all followed through on participation. All participants had to be biological fathers, and must have contact with their children.	*Themes* 1 emotional disengagement from one's children; 2 hospital as family disruption; 3 medication as straitjacket; 4 negative impact on one's memory; 5 pre-fatherhood aspirations; 6 fears for children, including fears of passing on psychosis; 7 impact of parenting on fathers themselves, including pride in father role; 8 support and understanding from children; 9 motivation to make positive changes to one's life.

continued

Table 7.1 Continued

Author and purpose	*Design*	*Data analysis*	*Sample*	*Findings*
			Must have a diagnosis of psychosis: schizophrenia, schizoaffective, or other psychotic disorder. All were white, aged 34–67 or older. All must be stable with regard to their mental state (i.e. patient on remission or maintenance treatment).	*Synthesis* Psychosis may directly and indirectly undermine father-child relationship as well as process of parenting. Fathers are particularly concerned about children inheriting psychosis. However, fathers with schizophrenia feel sense of pride in the father role, sense of purpose in their life, and pleasure in creation and development of life. Fathers also find that their children are motivation to change for better. *Recommendations* Treatment programs need to be sensitive to effects of fatherhood on psychosis and effects of a father's psychosis on mental health of his family. Parenting programs might help fathers with psychosis.

Fernandes (2009) To understand subjective experience of self by schizophrenics: What is their sense of themselves as they go through psychosis? How do they experience their illness? Is their experience of themselves transformed by psychosis?	Two interviews: participants asked about their history, subjective experience of their illness (up to 3 hours). Three theories of self explored (self as fragmented, divided, or ost). 20 minutes of meeting time was for building rapport. Interviews were semi-standardized. 4 of 5 were audiotaped.	Qualitative analysis based in psychodynamic theory. Content analyzed and compared to theories of self in schizophrenia (self as fragmented, divided, or lost). Phenomenological: meaning attached to phenomena of self through psychosis. Interviews were transcribed then data was reduced. Researcher attended to phraseology of answers and highlighted key phrases or metaphors used by participants. Four categorical codes were used: schizophrenia, subjective experience, self, and theories of self in schizophrenia.	*N* = 5 (1 excluded from study). 2 males, 2 females. Adults with a diagnosis of schizophrenia by qualified mental health practitioner (QMHP). Not currently psychotic or at risk. Must have diagnosis of schizophrenia or schizoaffective disorder. Ages 30s to 60s. 4 Caucasian, 1 African American. Most lived in major metropolitan area. Education carried from high school diploma to some college. 2 employed. 2 single, 1 divorced. None had children.	*Themes* Subjective experience of schizophrenia: • introduced items – All participants introduced problems of irregular sleep and difficulty concentrating. Sedation, dizziness, confusion, and difficulty remembering and tracking information. Others discussed housing. • responses to open-ended questions: none saw advantages to schizophrenia. Self: • self defined – Half of participants reported separateness from others or “my own being” as key aspects of the self. Many reduced the self into subparts. • associations to self – Understanding of dissociation, emotional conflict, anxiety, lack of control, and agitation. • participants’ selves – When they discuss their subjective experience of themselves, the majority mention having difficulty living in an unhealthy or chaotic society. None described a happy and whole self.

continued

Table 7.1 Continued

Author and purpose	*Design*	*Data analysis*	*Sample*	*Findings*
				Theories of self in schizophrenia: • whole self – Only one person said they were whole; she said it takes effort to achieve a whole self and establish inner peace. • fragmented self – All agreed this was accurate. • divided self – Most associated to some extent. • loss of self (when acutely psychotic). Most participants characterized themselves as "divided." They use a "false self" to interact with the world. This is why many with schizophrenia have trouble establishing trust. All participants were familiar with concept of a "loss of self," and felt they had been transformed by the disorder. *Conclusion* The difference between psychotic and non-psychotic individuals is likely one of quantity not quality. All participants find themselves characterized by disorganization, fragmentation, and false selves (at least temporarily). *Recommendations* Empathy and understanding will help with therapeutic rapport. We all have potential to experience the theories of self at some point in our lifetime.

Flanagan et al. (2012) To determine if personal, lived experience of schizophrenia is in line with diagnostic criteria provided by DSM-IV-TR and therefore whether or not updates are needed for criteria in DSM-5.	Interviews: 1 per participant of 30–60 minutes each. Interviews audiotaped and transcribed verbatim.	Descriptive/interpretive phenomenological analysis: 2 researchers read each transcript and developed themes. Themes were then brought to the larger group, and group themes and quotes/examples were decided upon.	*N* = 17. Participants recruited by poster at mental health center. $25 given for interview. Average age = 48. 71% female. 77% African American, 17% white, 6% Native American. 88% had at least high school degree. Diagnosis of schizophrenia or schizoaffective disorder.	Participants could relate to criteria listed in the DSM but felt description was incomplete. Missing common symptoms included: 1 strong emotional reactions to symptoms (“fear, sadness, embarrassment, and alienation” (p. 375); 2 individuals were not necessarily lacking in emotion but may have presented with flat affect because of internalized stigma and distraction by hallucinations; 3 interest in, but severe disruption of goal-directed behavior secondary to hallucinations (p. 375). Again, individuals were not necessarily unmotivated to set and reach goals but struggled with internalized stigma and exhaustion from hallucinations; 4 hiding experiences due to stigma, which as stated above can lead to appearance of flat affect, social withdrawal, and lack of drive to set and accomplish goals.

continued

Table 7.1 Continued

Author and purpose	*Design*	*Data analysis*	*Sample*	*Findings*
Forchuk et al. (2003) To understand subjective experience of recovery from psychosis from consumer/client perspective.	Face-to-face interview at multiple data points.	Authors refer to data analysis method as ethnographic and naturalistic. Leninger's phases of qualitative analysis were used to identity categories and themes. Researchers identified and listed descriptors that were developed into patterns, then synthesized into broad themes.	*N* = 10. Nonprobability, purposive sampling. Patients were sampled from a tertiary care psychiatric hospital and a general hospital. Utilized patients with ongoing problems related to symptoms of psychosis who were preparing to undergo an initial year of treatment with either clozapine or risperidone. Must have had symptoms of psychosis for at least 1 year. 7 male, 3 female. Ages 26–51 years. All white, all Canadian. Ethnic origins: 3 Italian, 2 Dutch, 1 English, 1 Irish, 1 Israeli, 2 mixed.	*Themes* 1 Individual's part in the process of beginning a new medication: • they were aware when medication were not working and sought involvement in the process. 2 Most troubling symptoms of illness: • auditory hallucinations and delusions, difficulties in sleeping and thinking. These symptoms were focus of patient's evaluations of effectiveness of medications. 3 Hopes: • over time, recovering patients evolved more complex hopes; changed from just wanting medication to work to wanting a job, wanting to live independently, etc. 4 Fears: • patients' biggest fears included stay in hospital for rest of their life, losing control over their behavior. 5 Current effects of medications: • effects of medication were split into 3 categories: no change, negative effects (feeling anxious, edgy, restless, etc.), and positive effects (symptom reduction).

				6 Relationships with staff: • patients placed high value on positive relationships with staff in recovery process. 7 Relationships with family: • all patients who improved reported improved relationships with family. *Synthesis of themes* A person's recovery from psychosis is process involving entire self. Begins with improvements in thinking and feeling and extends to series of reconnections with environment, including staff and family. Recovery is not a "cure" but is an attitude or stance affecting many life areas.
Gee et al. (2003) To determine impact of schizophrenia on "health related quality of life" (HRQoL).	Interviews (which ranged from 20–70 minutes). Use of grounded theory – the information from the one interview is analyzed before moving on to the next interview, so that information is "grounded" in knowledge gained from the population under study (p. 3). One interview per subject all by same psychologist.	Interviews recorded and transcribed verbatim. Recordings were then analyzed for themes.	*N* = 6. 3 males, 3 females. Mean age 23 years. Mean length of illness 12 years. Individuals with schizophrenia recruited through local health centers.	10 HRQoL areas identified: 1 barriers to relationships; 2 decreased behavioral control; 3 loss of opportunity within occupational roles; 4 financial constraints; 5 psychotic symptoms; 6 medication side effects and attitudes; 7 psychological response; 8 stigma; 9 concerns for future; 10 positive outcomes (3 felt yes, 3 felt no).

continued

Table 7.1 Continued

Author and purpose	*Design*	*Data analysis*	*Sample*	*Findings*
Gould et al. (2005) To explore "occupational" needs and interests of young men with schizophrenia. Authors define occupational as activities that are social, recreational, intellectual, or vocational.	Focus groups. Two groups were held, the first collected information and the second reviewed and checked information.	"Constant comparative method" (Glaser & Strauss, 1967). Sessions were audiotaped, transcribed verbatim, read independently by each researcher, then analyzed for similarities, differences, and any comments that stood out. Once categories emerged, they were used as chapters within a narrative format.	*N* = 4 (7 were recruited by recruitment posters, but only 4 attended). All males. Age 19–25 years with diagnosis of schizophrenia. Age of onset 16–18 years. Race was not noted. Education varied from 9th grade to university level.	A narrative of 5 "chapters" (p. 469): 1 "I remember when I was normal" (theme of loss). 2 "It's like your computer crashes." 3 "Coasting through life" (time of stillness, internal processing, and coping – a time to meet the needs of "being"). 4 "Try to remake that life as best you can" (focus changes to needs of "becoming", identification of needs, acknowledgement of need for support). 5 "Finally, I can move on with my life" (re-engagement and rebuilding with acceptance of and inclusion of diagnosis).
Humberstone (2002) To understand subjective experiences of people with schizophrenia living in highly staffed supported accommodation.	Semi-structured open-ended interview.	Grounded theory methodology	*N* = 13. Purposive sampling. All had diagnosis of schizophrenia and all were treated with antipsychotic medication. Selected from 12 different residential facilities in south and central Auckland. 10 males, 3 females. Duration of treatment 3–10 months.	Principle finding: • people living with schizophrenia in supported accommodation have wide range of experiences that can be categorized within rubric of "survival." It was a central concept that linked disparate data. Author calls unified social theory "a way to survive": participants saw themselves as survivors who needed to find unique ways to cope.

What had to be survived:

- psychosis: surviving the actual symptoms of abnormalities that impact their life;
- alienation: from friends and family, and being alone;
- basic life stuff: all had experiences of deprivation with respect to shelter, food acquisition, and physical safety. Many had been homeless and in prison.

Surviving health services:

- hospitals, medication, and in-patient and out-patient staff perceived as things to be survived rather than services that facilitated survival.

Survival strategies

Religion/God:

- For many, the omnipotence of God was the only thing more powerful than the psychosis. Their beliefs provide a sense of hope/meaning.

Family:

- Patients yearned for family members, especially due to separation.

Identity:

- The need to assert a unique, individual identity was way of surviving psychosis and its impact.

Author recommends

This study has implications for service development and clinical practice being based in this theory. Thus it makes argument for value of qualitative research for getting at things quantitative research cannot.

continued

Table 7.1 Continued

Author and purpose	*Design*	*Data analysis*	*Sample*	*Findings*
Jarosinski (2006) To understand personal experience of hallucinations, their meaning, and their connection to sense of self.	Heideggerian hermeneutic approach – seeking to understand the individual in multiple contexts (p. 41). Interviews, recorded, transcribed, and analyzed. Post-interview notes and a journal were kept and used to help identify themes.	Interviews (one with each subject of 45 to 60 minutes) recorded, transcribed and analyzed to find themes. Researcher plus team of 6 colleagues worked as hermeneutic circle to determine themes. Martin qualitative software was used to help in identifying themes. Four subjects verified themes.	$N = 12$ subjects with schizophrenia or schizoaffective disorder. 5 males, 7 females. Age 30–55 years, mean = 50 years. 6 African American, 6 Caucasian.	Main idea resulted as “A life disrupted: still lived,” “a pattern of survival and perseverance” (p. ix). 4 main themes under this idea were: 1 “Are they who they are?”: • trying to understand and find meaning in the hallucinations, fear, confusion. 2 “A not so certain life”: • living with a chronic disorder, loss, stigma, trying to find meaning. 3 “Finding strength in the broken places”: • small goals, one day at a time, a way to find meaning. 4 “I am still me”: • feeling that they remained themselves separate from the hallucinations.

Liu et al. (2012) To understand perceptions of Chinese patients with schizophrenia about their treatment, mental state, social relationships, and daily life throughout the psychotic episodes.	Face-to-face semi-structured interviews.	Comparative analysis.	$N = 16$. Purposive sampling. All had diagnosis of schizophrenia. All had previously been hospitalized, were in contact with mental health services and receiving antipsychotic medications at onset of study. Recruited from outpatient department of mental hospital in Shanghai. 5 men, 11 women. Ages 21–52 years (mean 34.4 years). 10 married, 3 divorced/separated, 3 single. 5 had bachelor's degrees or higher, 11 had high school or less. 8 employed, 3 students, 5 unemployed. Longest length of psychotic episode was 15 years, shortest was less than 1 year.	Identified three central themes: 1 Negative experiences: • experiences of hospitalizations; • confused past experience. 2 Sense of being powerless: • changes in self pessimism about the future; • a sense of being controlled. 3 Ambivalent therapeutic relationships: • different understanding of mental illness (did not believe that they were mentally ill, thought issues were related to stress, etc.); • boundary (were aware of professional boundaries between themselves and psychiatrists and felt that it was not true friendship).

continued

Table 7.1 Continued

Author and purpose	*Design*	*Data analysis*	*Sample*	*Findings*
McCann and Clark (2004) To understand how people with schizophrenia experience their illness.	Unstructured interviews: 1 per participant of 60–90 minutes each. Audio-recorded and transcribed. Transcriptions read twice and conclusions checked by second researcher.	Descriptive phenomenology.	$N = 9$. 5 men, 4 women.	*Three themes* 1 "Temporality" Symptoms of the disorder are unpredictable which leads to fear and lack of trust in future. This can lead to hopelessness and in turn self-harm or suicide (also noted are fear to leave house, decreased social contact, and decreased self-confidence). 2 "Relationality" How schizophrenia symptoms affect relationships, which can be positive, in support offered, or negative. Importance of spirituality noted. Nondisclosure due to stigma. 3 "Treatment" Medication side effects that harm body image including weight gain, impotence, lethargy. Medications made social and sexual (in males) relationships more difficult.

Ng et al. (2008) To attempt to understand what recovery means from the point of view of Chinese people with long-term schizophrenia living in Hong Kong.	3-hour focus group where participants were guided in a discussion by 4 local experienced psychiatrists.	Thematic content analysis based on grounded theory.	$N = 8$. Purposive sampling. Individuals recruited from Phoenix Clubhouse, rehabilitation facility operated by Department of Psychiatry, Queen Mary Hospital. Ages 18–65 years. All ethnic Chinese fluent in Cantonese. 4 men, 4 women. All taking antipsychotic medication and had had more than one psychotic episode in their life.	*Four categories* 1 Recovery as a multi-dimensional construct: • definition of recovery implies functional recovery. All subjects agreed that recovery implied more than symptomatic remission. Also means optimal functioning in other life domains. 2 Relationship of medication to recovery: • Most thought you had to have stopped medication to be recovered, but had different justifications for continued use of medication. 3 Sense of hopelessness and helplessness about recovery: • Most felt they had not fully recovered and lacked faith about possibility of doing so. Many did not understand their illness. 4 Factors that promoted recovery: • Most recognized that certain people could help them, including doctors, family members, etc. Role of family was viewed as especially important. *Central theme* Recovery is a sweet dream. It is idealized. Patients do not view recovery same way as doctors. Patients have idealized view of "regular people" and life after recovery. As if there are no problems.

continued

Table 7.1 Continued

Author and purpose	*Design*	*Data analysis*	*Sample*	*Findings*
				Conclusions of respondents Most believed that full recovery could not be achieved until they stopped medication and had a steady job. Support and care of family and friends were also vital, but sometimes problematic. Independent living is viewed differently in Chinese culture.
Phillips (2008) To describe, interpret, and understand meaning of and lived experience of hope for individuals diagnosed with schizophrenia.	In-depth interview.	Grounded theory.	*N* = 8 Hospitalized patients diagnosed with schizophrenia according to DSM. All residents of Hudson River Psychiatric Center in New York. Criterion sampling method. Ages 24–58 years. 4 Caucasians, 1 Jamaican, 3 African Americans. 6 males, 2 females.	*Main themes* Defining hope: • meaningful definitions from their own perspectives and not related to particular experience (i.e. having fun, waking up, wanting to succeed). Hope existed in the patients. Faith: • 4 out of 8 said that a faith in God or higher power is major source of hope. Important coping mechanism. Personal relationships: • 6 out of 8 said that maintaining relationships with others helped to instill hope, even within the hospital setting. Relationships with staff: • important for 7 out of 8 participants. Most spoke highly of staff.

Treatment:

- 7 out of 8 said hope was linked with treatment and programming offered at their facility. Recovery-oriented approaches. Many praised medication.

Work:

- many worked in a program at facility, others hoped to do so one day. It was a sense of purpose.

Helping others:

- 7 out of 8 said it was important to be able to help other residents and friends and family.

Independence:

- all 8 expressed hope they would leave hospital one day.

Other themes

Present orientation:

- many focused on day-to-day activities and found hope there.

Self-directed vs. other-directed:

- people wanted to define their own experiences.

Interactive person- vs. thing-oriented:

- they wanted to interact with others.

Conclusion

Hope still exists even amongst most persistently mentally ill populations and is essential factor in treatment and recovery. We must work to promote hope.

continued

Table 7.1 Continued

Author and purpose	*Design*	*Data analysis*	*Sample*	*Findings*
Phripp (1995) "To gain an insider's perspective of the everyday experience of living with schizophrenia in order to explore the impact of this experience on the sense of self" (p. 30).	6 in-depth interviews (audio-taped and transcribed), personal writing, and medical record reviews.	Findings coded and categorized. Categories examined for patterns or themes. Cases comparatively analyzed.	*N* = 3 individuals with diagnosis of schizophrenia (5 were recruited, 2 quit). Purposeful sample. 1 male, age 30 years; 2 females, ages 44 and 50 years. Ages of onset from 26–31 years. Recruited from mental health clinic in Canada where they each receive medication and supportive therapy. All have college degrees and are currently active with work, volunteer, or school.	Results were grouped into five categories per participant. "*Mary*" 1 "Breaking down: Am I schizophrenic?" • Mary felt breakdowns were brought on by stress, she used her family for support, and was suspicious of her diagnosis. 2 "Sleeping problem." • Felt her breakdowns stemmed from difficulty sleeping, and that this symptom was not given the weight or consideration by others that it deserved. 3 "Hearing voices." • Felt voices were separate from herself, in her head but real. Also had symptom of subvocalizations. 4 "Recovering." • Gaining some mastery over symptoms. Assisted by medications, family support, psychosocial support, persistence, occupation, and personal goals. 5 "Functioning but flawed." Note: Avoided being around other people with schizophrenia because she did not want to be like them (p. 51).

"Diane"

1 "A chemical imbalance: going for a crash."
   - Diane clearly felt her disorder was due to chemical imbalance and that getting medications worked out was best answer. Medications initially immobilized her. She would sit without motion or thought and unable to sleep.
2 "Fantasy."
   - Diane described having rich fantasy life throughout her childhood which her schizophrenia had altered, making it "all-consuming."
3 "Paranoia and perceptual changes."
   - Paranoia was insidious and difficult to distinguish disorder from reality. Perceptual changes were easier to see as from the disorder and served as warning signs to increase her medications to avoid the paranoia.
4 "Managing your illness."
   - Gaining a sense of self-control and functionality. Used medications, stress management, and lots of rest.
5 "Not like I probably might have been."
   - Diane reports judging herself by a "schizophrenia standard" to maintain positive outlook. She does not want to be seen from a strengths perspective, not pitied or patronized.

continued

Table 7.1 Continued

Author and purpose	*Design*	*Data analysis*	*Sample*	*Findings*
				She enjoys spending time with others with schizophrenia. She reports living with threat of reoccurring symptoms (p. 89). "*Alex*" 1 "Schizophrenia: a chronic illness." • understands that he has a chronic illness. 2 "In the schizophrenia." • loss of self, loss of control. Alex reports feeling he has no privacy and is being manipulated. 3 "Recovery." • feels recovery is never complete. Lives with threat of disorder overcoming and paralyzing him. Utilizes medications, family support, stress control, and lots of sleep. 4 "Lack of motivation." • hopelessness, suicidality, lack of control, fear.

5 “A different person – a different life” (p. 132).

Schizophrenia is a part of his identity but does not define him. Alex feels that schizophrenia has helped him to be less judgmental: “There is this infinity within each of us.”

Note: Alex liked the support groups but was cautious as group sharing had increased his anxiety and caused some symptoms.

Common themes

Psychotic episodes:

- overwhelming of self;
- loss of agency;
- sense of being controlled;
- not knowing what is real.

Recovery:

- ongoing process;
- continuum of acceptance;
- medication helps;
- active participation increases sense of agency;
- reconstructing identity to include the disorder and parts of self developing within limitations of the disorder;
- importance/significance of social interaction.

continued

Table 7.1 Continued

Author and purpose	*Design*	*Data analysis*	*Sample*	*Findings*
Powell (1998) To understand how individuals with schizophrenia experience their "symptoms" (p. 38), and to discover what techniques these individuals use to cope with symptoms, other than medication.	One-time interviews audiotaped and transcribed. Open-ended questions and demographics. "Personal experience and interpretive interactionist methods" (p. 44), "constant comparison technique" (p. 48).	Interviews recorded and transcribed. Analyzed for themes.	*N* = 33. Convenience sample recruited from self-help groups and non-profits. Ages 19–68 years. Mean age 36 years. 18 male, 15 female. Caucasian 51%, African American 27%, Hispanic 22%. All diagnosed with schizophrenia and on medications to help control symptoms.	Patterns found in symptom identification: • "internal pressure, external pressure, symptom dimensions, sense of self, and relationship to others" (p. 136). How participants evaluated symptoms "how unusual, how disruptive, and consequences" (p. 137). Symptom control strategies used "relational, interactive, physical, and structural" – medication alone was not enough (p. 138). Clear preference for "new" medications. Participants recalled experiences with healthcare providers as disempowering. Providers seemed misinformed and provided misinformation. Participants reported feeling stigmatized. Also discussed great feelings of loss and experience of time as different from the norm.

Roe et al. (2004) To determine personal coping styles in dealing with schizophrenia or related psychotic illness.	Semi-structured interviews beginning with hospital stays and running bimonthly for 1 year, then every 6 months for 2–3 years. Interviews were recorded. Interviewers composed summaries of each interview which were dictated and transcribed.	Based on verbatim transcripts of first post-hospital interview and then based on interviewer summaries of other interviews. Open-coding case analysis led to analyst-constructed categories (p. 124).	*N* = 43. Only 41 included in data analysis due to problems with recordings of 2 subjects' interviews. Recruited from hospitals associated with Yale University. Ages 20–39 years. 25 males, 18 females.	"Analyst constructed coping strategies most frequently mentioned" (p. 124). 1 Regulating activity, involvement, and external stimuli (not necessary for those who did not overschedule themselves initially). 2 Strategies of controlling symptoms (learning to give less concern to the voices and reality testing, also using mindfulness to observe the symptom and then choose how to react to it). 3 Determination and hope. 4 Changes in attitude and corrective experiences.
Sanseeha et al. (2009) To understand perception of self and of illness in individuals with schizophrenia, as well as family member perception.	In-depth interviews, reflective journaling, observation.	Data analyzed with Heidegger's hermeneutic phenomenology, "being in the world of the participant" (p. 307). Verbatim transcription. Triangulation interview methods.	*N* = 18 individuals with schizophrenia. Purposive selection from outpatient mental health clinic. Inclusion criteria: • free from psychiatric symptoms; • receiving mental health care; • over 18 years old; • spoke Thai; • lived with caregiver; • willingness to participate. *N* = 12 family members, determined by permission of subject. Participant ages of 24–57 years, mean of 35.6 years. All were Buddhists.	*Four themes* 1 Perceptions of mental illness: • chronic, need for medication and treatment. 2 Perceptions of cause: • supernatural powers (black magic or spiritual punishment for cultural violations), bad karma (blamed selves), or biological (genetic or trauma). 3 Perceptions of discrimination: • felt ashamed, isolated, rejected, distrusted. 4 Living with schizophrenia: • use of family support and Buddhist teachings for happiness – use of mindfulness, meditation, and prayer.

continued

Table 7.1 Continued

Author and purpose	*Design*	*Data analysis*	*Sample*	*Findings*
Shepherd et al. (2012) To determine personal experience of changes in schizophrenia over the "lifespan."	Semi-structured interviews of 45–60 minutes (1 per subject) and demographic questionnaire. 4 interviewers included 2 academics, 1 "consumer" (individual with schizophrenia), and 1 parent. 2 3-hour trainings for all interviewers. Interviews considered past, changes, current, and future thoughts on the disorder.	Interviews recorded, transcribed, and analyzed using "grounded theory techniques" "coding consensus, co-occurrence, and comparison" (p. 297).	*N* = 32. Roughly 41% females. Age 50 years and older, with mean of 56 years. Schizophrenia for 35 years (mean). Recruited from UCSD database.	Based on lifespan divisions of 1 (early course), 2 (middle course), and 3 (present and future outlook). 1 Contained losses/upheaval, confusion, and escapism (stage 1 was followed by a long transitional period). 2 Contained gaining insight, improvement in symptoms, development of self-management skills, and adaptations in social relationships. 3 Contained optimism/hope, acceptance/resignation, or despair.

Sung and Puskar (2006) To identify salient themes that characterize life experiences of college students with schizophrenia.	In-depth interviews employing semi-structured questionnaires.	Content of interviews were transcribed and a text was generated. Researchers then analyzed for recurring themes and categories of experience (phenomenological).	$N = 21$ individuals interested in and capable of reporting their experiences of schizophrenia. Convenience sample: recruited as subsample from group of 171 potential participants. Time frame: June to November 2002. Drew from 2 university hospitals in Korea. 13 male, 8 female. Ages 20–27 years; average age 23.1 years. Mean age when first diagnosed: 18.9 years. Average duration of illness: 52.5 months.	25 themes were ultimately identified, which were then grouped into six categories of experiences 1 Experiences of school life: • difficulty with academic performance, motivation loss with school life, feeling of isolation from peers, satisfaction with academic performance, urgent need for continuing academic performance. 2 Interactions with family: • contact deficiency, verbal interaction deficiency, conflict with family, support of family. 3 Interactions with friends: • loneliness in interaction with friends, difficulty making friends, withdrawal from friends, feeling comfortable around friends, seeking intimacy. 4 A mental illness: • denial of self-identification as a mental illness patient, despair due to mental illness, feeling of being out of touch with reality, accepting a mental illness, attaining new identity as a mental illness patient. 5 Everyday life: • loss of interest, loss of feeling of reality, maintaining a balanced lifestyle. 6 Social role performance: • powerlessness with social role performance, enhancing self-esteem, sense of belonging as a social member.

continued

Table 7.1 Continued

Author and purpose	*Design*	*Data analysis*	*Sample*	*Findings*
				Conclusion Most participants reported more negative than positive life experiences. Supports the need for treatment options that meet students' actual life experiences focusing on developmental characteristics and needs. Approaches could focus on counseling strategies to teach coping skills for psychotic symptoms and acceptance of the disease, education about medication compliance, use of self-help groups to make positive support, and psycho-education to promote resilience and recovery.
Suryani et al. (2013) To understand experience of auditory hallucinations of Indonesian people diagnosed with schizophrenia so as to inform provision of quality person-centered nursing care.	In-depth focused interviews. Each participant interviewed twice. First interview was to explore experiences of living with auditory hallucinations (45–60 minutes). Second interview was to provide opportunity for participants to review their respective transcript of interview (30– 40 minutes).	Phenomenological using Colaizzi's (1973) approach.	$N = 13$. Purposive sampling. Participants were recruited from an outpatient department of a mental health facility in Indonesia. All reported hearing voices. Comorbid disorders were excluded. 6 men, 7 women. Ages 19 to 56 years.	Four themes emerged from the study: 1 Feeling more like a robot than a human being: • individuals felt devoid of control or powerless to resist voice commands. 2 Voices of contradiction: • a point of confusion as voices contradicted one another and engendered feelings of doubt about what to do. Challenged the individual's personal integrity.

Individuals had been living with schizophrenia between 1 and 25 years.

3 Tattered relationships and family disarray:
   - relationships and family life imploded as the mental illness took grip of person's life; feelings of chaos as well as shame and inferiority.

4 Normalizing presence of voices as part of everyday life:
   - despite feelings of uncertainty generated by voices, participants normalized their hallucinations to be able to live with them. Sometimes ignore the voices, sometimes don't.

Conclusion
Experience of fear, apprehension, confusion, and uncertainty need to be incorporated into intervention models. Auditory hallucinations need to be re-conceptualized from formal clinical model to a human experience with sociocultural perspective.

continued

Table 7.1 Continued

Author and purpose	*Design*	*Data analysis*	*Sample*	*Findings*
Tooth et al. (2003) To understand, from a consumer perspective, what is important for recovery from schizophrenia. To understand how consumers define recovery. To compare findings to those in the literature.	2 "consumer" focus groups were used to formulate interview questions. Groups were recorded and transcribed. A 4-part interview process was used: first, an open question about recovery; second, semi-structured with questions from focus groups and literature; third, looking for "consumer" definition of recovery; fourth, standardized questionnaire on demographics and the "Structured Clinical Interview" (p. 71) which was also used to screen sample volunteers for schizophrenia.	First 3 parts of interviews were recorded, transcribed, and analyzed for common themes using the "Non-Numerical Unstructured Data Indexing Searching and Theorising (NUDIST) computer program for qualitative data analysis" (p. 72). Guba and Lincoln's criteria for qualitative research were applied (p. 72), and analysis was checked with each participant to confirm internal validity. Kappa-K coefficient of .86 was found in respect to the coding system.	*N* = 57. 42 males, 15 females. Individuals diagnosed with schizophrenia and who identified personally as "in recovery." Participants were reimbursed for participation. 82% on medication. 42% employed (including volunteer work).	*Results of interviews* Part 1: • "an active sense of self" (p. 72) is noted as the most common, important factor named in recovery. Social support was next factor noted. The numbing and fatigue inducing effects of medication were next listed as a challenge. After this, approximately 60% of participants listed health care professionals as a hindrance to their recovery. Part 2: • found that "understanding the illness" and spiritual beliefs were important for many in recovery process (p. 74). Part 3: • found that participants' definition of recovery frequently included self-determination/responsibility (table 5, p. 75). Part 4: • demographics used to determine homogeneity of sample.

Note 1: When parts 1 and 2 were combined (table 4, p. 75) the two most common factors reported as important for recovery were determination and understanding the illness. Next most noted factors were negative effects of medications and health care professionals, and after that, social supports (friends more so than family) were listed as important. Coming in just under this, in the 50th percentile range, was acceptance of medication, stigma, and spirituality.

Note 2: In discussion it is mentioned that participants were highly critical of the "biomedical approach" and that newer medications were not available to these participants.

Note 3: Also, the study was "unsuccessful" in its goal of forming a consumer's definition of recovery as participants' definitions lacked consistency, but also because participants saw themselves not so much as "in recovery" as just getting on with their lives.

continued

Table 7.1 Continued

Author and purpose	*Design*	*Data analysis*	*Sample*	*Findings*
Walton (1992) To develop a theory about experience of schizophrenia from Rogerian nursing science perspective. Walton (2000) (Represents the completed study.) To understand the social and relational impact of chronic schizophrenia on sufferers living in New Zealand. To answer the question: "What is it like to live with schizophrenia?"	Unstructured audiotaped interviews, and field notes. 57 hours of transcribed interview data, plus artworks and written material.	Heideggerian phenomenological study. Walton notes that she wants to use Van Manen's (1990) four fundamental lifeworld themes as a guide for reflection in the research process: lived space, lived body, lived time, and lived human relationships.	*N* = 10. Purposive non-random sample: most were recruited through a field worker, 3 self-selected. 7 men, 3 women. Ages 21–64 years. Some working in paid or voluntary capacity (occupations included artist, writer, academic, educator); others were unemployed. All participants had been diagnosed with schizophrenia at least 2 years prior. One had had his illness for 40 years. No distinction was made concerning diagnostic category. All living within the community; 4 were in supervised or supportive accommodation. All regularly took antipsychotic medication.	Six themes illustrate the impact of schizophrenia on an individual's interactions with others: 1 Living with the prejudice of others: • sense of injustice about being judged or pre-judged without an individual hearing, and the real consequences this can have (discrimination). 2 Being fearful of others: • whether real or imagined, finding people unpredictable and threatening. Even normal everyday experiences can feel threatening; 3 Feeling uncomfortable in the company of others: • less intense than fear yet more common among participants – difficulty socializing and establishing relationships. General feelings of unease regarding relationships. 4 Staying engaged with others in the world: • despite their difficulties, all made an effort to stay engaged with others in some way. Each had a circle of friends or family members with whom they made regular contact.

5 Depending on others for help:
   - health professionals had a lot of control over their lives. Most appreciated professionals who were honest, friendly, kind, and helpful, and did not appreciate those who were controlling.
6 Finding others who understand:
   - most support is found through others with the illness.

Conclusion
All participants found some of their relationships with others difficult. Some of this difficulty was due to prejudice; some was due to nature of the illness. However, overall, participants recognized importance of staying engaged with others in the world.

continued

Table 7.1 Continued

Author and purpose	*Design*	*Data analysis*	*Sample*	*Findings*
Yennari (2011) To understand "lived meaning" of diagnosis of schizophrenia, among and across individuals, specifically in regards to how they have been perceived and treated by others, and how they viewed themselves after being identified with the diagnosis.	Individual interviews.	Empirical phenomenological method developed by Amedeo Giorgi in 1970 with hermeneutic component. General themes observed across different descriptions were characterized as "shared constituents of the phenomenon under investigation" (p. 41). Edited description then organized to create general structure of phenomenon. Quotes were clustered. Themes for individual participants were noted and then compared across participants.	Individuals recruited to participate in this study met the following criteria: They were diagnosed by psychiatrist or psychologist as having schizophrenia, based on DSM-IV-TR criteria. They were adults of any age, men or women, born as American citizens or individuals who reside in the United States coming from Western culture backgrounds. Participants agreed or disagreed with their diagnosis, but were aware that they have or had been perceived by others as mentally ill. Participants were able to participate comfortably in all phases of research, including interacting with researcher, having interviews tape-recorded, and talking about their experiences of impact of diagnostic labeling.	Themes were grouped into two clusters: 1 The issue of living with the diagnostic label of schizophrenia: • impact of diagnostic labeling on identity (most would not accept it as labeling them); • concealment of the label in interactions with others (all had concealed it to some extent, i.e. referring to it as a depression); • facing ignorance (participants felt angry, hurt, misunderstood by others); • stigma (felt invalidated by other human beings, loss of friendships, etc.). 2 Specific to schizophrenia as a disorder with which participants struggled: • frightening onset of the illness; • role of spirituality in coping with the illness (about half said that they used it to cope); • tension between trust and mistrust in interpersonal (good and bad doctors) relationships; • medication side effects and noncompliance (all had had long history of medication use – trying different things, etc.); • perceptions of unhelpful and • beneficial aspects of treatment.

Participation was voluntary, informed, and confidential; participants were made aware that they had freedom to withdraw their participation at any time. Range of participants included individuals diagnosed with both reactive and process schizophrenia. The psychologist inviting clients to participate in this study made determination that potential participants were not cognitively impaired based on clinical judgment and diagnostic skills. *N* = 7. 5 male, 2 female. 4 African American, 3 white. Ages 26–58 years.	Findings indicate positive impact of spirituality on coping with schizophrenia, treatment adherence and satisfaction, and self-efficacy. Accounts demonstrate that illness of schizophrenia has personal and interpersonal consequences beyond those resulting from diagnostic labeling. Individuals did not want to be defined by illness. It was just one part of their being. Common experiences in journey of recovery: redefining the self, accepting one's illness, overcoming stigma, renewing hope and commitment, resuming control and responsibility, exercising citizenship, managing symptoms, being supported by others and being involved in meaningful activities, and expanded social rules.

Table 7.2 Themes from studies of people with schizophrenia

	Feelings of pain and loss	*Loss of sense of self*	*Experience of hallucinations*	*Disorientation*	*Faith/spirituality*
Anderson (2011)				Participants understand that their experience of reality is different and make an effort to test their perceptions.	
Baier (1995)			Hallucinations often originated from electronic media.	Participants experienced positive symptoms as distortions of reality and felt that awareness of this offered some insight.	
Baker (1996)	Individuals described feeling like a failure, both by letting themselves down and letting others down. Sense of loss based on losing a normal life and losing relationships. Pain, both in accompanying symptoms and resulting from symptoms (described as a low level of discomfort). Feeling worry and insecurity.	Individuals talked about losing control of their actions and their thoughts – not knowing what they would do or say.	When symptoms were at their worst, individuals found that they were disruptive and placing themselves in danger.	Individuals described feeling out of touch with reality and feeling "tormented" by their illness. Described their life as unpredictable and uncontrollable in regard to energies.	

Evenson et al. (2008)	Low self-esteem regarding impact of schizophrenia on role behavior (individuals felt like bad parents). Fear regarding passing on the psychosis. Shame regarding hospitalization and illness.		Describe delusions that family members are not related to you (children are not your children).	Schizophrenia negatively impacts memory.
Fernandes (2009)	Described sense of anxiety and lack of control, agitation regarding symptoms. Some reported feelings of shame from the direct symptoms or indirect consequences (Supplemental Security Income benefits). Feelings of depression.	Individuals described feeling separate from others and using a "false self" to interact with world. Feelings of disassociation and emotional conflict. Individuals did not feel "whole" – described themselves as either fragmented or divided. Individuals discussed the "loss of self" due to illness.	Described gradual onset of symptoms. Some can remember the moment when they first heard voices. Others thought they had a nervous breakdown which was an immediate onset of symptoms.	Difficulty concentrating. Described sedation, dizziness, confusion, and difficulty remembering and tracking information. Confused memories of psychotic episodes – disorganization.
Flanagan et al. (2012)	Participants struggled with internalized stigma.		Participants report being exhausted by hallucinations.	

continued

Table 7.2 Continued

	Feelings of pain and loss	*Loss of sense of self*	*Experience of hallucinations*	*Disorientation*	*Faith/spirituality*
Forchuk et al. (2003)	Patients expressed displeasure towards their introverted and withdrawn tendencies, which led to feelings of depression about situation. Patients described feelings of discouragement related to medications.		Individuals stated that the most troubling symptoms of their illness were auditory hallucinations and delusions. Patients described specific hallucinations that related to specific medications. Sometimes hallucinations tried to encourage them to harm someone.	Expressed difficulties thinking.	Spiritual changes as the result of disease.
Gould et al. (2005)		"I remember when I was normal" (p. 469).			
Humberstone (2002)	All had experienced deprivation as a result of their disease (homelessness, shelter, food acquisition). Sense of loss, loneliness, and isolation.	Original sense of identity is destroyed by schizophrenia (must be rebuilt). Sense of social and economic dislocation.	Hallucinations and delusions are something that must be "survived." Violence during hallucinations. Affective experience of psychosis is one of fear and distress punctuated by boredom. Two participants described current psychotic symptoms based on actual past threats to their physical safety.		Many viewed the omnipotence of God as the only thing more powerful than their psychosis. Spirituality provides a sense of hope and meaning. People with psychosis may have their spiritual beliefs intertwined or separate from their psychosis.

Jarosinski (2006)		Attempted to find sense of self separate from the hallucinations. "Are they who they are?" (p.ix).	Looked for meaning in hallucinations. Felt fear and confusion.		Participants report looking for meaning.
Liu et al. (2012)	Feeling of hopelessness and powerlessness regarding symptoms. Pessimism about future. Lower self confidence.	Described changes in self as a result of the illness – deficit and regression in occupational competency, academic ability, etc.	Many explained past psychotic experiences as interpersonal conflicts, temporary stress, or bad reactions caused by pressures in daily life. Described psychotic behavior as "abnormal."	Schizophrenia negatively impacts memory. Confused past experience with hospitalizations/ diagnosis. Anxiety regarding symptoms – not knowing what is going on with the body.	Reach out to spiritual methods (traditional Chinese) to cure the disease.
McCann and Clark (2004)	Decreased self-confidence was noted. Side effects of medications led to negative self image.				Importance of spirituality noted.
Ng et al. (2008)	Sense of hopelessness and helplessness about recovery. Sense of defeat.			Many subjects expressed confusion about what exactly they were suffering from.	

continued

Table 7.2 Continued

	Feelings of pain and loss	*Loss of sense of self*	*Experience of hallucinations*	*Disorientation*	*Faith/spirituality*
Phillips (2008)					4 out of 8 said that faith in God or higher power was a major source of hope. Important coping mechanism. Belief in God allows individuals to cope with disappointment, limitations, and challenges related to treatment.
Phripp (1995)	Participant reports that to preserve self-image she judges herself by schizophrenia standard.	Participant describes loss of sense of self as "in the schizophrenia" (p. 132). Feeling he has no privacy and is being manipulated. Psychotic episodes felt like an overwhelming of self with loss of agency.	Hallucinations reported as hearing voices within your head but feeling they were separate from you.	Participants report feeling that time passed differently as a symptom of schizophrenia. Difficulty distinguishing the disorder from reality, which led to paranoia.	
Powell (1998)		Expressed concern over sense of self.			
Roe et al. (2004)			Participants reported that learning to give less concern to the voices was important for recovery.	Participants made use of reality testing.	Use of mindfulness to control symptoms and cope.

Sanseeha et al. (2009)	Participants felt discriminated against. They felt ashamed and rejected.				Participants used Buddhist teachings, mindfulness, meditation, and prayer for coping.
Sung and Puskar (2006)	Described dissatisfaction with performance in life areas (academics) based on illness. Feelings of deficiency. Loss of motivation. Despair. Loss of interest in activities. Loss of self-confidence.	Individuals described loss of self as result of their illness (defined as being out of touch with reality).		Difficulty concentrating.	
Suryani et al. (2013)	Intense fear regarding psychosis. Feeling of incapacitation/ helplessness. Feelings of shame and inferiority.	Individuals described feeling more like a robot than a human being. Confusion over proper behavior (due to voices) challenged individual's personal integrity.	Individuals felt powerless to resist voice commands. Voices and hallucinations contradicted one another. Individuals tried to normalize presence of voices as part of everyday life (sometimes ignoring voices or pretending hallucinations are normal).	Contradiction in voices leads to feelings of doubt and confusion about what to do.	
Tooth et al. (2003)					Importance of spirituality noted.

continued

Table 7.2 Continued

	Feelings of pain and loss	*Loss of sense of self*	*Experience of hallucinations*	*Disorientation*	*Faith/spirituality*
Walton (1992, 2000)			Describes hallucinations related to people – such as imagining people shouting at them.	Even everyday experiences can feel threatening – finds people unpredictable and scary.	Some spoke of utilizing churches and spirituality as a means of support.
Yennari (2011)		Diagnostic label affects an individual's sense of identity – individuals did not want to be defined by it. Individuals described being deceptive about their illness/identity to others. Individuals tried to redefine the self.	Described onset of hallucinations/delusions as extremely frightening. Not being able to control one's mind. Some denied negative experience of hallucinations.		Role of spirituality in coping with the illness (50%). Studies indicate that spirituality has positive impact. Religious faith as a source of altruism/ unselfish giving. God gives encouragement and hope. Religious faith as protection.

References

Anderson, L. (2011). *African American males diagnosed with schizophrenia: A phenomenological study* (Unpublished doctoral dissertation). Virginia Commonwealth University, Richmond, Virginia.

APA (American Psychiatric Association). (2013). *Diagnostic and statistical manual of mental disorders* (5th edn.). Arlington, VA: Author.

Baier, M. (1995). *The process of developing insight and finding meaning within persons with schizophrenia* (Unpublished doctoral dissertation). Saint Louis University, Saint Louis, Missouri.

Baker, C. (1996). Subjective experience of symptoms in schizophrenia. *Canadian Journal of Nursing Research*, *28*(2), 19–35.

Beecher, B. (2009). The medical model, mental health practitioners, and individuals with schizophrenia and their families. *Journal of Social Work Practice*, *23*(1), 9–20.

Berlin, S. B. (2002). *Clinical social work practice: A cognitive-integrative perspective*. New York: Oxford.

Bond, G. R., and Drake, R. E. (2012). Making the case for IPS supported employment. *Administration and Policy in Mental Health and Mental Health Services Research*, *41*(1), 69–73. doi:10.1007/s10488–012–0444–6.

Burns, T. (2010). The rise and fall of assertive community treatment? *International Review of Psychiatry*, *22*(2), 130–137.

Coldwell, C., and Bender, W. (2007). The effectiveness of assertive community treatment for homeless populations with severe mental illness: A meta-analysis. *American Journal of Psychiatry*, *164*, 393–399.

Dietrich, M., Irving, C., Park, B., and Marshall, M. (2010). Intensive case management for severe mental illness. *Cochrane Database of Systematic Reviews 2010*, *10*, CD007906. doi: 10.1002/14651858.CD007906.pub2.

Eklund, M., Hermansson, A., and Hakansson, C. (2012). Meaning in life for people with schizophrenia: Does it include occupation? *Journal of Occupational Science* *19*(2), 93–105.

Evenson, E., Rhodes, J., Feigenbaum, J., and Solly, A. (2008). The experience of fathers with psychosis. *Journal of Mental Health*, *17*(6), 629–642.

Fernandes, N. J. (2009). *The subjective experience of self in schizophrenia: a phenomenological study* (Doctoral dissertation). Retrieved from ProQuest Dissertations and Theses Global (3405284).

Flanagan, E., Solomon, L., Johnson, A., Ridgway, P., Strauss, J., and Davidson, L. (2012). Considering DSM-5: The personal experience of schizophrenia in relation to the DSM-IV-TR criteria. *Psychiatry*, *75*(4), 375–386.

Forchuk, C., Jewell, J., Tweedell, D., and Steinnagel, L. (2003). Reconnecting: The client experience of recovery from psychosis. *Perspectives in Psychiatric Care*, *39*(4), 141–150.

Frankel, A. J., and Gelman, S. R. (2011). *Case management: An introduction to concepts and skills*. Chicago: Lyceum.

Gee, L., Pearce, E., and Jackson, M. (2003). Quality of life in schizophrenia: A grounded theory approach. *Health and Quality of Life Outcomes*, *1*(31), 1–11.

Gould, A., DeSouza, S., and Rebeiro-Gruhl, K. (2005). And then I lost that life: A shared narrative of four young men with schizophrenia. *British Journal of Occupational Therapy*, 68(10), 467–473.

Griffiths, C. A. (2006). The theories, mechanisms, benefits, and practical delivery of psychosocial educational interventions for people with mental health disorders. *International Journal of Psychosocial Rehabilitation*, *11*(1), 21–28.

Gunnmo, P., and Bergman, H. F. (2011). What do individuals with schizophrenia need to increase their well-being. *International Journal of Qualitative Studies on Health and Well-being*, 6(11), 1–11.

Harley, E. W., Boardman, J., and Craig, T. (2012). Friendship in people with schizophrenia: A survey. *Social Psychiatry and Psychiatric Epidemiology*, *47*(8), 1291–1299.

Heald, A. (2010). Physical health in schizophrenia: A challenge for antipsychotic therapy. *European Psychiatry*, *25*(Supp. 2), S6–S11.

Hewitt, J., and Coffey, M. (2005). Therapeutic working relationships with people with schizophrenia: Literature review. *Journal of Advanced Nursing*, *52*(5), 561–570.

Humberstone, V. (2002). The experience of people with schizophrenia living in supported accommodation: A qualitative study using grounded theory methodology. *Australian and New Zealand Journal of Psychiatry*, *36*(3), 367–372.

Jarosinski, J. (2006). *A life disrupted; still lived* (Unpublished doctoral dissertation). Virginia Commonwealth University, Richmond, Virginia.

Johnson, J., Gooding, P., and Tarrier, N. (2008). Suicide risk in schizophrenia: Explanatory models and clinical implications, the Schematic Appraisal Model of Suicide (SAMS). *Psychology and Psychotherapy: Theory, Research and Practice*, *81*(1), 55–77.

Jones, C., Hacker, D., Cormac, I., Meaden, A., and Irving, C. B. (2012). Cognitive behaviour therapy versus other psychosocial treatments for schizophrenia. *Cochrane Database of Systematic Reviews 2012*, *4*, CD008712. doi:10.1002/14651858.CD008712.pub2.

Kidd, S. A., George, L., O'Connell. M., Sylvestre, J., Kirkpatrick, H., Browne, G., et al. (2011). Recovery-oriented service provision and clinical outcomes in assertive community treatment. *Psychiatric Rehabilitation Journal*, *34*(3), 194–201.

Kirsh, B., and Cockburn, L. (2007). Employment outcomes associated with ACT: A review of ACT literature. *American Journal of Psychiatric Rehabilitation*, *10*(1), 31–51.

Komossa, K., Rummel-Kluge, C., Hunger, H., Schwarz, S., Bhoopathi, P. S., Kissling, W., et al. (2010). Ziprasidone versus other atypical antipsychotics for schizophrenia. *Cochrane Database of Systematic Reviews 2009*, 4, CD006627. doi:10.1002/14651858.CD006627.pub2.

Komossa, K., Rummel-Kluge, C., Schmid, F., Hunger, H., Schwarz, S., Srisurpanont, M., et al. (2010). Quetiapine versus other atypical antipsychotics for schizophrenia. *Cochrane Database of Systematic Reviews*, doi:10.1002/14651858.CD006569.pub3.

Komossa, K., Rummel-Kluge, C., Schwarz, S., Schmid, F., Hunger, H., Kissling, W., et al. (2011). Risperidone versus other atypical antipsychotics for schizophrenia. *Cochrane Database of Systematic Reviews 2011*, 1, CD006626. doi:10.1002/14651858.CD006626.pub2.

Kurtz, M., and Mueser, K. (2008). A meta-analysis of controlled research on social skills training for schizophrenia. *Journal of Consulting and Clinical Psychology*, *76*, 491–504.

Leucht, S., Corves, C., Arbter, D., Engel, R., Chunbo, L., and Davis, J. (2009). Second-generation versus first-generation antipsychotic drugs for schizophrenia: A meta-analysis. *Lancet*, *373*, 31–41.

Leucht, S., Tardy, M., Komossa, K., Heres, S., Kissling, W., and Davis, J. M. (2012). Maintenance treatment with antipsychotic drugs for schizophrenia. *Cochrane Database of Systematic Reviews 2012*, *5*, CD008016. doi:10.1002/14651858.CD008016.pub2.

Liberman, R. P. (2012). Phase-specific recovery from schizophrenia. *Psychiatric Annals*, *42*(6), 211–217.

Liu, L., Ma, X., and Zhao, X. (2012). What do psychotic experiences mean to Chinese schizophrenia patients? *Qualitative Health Research, 22*(12), 1707–1716.

Lobos, C. A., Komossa, K., Rummel-Kluge, C., Hunger, H., Schmid, F., Schwarz, S., et al. (2010). Clozapine versus other atypical antipsychotics for schizophrenia. *Cochrane Database of Systematic Reviews 2010, 11*, CD006633. doi:10.1002/14651858.CD006633.pub2.

Marshall, M., and Lockwood, A. (2011). Assertive community treatment for people with severe mental disorders. *Cochrane Database of Systematic Reviews 2011, 4*, CD001089. doi:10.1002/14651858.CD001089.pub2.

McCann, T., and Clark, E. (2004). Embodiment of severe and enduring mental illness: Finding meaning in schizophrenia. *Issues in Mental Health Nursing, 25*, 783–798.

Meade, M. O., and Richardson, W. S. (1997). Selecting and appraising studies for systematic review. *Annals of Internal Medicine, 127*(7), 531–537.

Miller, S. D., Duncan, B. L., and Hubble, M. A. (2005). Outcome-informed clinical work. In J. C. Norcross, and M. R. Goldfried (Eds.), *Handbook of psychotherapy integration* (2nd edn.) (pp. 84–102). New York: Oxford University Press.

Mueser, K. T., Bond, G. R., Drake, R. E., and Resnick, S. G. (1998). Models of community care for severe mental illness: A review of research on case management. *Schizophrenia Bulletin, 24*, 37–74.

Newton-Howes, G., and Wood, R. (2013). Cognitive behavioural therapy and the psychopathology of schizophrenia: Systematic review and meta-analysis. *Psychology and Psychotherapy: Theory, Research and Practice*, 86, 127–138.

Ng, R., Pearson, V., Lam, M., Law, C., Chiu, C., and Chen, E. (2008). What does recovery from schizophrenia mean? Perceptions of long-term patients. *International Journal of Social Psychiatry, 54*(118), 118–130.

Noblit, G. W., and Hare, R. D. (1988). *Meta-ethnography: Synthesizing qualitative studies*. Newbury Park, CA: Sage.

Park, M. M., Zafran, H., Stewart, J., Salsberg, J., Ells, C., Rouleau, S., et al. (2014). Transforming mental health services: A participatory mixed methods study to promote and evaluate the implementation of recovery-oriented services. *Implementation Science*, 9(1), 1–21

Pharoah, F., Mari, J. J., Rathbone, J., and Wong, W. (2010). Family intervention for schizophrenia. *Cochrane Database of Systematic Reviews 2010, 12*, CD000088. doi: 10.1002/14651858.CD000088.pub3.

Phillips, J. K. (2008). *The experience of hope in those diagnosed with schizophrenia: A qualitative study* (Doctoral dissertation). Available from ProQuest Dissertations and Theses Global (3338144).

Phripp, T. (1995). *Not like I might have been* (Unpublished Master's Thesis). Queen's University, Kingston, Ontario, Canada.

Pitschel-Walz, G., Leucht, S., Bauml, J., Kissling, W., and Engel, R. (2001). The effect of family interventions on relapse and rehospitalization in schizophrenia: A meta-analysis. *Schizophrenia Bulletin, 27*, 73–92.

Powell, J. (1998). *Living with schizophrenia outside mental health provider's conceptualizations: An abyss of misunderstanding and marginalization* (Unpublished doctoral dissertation). University of Wisconsin-Milwaukee, Milwaukee, Wisconsin.

Reindal, S. M. (2008). A social relational model of disability: A theoretical framework for special needs education? *European Journal of Special Needs Education, 23*(2), 135–146.

Roberts, A. R. (Ed.) (2009). *Social workers' desk reference* (2nd edn.). New York: Oxford University Press.

Roe, D., Chopra, M., and Rudnick, A. (2004). Persons with psychosis as active agents interacting with their disorder. *Psychiatric Rehabilitation Journal, 28*(2), 122–128.

Sanseeha, L., Chantawan, R., Sethabouppha, H., Disayavanish, C., and Turale, S. (2009). Illness perspectives of Thais diagnosed with schizophrenia. *Nursing and Health Sciences, 11*, 306–311.

Shepherd, S., Depp, C., Harris, G., Halpain, M., Palinkas, L., and Jeste, D. (2012). Perspectives on schizophrenia over the lifespan: A qualitative study. *Schizophrenia Bulletin, 38*(2), 295–303.

Smolak, A., Gearing, R. E., Alonzo, D., Baldwin, S., Harmon, S., and McHugh, K. (2013). Social support and religion: Mental health service use and treatment of schizophrenia. *Community Mental Health Journal, 49*(4), 444–450.

Stahl, S. M. (2013). *Stahl's essential psychopharmacology: Neuroscientific basis and practical application*. Cambridge: Cambridge University Press.

Stein, L. I., and Test, M. A. (1980). Alternative mental hospital treatment: I. Conceptual model, treatment program, and clinical evaluation. *Archives of General Psychiatry, 37*, 392–397.

Substance Abuse and Mental Health Services Administration. (2009). *Evidence-based practices: Shaping mental health services toward recovery*. Retrieved from www.innovations.ahrq.gov/content.aspx?id=313.

Sung, K., and Puskar, K. (2006). Schizophrenia in college students in Korea: A qualitative perspective. *Perspectives in Psychiatric Care, 42*(1), 21–32.

Suryani, S., Welch, A., and Cox, L. (2013). The phenomena of auditory hallucination as described by Indonesian people living with schizophrenia. *Archives of Psychiatric Nursing, 27*, 312–318.

Thornicroft, G., Brohan, E., Rose, D., Sartorius, N., and Leese, M. (2009) Global pattern of experienced and anticipated discrimination against people with schizophrenia: A cross-sectional survey. *The Lancet, 373*(9661), 408–415.

Tooth, B., Kalyanasundaram, V., Glover, H., and Momenzadah, S. (2003). Factors consumers identify as important to recovery from schizophrenia. *Australasian Psychiatry, 11*, 70–77.

Tsang, H., Leung, A., Chung, R., Bell, M., and Cheung, W. (2010). Review on vocational predictors: A systematic review of predictors of vocational outcomes among individuals with schizophrenia. An update since 1998. *Australian and New Zealand Journal of Psychiatry, 44*, 495–504.

van Os, J., Rutten, Bart P. F., and Poulton, R. (2008). Gene-environmental interactions in schizophrenia: Review of epidemiological findings and future directions. *Schizophrenia Bulletin, 34*(6), 1066–1082.

Walsh, J. (2010). *Psychoeducation in mental health*. Chicago: Lyceum.

Walsh, J. (2013). *The recovery philosophy and direct social work practice*. Chicago: Lyceum.

Walton, J. (1992). The lived experience of schizophrenia. *Rogerian Nursing Science News: Newsletter of the Society of Rogerian Scholars, 4*(3), 5–6.

Walton, J. (2000). Schizophrenia and life in the world of others. *Canadian Journal of Nursing Research, 32*(3), 69–84.

Xia, J., Merinder, L. B., and Belgamwar, M. R. (2011). Psychoeducation for schizophrenia. *Cochrane Database of Systematic Reviews 2011*, 6, CD002831. doi:10.1002/14651858.CD002831.pub2.

Yennari, A. (2011). *Living with schizophrenia: A phenomenological investigation* (Doctoral dissertation). Available from ProQuest Dissertations and Theses Global (3465900).

8 The lived experience of women with depression

Depression continues to be one of the leading causes of disease burden for women (Üstün et al., 2004). Prevalence rates have remained consistent across the life span with women experiencing major depression about twice as often as men beginning in adolescence (Craighead et al., 2007; Kessler, Chiu et al., 2005; Piccinelli and Wilkinson, 2000; Richards, 2011). There are various explanations put forward for this gender discrepancy, including hormonal changes (Desai and Jann, 2000); rumination as a coping strategy (Nolen-Hoeksema, 2002); higher rates of sexual abuse (Bolen and Scannapieco, 1999); greater interpersonal stress (Girgus and Nolen-Hoeksema, 2006); lower appreciation and pay for women's work, and role overload (Le et al., 2003). These various reasons have been studied quantitatively, but qualitative research may further illuminate women's experience of depression and provide insights into how women cope and recover, and discover what is helpful about treatment.

Applying the search process and terms with the assistance of a reference librarian as described in Chapter 2, inclusion criteria produced a total of 24 studies with 574 participants between 1984 and 2014. Most of the studies were unpublished as dissertations. The adult women (over the age of 18) were Caucasian, African-American, or Latina. The majority of subjects were recruited from outpatient health clinics or through flyers, public advertisement, and word of mouth. Most of the studies involved individual interviews as a data collection method. See Table 8.1.

Themes

The themes that were formulated from the 25 studies involved the following: (1) experience of depression; (2) attributions about depression; (3) coping efforts; and (4) treatment.

Experience of depression

Women who are depressed, at least those in the US studies, described depression as a biopsychosocial phenomenon.

Biological

Participants often discussed the physical manifestation of depression as physical with respondents reporting sleep issues, problems with energy and fatigue, changes in appetite, and actual physical pain and disorders (Ashby, 2014; Hodge, 1994; Poleshuck et al., 2013). Physical symptoms included jaw and back pain (Ashby, 2014), irritable bowel syndrome (Poleshuck et al., 2013), nausea, cramps, and rapid heartbeat (Jones, 2010). As an example, a woman in Moreta (2007) described chest pain: "The pain in my chest, which I never had before, I am used to being sad and crying but I had never had [this feeling] so bad that it started to be a physical thing" (p. 71). Women in the Nicolaidis' studies (Nicolaidis et al., 2008, 2010, 2011) saw depression, intimate partner violence, and physical problems as being interrelated, with depression leading to physical problems over time.

Psychological

Under the psychological manifestation of depression, many DSM related symptoms, such as sadness and crying, were revealed by participants (Howe, 2009; Jones, 2010). Shame was more common than the symptom of guilt listed in the DSM, and encapsulated experiences, such as worthlessness, feeling like a bad person, unlovability, inadequacy, incompetence, lack of value, and self-blame (Ashby, 2014; Cassidy, 2007). Being "different" from others was also described, and was seen, at least in Cassidy (2007), as being related to the isolation that was also common (reported in "Social"). One participant reported: "Depression is isolating and I think that heightens the feeling different. Or the feeling different heightens the isolation" (Cassidy, 2007, p. 82).

Other psychological experiences of depression involved feeling overwhelmed (Ashby, 2014; Poleshuck et al., 2013; Schneider, 1991) and anger and irritability (Ashby, 2014; Jones, 2010; Poleshuck et al., 2013; Schneider, 1991). One woman said: "I snap. I get up and I just I just snap…" (Poleshuck et al., 2013, p. 8).

Women also reported a sense of loss of control. One participant stated: "Yeah, it's out of my control, and it is very frustrating. I mean, I've done everything I can do about it, and I've tried and tried and tried" (Jones, 2010, p. 11). Another pointed out: "I think that's part of the problem as far as emotionally because I never, no matter how hard I try, it never feels like I get everything under control" (Hodge, 1994, p. 136).

Worsening some of the psychological reaction was the stigma women faced. Being thought "crazy," "weak," or "flawed" were mentioned (Ashby, 2014). One participant in Moreta (2007) said: "No, I didn't accept it [her diagnosis], because … a lot of people have the same impression that I did, that I thought that is for crazy people, it is for people in institutions, and who are really weak" (p. 90).

Social

As well as biological and psychological aspects, there was also a social component to the experience of depression. Many people spoke of loneliness, isolation, and social withdrawal (Ashby, 2014; Cassidy, 2007; Hodge, 1994; Jones, 2010; Poleshuck et al. 2013; Steen, 1991), difficulty forming intimate relationships (Schneider, 1991), and lack of support (Hodge, 1994). One woman described: "I had nobody. It was a really isolating feeling" (Jones, 2010, p. 50). Another said: "I always wanted to be alone, I didn't want to be around people, I didn't want to talk to anybody, and I felt very lonely" (Moreta, 2007, p. 67). Atanmo-Strempek (2014) spoke about feeling isolated from the church they attended due to depression. Participants in Jack (1984) talked about either feeling isolation or being subordinate in marriage and losing the self. The choice seemed to be between being lonely and being passive.

Under the social aspect were also the reactions that other people had to depression in women and the negative stigma they experienced. In Lazear, Pires, Isaacs, Chaulk, and Huang (2008), a participant stated: "When I told my mother that I thought I had depression, she said, 'Oh, you're so weak. I had three kids and I walked to the river to carry water the day after birth.' Everybody just dismissed my feelings" (p. 131). In Waite and Killian (2008), women thought that friends and family would disapprove of them if they knew that they had depression: "It's hard because many people look down on you when you say you have a mental problem. Not many people know about my depression and I am keeping it that way" (p. 191). Webster (2005) further discussed that the stigma of having depression caused friends to distance themselves. One participant stated: "[Depression is] really difficult to deal with. Family, friends, you kind of don't know where you stand anymore.... I've had situations where people purposely pull back from me because I've been going through such a hard time" (p. 134).

Attributions given for depression

As well as the suffering of depression and negative stigma, another major theme was the attributions or explanations women gave to make meaning of their depression. Although a variety of reasons were put forward, for many of the women studied, depression was perceived as having emerged from some type of event or life situation, such as a difficult family background, trauma, illness, poverty, or interpersonal issues (Jack, 1984). Violence – both in childhood and adulthood – was a common theme in studies (Caplan and Whittemore, 2013; Clarke and Amerom, 2008; Nicolaidis et al., 2010; Schneider, 1991; Waite and Killian, 2009). One woman described:

> I couldn't leave my room; I totally withdrew from everything. That was the only time [after a rape] in my life I ever felt what you might say is suicidal-like. I just didn't want to go on because I just didn't feel like there was anything left.
>
> (Hodge, 1994, p. 141)

In general, women didn't see depression as arising from individual factors, such as genetics or some flaw within them, but instead, as resulting from stressful relationships, events, or life circumstances.

Coping with depression

Another major theme involved how women coped with depression. A multitude of possible coping methods were mentioned, some potentially harmful, such as substance abuse (Ashby, 2014; Poleshuck et al., 2013), and some that could be considered beneficial, such as informal support. Among the myriad activities indicated, the only type of coping that coalesced into its own category involved spiritual or religious coping (Ashby, 2014; Atanmo-Strempek. 2014; Cassidy, 2007; Howe, 2009; Waite and Killian, 2008; Weathersby, 2008). Faith, prayer, reading the Bible, mindfulness, and belief in God, although not attendance at religious institutions per se, were named as a way to gain strength and hope. In an all-Latina sample, many participants thought that faith and prayer were more effective than psychotherapy (Caplan and Whittemore, 2013). In Perez (2013), a woman described: "I'm a Christian and I believe that there is hope and that this trial and tribulation that I may be going through will come to an end" (p. 56). Soto (2011) also had participant quotes representative of these views: "I would have become crazy or I wouldn't have moved forward if it wasn't for the faith that I have in God" (p. 75) and "In my depression, I kept thinking and thinking … but when I cried out to God he was there and I felt it, I could feel the strength in my life" (p. 80). Notably, when mentioned, religious leaders were not viewed as a source of help (Atanmo-Srempek, 2014; Caplan and Whittemore, 2013).

Treatment

Treatment was a major theme and within it were subthemes: psychotherapy; medication; and barriers to treatment.

Psychotherapy

In most studies that mentioned psychotherapy, the experience was seen as positive with the following benefits: the fostering of hope; accurate information about depression (Marsach Wood, 2008); the development of insight; the creation of change; and a sense of safety and acceptance (Caplan and Whittemore, 2013). Therapists validated women's experiences, as one participant indicated: "To have somebody that is like really focusing on them and making them feel like they are the only person that matters in that moment, it definitely helps" (Marsach Wood, 2008, p. 54). There was also mention of a preference for psychotherapy over medication (Clarke and Amerom, 2008) since that gave them coping skills to deal with life circumstances (Marsach-Wood, 2008).

However, the experience of psychotherapy was not uniformly positive (Caplan and Whittemore, 2013). For instance, in Webster (2005), all women reported learning things from therapy, but over time the benefits dissipated. Similarly, in Hodge (1994) most women who had tried therapy briefly did not continue. One participant reported: "I felt like counseling didn't help because … they sat there and tried to tell me what my problem was" (p. 141). Poleshuck et al.'s (2013) African-American sample of women also thought that therapists could be dismissive of client preferences: "I didn't like nobody like telling me what … I need to do and what's wrong for me and what's right for me.… So that's why I never kept going."

In Poleshuck et al.'s (2013) study, some of the complaints about therapy was that it left them too exposed and vulnerable, especially weighed against the inability of such treatment to change past or current life circumstances. Participants also expressed distaste at being left vulnerable to abandonment when their providers, who were often interns or trainees, left the agency for other opportunities.

Medication

Other participants discussed the use of medication as an aspect of their experience of coping with depression. Medication was seen as potentially helpful in allowing women to feel better and to do what needed to be done. As one woman described: "So there is a feeling [with medications] that I can cope, and optimism. I can get up in the morning and I don't dread the day" (Webster, 2005, p. 146).

In general, there was more dissatisfaction expressed about the use of medication. Concerns about side effects were named (Nicolaidis et al., 2008, 2010, 2011), especially weight gain (Moreta, 2007). For instance, a participant explained:

> The medications made me gain weight. And now I have complications from being heavy, it's awful. I just have complications medically that I wouldn't have if I hadn't gained weight, and it certainly doesn't make me feel good about myself.
>
> (Moreta, 2007, p. 137)

Participants also expressed concerns about lack of information of how medication worked, whether they were on the right medication, and how long they were supposed to be on it (Lazear et al., 2008). As one woman stated: "My primary care physician didn't have any answers" (Marsach-Wood, 2008, p. 80). The African-American participants in Poleshuck et al. (2013) also disliked pressure to take medication when that was not their preference.

In Waite and Killian (2009), women only took medication as a last resort and discontinued it when they felt better. As one participant stated: "Medication can work, but I don't think they really tell you what that stuff does to your body. I don't want to be dependent on any drugs to be able to live my life" (p. 329). Concerns about dependency and addiction were also named as reasons that people would not take medication, described in the following section.

Barriers to treatment

One umbrella topic that emerged was what acted to prevent women from seeking services. Like the theme of coping strategies, there was a multitude of reasons given, such as fear of personal concerns being dismissed, worry about becoming dependent on medication, lack of family support, the vegetative symptoms of depression or other mental health symptoms, such as anxiety, precluding their getting to treatment, and lack of transportation. In Poleshuck et al. (2013), some of the reasons had to do with what participants experienced as negative interactions in the past, described earlier.

Negative stigma acted to prevent other women from accessing services (Lazear et al., 2008; Moreta, 2007):

> Maybe, you know, it is because of the time that I grew up, there was still this thing of crazy people go to a psychiatrist, and normal people should just be able to pull themselves up, you know. And, you shouldn't need to go to see a therapist and you shouldn't need to take medication.
>
> (Moreta, 2007, p. 89)

This negative stigma was also seen in Lazear et al. (2008) in which women felt as if they would be labeled "crazy" if they sought professional help. As one participant described:

> I cried secretly because I didn't want to seem like I was crazy. I asked my mother and mother-in law, but they just kept saying, "Be strong. We've had so many children and we're fine. So you'll get over it."
>
> (p. 131)

In studies with women who were of ethnic minority, reasons had to do with discrimination in terms of perceived attitudes or treatments from providers (Lazear et al., 2008; Nicolaidis et al., 2010). In the African-American sample studied in Nicolaidis and colleagues, there was mistrust of healthcare as a "white" system. One participant stated: "If somebody that's White come in with the same case, they're 'Oh, what's the matter?'... Where I have a question or a concern ... they could care less" (Nicolaidis et al., 2010, p. 1472). In a sample of women who had breast cancer and depression, most women were not offered mental health services or asked about their mental health status (Weathersby, 2008). As one participant stated: "I don't think people look at Black people and think about mental health" (p. 130).

In general, concrete reasons, such as affordability, availability of services, and lack of transportation and childcare, were not named as barriers. Instead, people suffered from negative stigma and experiences with treatment and the meaning it had for women. They also were turned off services because of perceived discrimination and bias against them by service providers.

Discussion and implications for practice

In this section, major findings of the meta-synthesis are described, along with their practice implications. In their narratives, women described considerable suffering associated with depression. They elaborated on some of the DSM-defined symptoms of depression, such as problems with sleep, fatigue, and feelings of sadness, but participants also went beyond these symptoms to discuss other significant symptoms – anger and irritability, feeling overwhelmed and isolated, with a loss of control. Participants also talked about shame, which went beyond the guilt that is cited as a symptom in the DSM. This shame encapsulated experiences such as feeling like a bad person, weakness, unlovability, inadequacy, incompetence, lack of value (Ashby, 2014), and self-blame (Cassidy, 2007). Being "different" from others was also described, and can be viewed as related to the sense of shame that these women felt, that they were not like other people. Given such feelings, the isolation that resulted was common, and descriptions were much more poignant than the symptom of social withdrawal listed in the DSM. Women faced a profound sense of disconnection and loneliness.

One practice implication from this finding is to listen for – and ask about – these various aspects to the experience of depression. Although the diagnosis is constrained by DSM (in the US) and ICD criteria, women's (and possibly also men's) experience is richer and more nuanced than the criteria would allow for. Providing validation of and normalizing these various experiences would help women feel understood and accepted, an important benefit of psychotherapy named in this study.

Although the literature on depression has discussed the tendency of older adults to describe depression in physical terms (Fiske et al., 2009), and the tendency of people from ethnic minority groups to experience mental health problems in somatic ways (Kirmayer and Young, 1998), in the meta-synthesis this was a more widespread phenomenon. The interrelationship between depression and physical conditions seems to imply that medical practitioners should be screening for depression in women that they see. For example, in Poleshuck et al. (2013), women did not describe themselves as "depressed," even though they screened in the clinical range of a standardized depression measure.

As well as describing the anguish of depression and this negative stigma, women attributed the external context as reasons for their depression. The literature has hypothesized as a possible reason for higher rates of depression among women that they are more vulnerable to certain stressful life events (Girgus and Nolen-Hoeksema, 2006; Le et al., 2003), and this seemed to be borne out in the meta-synthesis. In this cross-section of studies, environmental events, especially trauma, were often given as reasons for depression, An implication is that treating trauma and its aftermath would be important for helping women with such histories and depression.

Further, interpersonal therapy, in particular might be an approach that women with depression find amenable given the fact that they have often suffered from abuse, loss, and abandonment in their relationships (Weissman et al., 2000). Interpersonal therapy is a relatively brief psychodynamic intervention (approximately 12 sessions) focusing on how interpersonal problems have contributed to depression. Intervention focuses on significant role transitions, grief processes, and interpersonal disputes or deficits.

Attribution theory posits that one's belief that problems are due to qualities internal to the self, stable over time, and globally consistent across situations tend to be related to psychological problems, such as depression (Seligman et al., 1988). In their study, Lebowitz et al. (2013) found that people who attributed their depression to genetic reasons caused people to feel more pessimistic about recovery. Aside from a one-off mention, women did not talk about internal causes of depression, such as genetics. Although attribution theory would suggest that women may feel more hopeful as a result, the fact that the trauma had often occurred in childhood and had sometimes repeated itself in adulthood and that women continued to face other environmental stressors, such as poverty and interpersonal problems, seems to indicate that the theory might not hold up for these women. The sense of being overwhelmed and out of control might have resulted from facing these chronic life circumstances.

Although women in the meta-synthesis tried to use various coping strategies, there was no consistency to these except for spiritual beliefs and practices. This is a unique finding to emerge from this qualitative research. Providers can sensitively explore women's belief systems and practices in order to find out whether a spiritual connection can be part of an approach to manage depression. There has also been a new movement within the therapeutic field to use mindfulness as an adjunctive to cognitive-behavioral approaches for depression, and studies have indicated the effectiveness of mindfulness-based cognitive-behavioral therapy in preventing depression relapse (Piet and Hougaard, 2011). Women with a spiritual bent, particularly, may find this approach compatible and helpful, although other spiritual practices, particularly prayer, were named as beneficial.

Finally, practitioners should pay special attention to the participant women's views of treatment. Many women found talk therapy to be helpful; however, there were also dissatisfactions named. The perception that there was discrimination against clients of color was a concern that arose in the meta-synthesis. It is critically important that any overt or covert discrimination or bias be uncovered and addressed so that people receive equality of services.

Other agency barriers also need to be addressed. The finding in Poleshuck et al. (2013) that women felt abandoned and distrustful of further services when interns or trainees left means that vulnerable and impoverished clients should not always be assigned to those in training because of their lack of inability to pay. Clear parameters around the length of the relationship and the trainee's role in the agency need to be set at the start of services, and a co-counseling role with a permanent staff member is preferred.

Although a basic tenant of counseling is non-judgemental support and acceptance, women sometimes seemed to feel as though their preferences were disregarded. A solution-focused approach might be helpful in this regard. Solution-focused therapy has, as its main premise, that clients' preferences and goals determine the course of treatment. Clients' strengths and resources are activated in service of these goals (de Jong and Berg, 2012). Solution-focused therapy also emphasizes that clinicians should routinely ask how clients cope with difficulties, such as depression. This technique serves several purposes: it reinforces client resources, gives credit to clients for being active problem-solvers in their own lives, and it also gives the implicit message that clients are the experts in what is helpful to them.

Medication was often used; however, again there concerns about lack of information and side effects. Although medical providers should make more efforts to provide education, mental health and social service providers that are not able to prescribe can also provide education and information, explore and process concerns about medication, and act as an advocate and broker to those that do prescribe medication.

Table 8.1 Methodological features of studies and findings from studies of women with depression

Author and purpose	*Methodology, method, and analysis*	*Sampling*	*Findings*
Ashby (2014) "To develop a grounded theory that explains the process that women experience as they move through depression and recovery" (p. 37).	Grounded theory with constructivist research paradigm. Semi-structured interviews; 30 interviews from 18 participants: some asked to do second follow-up interview. Open coding, then axial coding, then selective coding.	*N* = 18. Purposive sampling with 5 criteria: 1 women experienced depression between ages 18 and 80; 2 living in Salt Lake County; 3 told by healthcare providers they had depression; 4 self-identified as recovered or in recovery; 5 willing to share their experience and spoke English. Theoretical sampling used to continue research. Recruited through social media, printed flyers, and word of mouth. Demographics: Most women in twenties and thirties. 15 white, 2 Hispanic, 1 black. Most college or graduate degree. 10 single, 6 in relationship, 2 divorced. 10 Mormon, 3 other Christian, 5 spiritual.	*Reported depression triggers* • Biological: chemical imbalance, family history, and hormonal disruptions. • Environmental: childhood abuse, sexual trauma, parents' divorce, death of a loved one, caregiving, and relationship issues. • Stressful life events: medical issues, faith crises, and work or school demands. • Feelings of shame: high expectations of self and/or others; dismissal of thoughts, emotions, needs by others. *Reported effects of depression* • Physical health: appetite, sleeping, energy, physical pain. • Emotional health: "dark, stressed, anxious, overwhelmed, angry, defeated, out of control." • Social health: isolated and withdrawn from others; felt very alone; few friends and social anxiety. • Spiritual health: disconnected from spiritual source of strength. *Reported coping mechanisms* • Numbing: disordered eating, substance abuse, sleep, self-injury, shopping, and sex. • Controlling perception of self and others' perception of self. • Reaching out to others: used by a few but usually not the first coping mechanism tried.

			Turning points for deciding to seek help
			• Exhibiting behaviors inconsistent with values and personality.
			• Reaching an emotional breaking point.
			• Encouragement from family and friends.
			Receiving a diagnosis
			• Empowered by being able to label what they were experiencing as a disease.
			• Discouraged because diagnosis suggested they were weak or flawed.
			Reported treatment experiences
			• Methods used: family/friends support, therapy, medication, self-help, changing environment, exercise and diet.
			• Barriers to recovery:
			  • limited understanding of depression;
			  • lack of empathy and support from others;
			  • women attempted to control emotions.

Atanmo-Strempek (2014) To explore "the lived experiences of African American women who are active churchgoers and the relationship among religiosity and depression" (p. 12).	Holistic case study approach. Demographic questionnaire, Beck Depression Inventory-II, and semi-structured interviews. Themes analysis and coding.	*N* = 6. Purposive sampling. Women ages 18–65 years who self-identify as African American and attend church 3–5 times a month. Recruited from 4 churches in urban area of northeastern US. Varying levels of age and education. 2 employed, 4 unemployed. 2 single, 2 married, 1 separated, 1 widowed.	*Experience of symptoms* • Isolated from others in church: withdrawal from activities and participation. • Lack of support for feelings of being judged and mistrusted by church. • Experienced anger, isolation, sadness, insomnia, emotional hurt/pain, becoming withdrawn, and losing interest in previously enjoyed activities. • Rejection: social isolation, being ignored, abandonment, denied assistance, excluded, and shunned. *Ways they cope* • Christian religious beliefs including reading Bible and prayer. • Church provided sense of hope.

continued

Table 8.1 Continued

Author and purpose	*Methodology, method, and analysis*	*Sampling*	*Findings*
Besson (2012) To examine experiences of African American females receiving psychotherapy from white clinicians. Ensuring cultural sensitivity within treatment of depression in 12-week intervention program.	Transcendental/psychological phenomenological approach with mixed-method concurrent-nested design. Semi-structured interview. Phenomenological data analysis.	$N = 6$. Purposive sampling. Black women between 25 and 55 years experiencing depression.	1 Preconceptions of the group and facilitators. 2 Critical incident. 3 Process of healing. 4 Therapeutic qualities of facilitators. 5 Cultural differences not a barrier to connecting to facilitators. 6 Therapeutic gains.
Caplan and Whittemore (2013) "To explore barriers to treatment engagement, and to examine how childhood adversity and gender-based violence (GBV) contribute to lack of perceived support for treatment engagement" (p. 412).	"Qualitative descriptive methodology" (p. 412). Individual interviews. Code themes into categories created by content analysis.	$N = 12$ Latina females. "The sample was part of a larger study ($N = 67$) that examined the efficacy of a diabetes prevention program provided by visiting nurses to adults at-risk for type 2 diabetes who were living in a subsidized housing community (Whittemore, Rosenberg, & Jeon, 2013)" (p. 413). Convenience sample. Participants were eligible for this sub-study if they scored above the criterion score of 16 on the Center for Epidemiologic Studies Depressive Scale (CES-D; Radloff, 1977) at one of the data collection points.	Gender-based violence and childhood adversity, most had exposure in childhood and adulthood to abuse (traumatic experiences). Strength and self-reliance (handling it on their own). Some people found psychotherapy helpful but about half did not. For some participants, faith in God and prayer were seen as more effective than therapy in treating depression. Non-disclosure about abuse and lack of engagement with service providers for it was seen as carrying over to depression treatment as well. Religious leaders or formal institutional religion were not viewed as a source of help. Negative experiences with therapists. One-third of participants would not seek help due to fears about medication (being drugged, being addictive, therapists who relied upon medication).

Cassidy (2007) To better understand the relationship between sociocultural factors and sexual orientation in the etiology of depression: "two questions that guided my inquiry (a) 'How do lesbians experience and manage depression?' and (b) 'What is the role of marginalization in lesbians' experiences with, and management of, depression?'" (p. 75).	Thematic analysis. Semi-structured interviews and demographic handouts. Thematic and coding data analysis.	$N = 20$. Self-identified lesbians who self-reported at least one depressive episode. Purposive sampling Flyers posted in "lesbian friendly" bookstores and cafes, and on social media.	Sociocultural context of difference. The myth of control. (Re)positioning difference. Locating my self as different. Identifying my difference. Trying to manage. Normalizing. Distracting myself. Escaping my pain. Making my pain real. Conclusion. Recognizing the need for change. Working with my difference. Looking for help. (Re)locating the problem. Working through stuff. Making connections. Having epiphanies. Addressing the problem. Renaming it. Framing it. Managing it. Critical awareness. (Re)locating (my) difference. Creating a supportive environment. Attending to life. Looking out for what I need. Contextualizing my experiences. Taking what's mine and letting go of the rest.

continued

Table 8.1 Continued

Author and purpose	*Methodology, method, and analysis*	*Sampling*	*Findings*
Clarke and Amerom (2008) To compare internet blogs of men and women who self identify as depressed.	Qualitative content analysis. Anonymous self-reported blogs. Selective coding for data analysis.	*N* = 90. 45 women, 45 men. Quota sample. Participants self identify as depressed, and describe their experiences relating to depression in their blogs.	Women are more likely to discuss psychotherapy and self help in depression blogs. Acceptance of bio-medicalization of depression: • women are more skeptical of treatment providers and formal diagnoses, citing doctor's ties to pharmaceutical companies and physician qualifications. Women are more likely to seek alternative treatment options and feel disempowered by lack of treatment options. Causes of depression: • women associated depression with problems with interpersonal relationships. Women believed an abnormal childhood and family experiences to be the root cause of depression. Violence: • Women infrequently discussed violence in their blogs. If they did, it was limited to self-harm behaviors. Suicidal thoughts were not a major theme for women.

Hodge (1994) To explore the causes of the 2:1 ratio of females to males with depression and the reasons women are depressed.	Ethnomethodology informed by feminist theory. Inductive and exploratory unstructured interviews. Inductive data analysis.	$N = 7$. Young adult women.	Violence. Self image. School demands. Lack of support from parents. Obligations. Overcoming paralysis. Putting up a façade. Physical symptoms. Lack of control. Isolation. Relationships. Therapy.
Howe (2009) To examine perceptions of relationship between social support and depression among African American women living with systemic lupus erythematosus (SLE) and to explore relationship among depression, social support, and frequency and intensity of SLE flares.	Grounded theory. Semi-structured interviews.	$N = 10$. Purposive sample of African American women 30–50 years old with lupus and mild–severe depression via the Beck Depression Inventory – from two support groups in a large city.	1 Challenges of living with SLE and depression. 2 Coping strategies for managing SLE and depression. 3 Perception of social support.

continued

Table 8.1 Continued

Author and purpose	*Methodology, method, and analysis*	*Sampling*	*Findings*
Jack (1984) To examine women's personal experiences of depression, and the cognitive schemas that guide a woman's thinking about "self and self-evaluation, care, her roles of wife and mother, and her future options" (p. 8). Also, to examine how a woman's understanding of self, morality, and social role contributes to the dynamics of depression.	2-year longitudinal, exploratory study. Oral, intensive, and semi-structured interviews with a descriptive approach. Data analysis occurred on a descriptive and theoretical level, based on Bowlby's theory of attachment and Gilligan's theories of self and morality. Themes emerged from data in grounded theory.	$N = 13$. Purposive sampling (referral based, researcher strategically picked referral sources). Age range 19–55 years. Socioeconomic status ranged from poverty (on welfare) to upper class. 9 of women have children, only 1 woman was not married when first interviewed. 4 depressed female patients randomly selected by Whatcom County Counseling and Psychiatric Clinic; 5 women selected from local fundamentalist churches (Christian Reformed Church); 4 pregnant women referred by two obstetricians.	1 Women describe their relationships as the "cause" of their depression (inhibited communication, financial dependence, and emotional coldness). 2 Self-evaluation is guided by thought processes of how one "should" care for others (Gilligan's morality of care). 3 Women experience loss of self. 4 Sees future as either subordination in marriage or isolation because of loss of "authentic self." 5 Active appearance of passiveness and submissiveness in relationship. 6 Changing women's understanding of care and role, and their relationships, coincides with less depressive symptoms.

Jones (2010) To explore lived experience of depression in female collegiate athletes.	Phenomenology. In-depth, unstructured interviews. Analyzed using phenomenological research methods to generate a thematic analysis.	$N = 10$. Purposive sampling. Participants recruited through local, San Jose, CA, US Division I collegiate athletic programs. Criteria for inclusion in study were: a being current or former female collegiate athlete; and b self-identifying as having experienced depression.	Revealed one ground (role of sport) and four general categories: • weariness; • self-doubt; • feeling out of control; • nowhere to go.
Lazear et al. (2008) To describe experiences of women with depression and young children living in low-income communities who are ethnically and culturally diverse.	Qualitative ethnographic. Focus groups.	$N = 138$ women. 15 focus groups. Average age 30 years. Number of children of each participant ranged between 1 and 10, average age child, 6 years. Only half of participants opted to answer questions about marital status: 75% of women reported being married.	*Social risk factors* • Domestic violence. • Isolation. • Language barriers. • Difficulties with schools and public systems. • Lack of access to high quality and culturally competent mental health and medical services. *Reliance on informal systems of care to deal with depression* • Friends. • Family. • Peers. *Women did not seek services from mental health providers* • Lack of insurance. • Stigma. • Cultural beliefs. • Attitudes of providers,

continued

Table 8.1 Continued

Author and purpose	*Methodology, method, and analysis*	*Sampling*	*Findings*
Marsach-Wood (2008) To explore rate at which guideline concordant care for depression combining psychotherapy and psychopharmacology as recommended treatment is occurring. Also, personal experiences of women seeking depression in primary care settings was explored.	Mixed method concurrent triangulation design research study including qualitative and quantitative methods. Semi-structured questionnaire and select in-depth interviews. Qualitative data analysis through identifying interrelated conceptual thematic material.	*N* = 40 overall; *N* = 10 in-depth interviews. Selection: based on their availability in response to advertisements requesting participants. Women age 18 to 65 years with primary care doctor treating depression in several PA townships.	1 Symptoms that brought them to treatment. 2 Physician interaction and expectations. 3 Expectations satisfied. 4 Prescribed an SSRI. 5 Prescribed psychotherapy. 6 Stressful life events. 7 Feelings about efficacy and success rate of medications alone. 8 Feelings about success rate of combined treatment. 9 Suggestions for study and for improving primary care services.
Moreta (2007) To better understand personal experiences which lead women to seek treatment for depression relatively soon after their symptoms begin.	Grounded theory. Semi-structured interviews. Data analysis with open coding.	*N* = 9. Purposive sampling based on advertisement respondents who met inclusion criteria. All respondents were residents of Brooklyn, NY.	Stressors leading to seeking treatment: • affective, cognitive, and physical symptoms; • gaining awareness; • relationships; • uninformed decision making.

Nicolaidis et al. (2008) Nicolaidis et al. (2010) Nicolaidis, Perez et al. (2011) To explore different groups of women's "beliefs, attitudes, and recommendations regarding depression and depression care, with a special focus on the impact of gender, ethnicity, violence, and social stressors" (Nicolaidis, Perez et al., 2011, p. 1131).	Grounded theory. Community-based participatory research approach. Focus groups formed from 3 different populations of interest: general English-speaking, African American, and Latina. Thematic analysis using an inductive approach at a semantic level, with an essentialist paradigm.	*General English speaking sample* N = 23. Iterative recruitment approach. Women recruited through survey from internal medicine clinic; English-speaking only. 22 white, 1 Native American. Older than other eligible non-participants. *Latina sample* N = 31. Recruited by word of mouth and flyers. Women had to be 18+ years and consider themselves Latina/Hispanic, speak Spanish, score 15 or higher on PHQ-9, and have history of intimate partner violence (IPV). Most women early middle-aged, low income, less than high school education; over half unemployed *African American sample* N = 30. Women had to be 18+ years and consider themselves African American, speak English, score 15 or higher on PHQ-9, and have history of IPV.	Life stressors affecting well-being: • childhood sexual abuse; • emotional, physical, and sexual abuse from partners; • difficult relationships with family; • poverty; • immigration status. Depression as result of keeping things hidden inside: • inability to talk; • led to physical illnesses. Themes around depression care: • needed to be heard to be able to heal; • felt they couldn't talk to health care professionals because their experiences wouldn't be validated; • desire for health information; • wanted depression treatment that addressed real life needs; • negative attitudes towards antidepressants, mainly due to side effects; • negative experiences with healthcare attributed to lack of insurance or class issues; • need for health professionals to know about their current and past abuse history to effectively treat their health needs; • trust and desire for respect major factors women wanted in providers; • intergenerational messages to avoid health care; • mistrust of health care system as a "white" system and negative experiences attributed to racism;

continued

Table 8.1 Continued

Author and purpose	*Methodology, method, and analysis*	*Sampling*	*Findings*
		Most low income, mixed education levels, almost half without insurance and unemployed.	• in therapy/counseling, wanted staff that were same gender and race as themselves. Comorbidity of depression with other issues: • physical symptoms, mental health, substance abuse, and IPV all interrelated and cannot be considered separately.
Perez (2013) To study use of "hope" as factor in studying women recovering from major depression.	Phenomenological guided by Streubert's method. Open-ended interviews. Interviews coded for themes.	$N = 11$. Purposive sampling was used to recruit from Mood Disorders support group of NYC and Maimonedes Community Mental Health Center Outpatient Department of Brooklyn, NY. Women recruited were of varied ethnic/racial and religious backgrounds, ages 24–37 years.	Hope: Self, spiritual, interpersonal connections. Belief in a better future. Vital life energy. Fostered in caring connections. Diminished in distress. Apprehending essential relationships.

Pietiers and Heilemann (2010) To explore perspectives of 12 Latina women seeking to enter therapy for depression.	Grounded theory. Individual, in-depth structured interview. Constructionist grounded theory techniques used to analyze data.	$N = 12$. Participants recruited via flyers. Latina women eligible for low-income services. Average age 29 years. Born or lived in US prior to age 18.	Put needs of others before their own. Feeling time limited: not enough time to deal with problems. Positive motivators: • urgency; • inspiration to be better parent; • desire for better life; • internal motivations; • supportive peers; • flexible therapy appointments. Painful motivators: • feeling alone and can't manage the burden of depression; • symptoms of depression; • realizing they don't like the person they are becoming while depressed; • break-ups with partners; • old coping strategies no longer effective; • previously unfulfilling therapeutic encounters.

continued

Table 8.1 Continued

Author and purpose	*Methodology, method, and analysis*	*Sampling*	*Findings*
Poleshuck et al. (2013) To better understand the barriers that low-income and African American women face with regards to delivery of mental health treatment. Interested in "determining what factors regarding their experiences of symptoms associated with depression and uptake of psychotherapy were most relevant for women's health clinic patients specifically" (p. 2).	Thematic content analysis approach utilizing a group consensus process. PHQ-2 questions (Kroenke, Spitzer, & Williams, 2001; Spitzer, Kroenke, & Williams, 2000) to identify women currently experiencing symptoms of depression and to evaluate perspectives about psychotherapy (p. 2).	N = 23. Age 18–49 years. Median age 32.87 years. African American or black 60.9%, Caucasian or white 30.4%, Latina or Hispanic 4.3%, other 4.3%. Annual income reported as less than $10,000 by 65.2%, as between $10,000 and $19,000 by 21.7%, as greater than $19,000 by 8.6%. Random Sampling screened with the PHQ-2 (Kroenke, Spitzer, & Williams, 2001; Spitzer, Kroenke, & Williams, 2000) (p. 2). Women attending routine gynecological appointments for care at a university hospital-based health clinic for insured patients (p. 2).	Did not generally describe as "depression" (and denied it), even though had elevated depression scores. Were more likely to describe their symptoms as social withdrawal, being overwhelmed, suffering from physical symptoms, and anger/irritability. Some women coped by means of: • socializing; • music; • drugs. Negative therapy experiences: Therapy felt invasive and too personal without being viewed as having accompanying benefit ("it won't change anything"). Felt too vulnerable in therapy to therapists who might betray, cause harm, or abandon them (high turnover among clinicians), dismissive of client preferences. Despite these risks, did see benefits to therapy: • feel sense of safety and acceptance; • develop insight. Attitudes toward medication were similar to experiences of therapy – didn't want to be pushed into taking medication when it didn't seem like right course of action. Negative attitudes toward providers based on prior experiences with therapy.

			Didn't see a benefit (didn't change anything, didn't help them feel better). Symptoms of the depression (vegetation) and other mental health problems (fear of using public transportation, substance abuse).
Polusny (2000) "To explore the lived experiences of clinical depression for women in the context of their social relations and environment" (p. 292). In hope of better understanding these lived experiences to help prevent childhood abuse and racism, provide relief from economic hardships, encourage early diagnosis, and provide safe and effective treatment. "Second purpose was to share this experience with public health nurses (PHNs) who are in a position to alleviate the social and environmental conditions that perpetuate excess morbidity from depression in women" (p. 293).	Phenomenological method, grounded theory, utilizing Spiegelberg's synthetic analysis (1971). Intensive, depth interviews conducted in environment that was comfortable to participant (home, nearby restaurant, work cafeteria). Interviews focused on women's mental health history and significant relationship history. Interviews tape-recorded and transcribed using ethnography data management (p. 294). Imaginative variation was used to evaluate each cluster of themes for its essential necessity in relation to each case.	Convenience sampling. *N* = 24 (12 dyadic). Diverse population. Flyer distributed to 3 outpatient mental health clinics in central urban areas in large midwestern city. Age 25–44 years; criteria, diagnosed with clinical depression. Mostly white, working class people with traditional lifestyles, conservative politics. Majority of participants were single, and earned less than $20,000 per year. Each volunteer nominated a close friend to participate in study as well (snowball sampling). 5 friends were depressed at time of study or had experienced it in past, 7 friends had no history of clinical depression.	All participants reported having experienced depression in some form. Participants who were depressed or had experienced depression would quit school, change jobs, or withdraw from social contact in attempt to control moods. Failures at controlling their moods towards happiness would result in self-medication through drugs, alcohol, or suicide. Non-depressed women perceived sadness as controllable. Sadness was not perceived by these women as a character flaw or deserving of punishment. Did not understand why their depressed friends couldn't just "do something" about their problems (p. 296). *Themes* • withdrawal from social contact; • dissonance in social relations and environment; • felt stigmatized; • lack of financial resources; • decision to seek care was a turning point; • lack of financial resources; • feelings of isolation; • connectedness; • harmony; • sexual violence; • feelings of sadness.

continued

Table 8.1 Continued

Author and purpose	*Methodology, method, and analysis*	*Sampling*	*Findings*
Schneider (1991) "To supplement external-perspective descriptions offered by standard psychopathologies of women's experiences with depression, by taking a feminist perspective and analyzing common themes" (Abstract).	Emancipatory research, semi-structured individual and group interviews that were transcribed, chronological narrative. Used three validity criteria from John Kotre (1984).	$N = 4$. Convenience sampling of women who had been diagnosed with Major Depression or Dysthymic Disorder within two years prior to study, and been treated in an inpatient psychiatric unit of community hospital or at community mental health center in small midwestern town (strong Appalachian influence). Women were between ages of 25 and 65, and white.	"All participants reported some degree of emotional, physical, and sexual abuse" (Abstract). Low self-esteem, a need to maintain control, lack of perceived safety, and difficulty forming intimate relationships. Breaking isolation of depression was seen as most healing of their experiences. Anger, out of control (helplessness), problems with marriage, unmet needs (security, trust recognition), low self-esteem, history of abuse, and need for control.
Soto (2011) To explore Latina women's use of religion and spirituality in coping with depression and whether their religious and spiritual beliefs and practices were incorporated into psychotherapy.	Phenomenological. Open-ended interviews.	$N = 8$. Convenience sample of Latina women diagnosed with depression who were native to US or born outside of mainland US in Spanish-speaking country, recruited in Massachusetts through clinics via word of mouth or flyers. All were residents of Latin origin, not Spain or Brazil.	Spiritual responses to life challenging events. Role of faith in responding to life challenges. Feeling strengthened by God. Moments of doubting one's faith or doubting in God. Religious and spiritual beliefs and practices in coping with life challenges. Religious beliefs in coping with emotional suffering. Religious practices in coping with emotional challenges.

			Interpretation of visions and premonitions. Incorporating religion and spirituality into psychotherapy. Who initiated discussion of religion and spirituality. Participants reported that spiritual activities and beliefs help them cope with both life events that caused depression and depression itself.
Steen (1991) To describe structure and meaning of experience of recovering from clinical depression for middle-aged white women in two midwestern states.	Descriptive, exploratory study (natural inquiry research). Phenomenological method, unstructured, in-depth, audio-tape recordings of personal interviews (open-ended questions); at least hree interviews conducted with each participant. Data analysis: using Spiegelberg's (1976) 8-step protocol.	$N = 22$. Purposive sampling. All the women had been clinically depressed and were in recovery stage based on their scores for Beck Inventory. White women, between the ages of 40 of 55, high school educated, born in US, had been treated for clinical unipolar depression within last 5 years. Recruiting informants: Self-referral by way of advertisement published in variety of organization's newsletters in Austin, Texas and Kansas City, Missouri. (Some informants referred by psychiatric nurse therapists who were aware of study.)	1 Existential alienation/pain (aloneness, abuse, damaged self-esteem). 2 Crises of adulthood (feelings and coping). 3 First turning point (making connections and treatment experiences). 4 Second turning point (becoming an agent and becoming a succorer). 5 Becoming a gardener (cultivating the self).

continued

Table 8.1 Continued

Author and purpose	*Methodology, method, and analysis*	*Sampling*	*Findings*
Waite and Killian (2008) To explore health beliefs of African American women and depression to improve insight into treatment decisions. Waite and Killian (2009) "To better understand how a cohort of low-income African American women from a nurse-managed health care center viewed depression" (p. 325).	Kleinman's explanatory model of illness. Focus group interviews. Constructs of Health Belief Model used to analyze data.	$N = 14$ women. Purposive sample recruited from community nurse managed health center. African American women with diagnosis of depression. Average age 45.	Women believed they weren't susceptible to depression. Women didn't recognize severity of depression till it significantly interfered with daily functioning. Women acknowledged depression requires treatment. Treatment type correlated with perceived severity of depression. Barriers to treatment: • mistrust of medical professionals; • denial of depression; • limited knowledge regarding etiology of depression; • stigma associated with depression; • lack of financial resources for treatment. Women were prompted to seek treatment by physical symptoms or external reminders like media coverage of depression. Cause of depression: • traumatic events: childhood molestation, rape and violence; • stressful life circumstances: lack of income or lack of resources to meet needs of children; • poor health; • style of coping: how they coped with stress; • chemical imbalance.

			Symptoms: • detachment: disconnected from self and others; • ill ease: not feeling well, feeling weary; • weakness: affected every aspect of self. Cure and control of depression: • women unsure if it could be cured, just controlled; • individual focus on managing it. Treatment: • therapy and medication not seen as viable first step; • effective treatment: prayer, exercise, yoga, meditation; • medication only taken as last resort and discontinued as soon as woman felt better; • treatment only effective if women took active part in caring for themselves; • needed faith: connection and belief in a higher power.
Weathersby (2008) To understand social psychological and social structural processes of African American women with breast cancer experiencing depressive symptoms.	Grounded theory. Unstructured interviews. Data analysis using constant comparison method.	$N = 9$. Purposeful sampling. Then theoretical sampling of African American women with breast cancer experiencing self-defined depressive symptoms currently or in the past, age 40 years or older, recruited by word of mouth, breast cancer support groups, and African American churches.	Transcending the now: • relying on faith; • being strong; • seeking support; • dealing with life too; • enduring breast cancer.

continued

Table 8.1 Continued

Author and purpose	*Methodology, method, and analysis*	*Sampling*	*Findings*
Webster (2005) To explore what women learn about coping from major depression and other difficult life challenges.	Qualitative. Two in-depth, cross-sectional interviews. Modified narrative analysis; initial coding and focused coding.	*N* = 15. Combination of convenience and snowball sampling used to select women between ages of 30 and 50 years who had experienced major depression at some point in their lives. 87% white, 7% black, 7% Asian American.	Coping skills: • close relationships; • work/school; • physical health; • spirituality; • mastery; • therapy. Barriers: • substance abuse; • lack of resources; • conflictual relationships.

References

Beck, A. T., Rush, A. J. Shaw, B. F., and Emery, G. (1979). *Cognitive therapy of depression*. New York: Guilford.

Bolen, R. M., and Scannapieco, M. (1999). Prevalence of child sexual abuse: A corrective metanalysis. *Social Service Review*, *73*(3), 281–313.

Bronfenbrenner, U. (1995) Developmental ecology through space and time: A future perspective. In P. Moen, G. H. Elder, and K. Luscher (Eds.), *Examining lives in context.* Washington, D.C.: American Psychological Association.

Corcoran, J., Brown, E., Davis, M., Pineda, M., Kadolph, J., and Bell, H. (2013). Depression in older adults: A meta-synthesis. *Journal of Gerontological Social Work*, *56*, 509–534.

Craighead, W. E., Sheets, E. S., Brosse, A. L., and Ilardi, S. S. (2007). Psychosocial treatments for major depressive disorder. In P. E. Nathan, and J. M. Gorman (Eds.), *A guide to treatments that work* (3rd edn.). New York: Oxford University Press.

Cuijpers, P., Geraedts, A., Van Oppen, P., Andersson, G., Markowitz, J., and Van Straten, A. (2011). Interpersonal psychotherapy for depression: A meta-analysis. *The American Journal of Psychiatry*, *168*(6), 581–592.

De Jong, P., and Berg, I. K. (2012). *Interviewing for solutions* (4th edn.). Boston, MA: Brooks Cole.

Desai, H. D., and Jann, M. W. (2000). Major depression in women: A review of the literature. *Journal of the American Pharmaceutical Association* [Washington, D.C.: 1996], *40*(4), 525–537. Retrieved from http://search.ebscohost.com.proxy.library.vcu.edu/login.aspx?direct=true&AuthType=ip,url,cookie,uid&db=fyh&AN=MED-10932463&site=ehost-live&scope=site.

Finlayson, K. W., and Dixon, A. (2008). Qualitative meta-synthesis: A guide for the novice. *Nurse Researcher*, *15*(2), 59–71.

Fiske, A., Wetherell, J. L., and Gatz, M. (2009). Depression in older adults. *Annual Review of Clinical Psychology*, *5*, 363–389.

Girgus, J. S., and Nolen-Hoeksema, S. (2006). Cognition and depression. In C. L. M. Keyes and S. H. Goodman (Eds.), *Women and depression: A handbook for the social, behavioral, and biomedical sciences* (pp. 147–175). New York: Cambridge University Press. doi:10.1017/CBO9780511841262.009.

Kessler, R. C., Chiu, W. T., Demler, O., and Walters, E. E. (2005). Prevalence, severity, and comorbidity of twelve-month DSM-IV disorders in the National Comorbidity Survey Replication (NCS-R). *Archives of General Psychiatry*, *62*(6), 617–627.

Kirmayer, L. J., and Young, A. (1998). Culture and somatization: Clinical, epidemiological, and ethnographic perspectives. *Psychosomatic Medicine*, *6*, 420–430.

Le, H., Muñoz, R. F., Ippen, C. G., and Stoddard, J. L. (2003). Treatment is not enough: We must prevent major depression in women. *Prevention and Treatment*, *6*(1) (no pagination). doi: http://dx.doi.org.proxy.library.vcu.edu/10.1037/1522-3736.6.1.610a.

Lebowitz, M., Ahn, W. K., and Nolen-Hoeksema, S. (2013). Fixable or fate? Perceptions of the biology of depression. *Journal of Consulting and Clinical Psychology*, *81*, 518–527.

Meade, M. O., and Richardson, W. S. (1997). Selecting and appraising studies for a systematic review. *Annals of Internal Medicine*, *127*, 531–537.

Noblit, G. W., and Hare, R. D. (1988). *Meta-ethnography: Synthesizing qualitative studies*. Newbury Park, CA: Sage Publications.

Nolen-Hoeksema, S., and Harrell, Z. A. (2002). Rumination, depression, and alcohol use: Tests of gender differences. *Journal of Cognitive Psychotherapy*, *16*(4), 391–403. doi:10.1891/jcop.16.4.391.52526.

Piccinelli, M., and Wilkinson, G. (2000). Gender differences in depression: Critical review. *British Journal of Psychiatry, 177*, 486–492.

Piet, J., and Hougaard, E. (2011). The effect of mindfulness-based cognitive therapy for prevention of relapse in recurrent major depressive disorder: A systematic review and meta-analysis. *Clinical Psychology Review, 31*, 1032–1040.

Richards, D. (2011). Prevalence and clinical course of depression: A review. *Clinical Psychology Review, 31*(7), 1117–1125.

Seligman, M. E. P., Castellan, C., Cacciola, J., Schulman, P., Luborsky, L., Ollove, M., et al. (1988). Explanatory style change during cognitive therapy for unipolar depression. *Journal of Abnormal Psychology*, 97(1), 13–18.

Üstün, T. B., Ayuso-Mateos, J. L., Chatterji, S., Mathers, C., and Murray, C. J. L. (2004). Global burden of depressive disorders in the year 2000. *British Journal of Psychiatry, 184*(5), 386–392.

Weissman, M., Markowitz, J., and Klerman, G. (2000). *Comprehensive guide to interpersonal psychotherapy*. New York: Basic Books.

Included studies

Ashby, S. (2014). *A grounded theory analysis on depression and recovery among women* (Order No. 3643841). Available from ProQuest Dissertations and Theses Global. Retrieved from http://search.proquest.com.proxy.library.vcu.edu/docview/1634512743?accountid=14780.

Atanmo-Strempek, D. (2014). *No longer silent: African american women speaking up on depressive symptoms and religion* (Order No. 3671051). Available from ProQuest Dissertations and Theses Global. Retrieved from http://search.proquest.com.proxy.library.vcu.edu/docview/1645957177?accountid=1780.

Besson, D. D. (2012). *Therapy experiences of depressed black women receiving culturally sensitive treatment delivered by white clinicians: A phenomenological study* (Order No. 3524232). Available from ProQuest Dissertations and Theses Global. Retrieved from http://search.proquest.com.proxy.library.vcu.edu/docview/1071045039?accountid=14780.

Caplan, S., and Whittemore, R. (2013). Barriers to treatment engagement for depression among Latinas. *Issues in Mental Health Nursing*, 34(6), 412–424.

Cassidy, R. L. (2007). *(Re)positioning difference: Lesbians' management of depression* (Order No. 3266954). Available from ProQuest Dissertations and Theses Global. Retrieved from http://search.proquest.com.proxy.library.vcu.edu/docview/304731575?accountid=14780.

Clarke, J., and van Amerom, G. (2008). A comparison of blogs by depressed men and women. *Issues In Mental Health Nursing*, 29(3), 243–264.

Hodge, D. M. (1994). *Young adult women and the social construction of depression: A qualitative study* (Order No. 9420966). Available from ProQuest Dissertations and Theses Global. Retrieved from http://search.proquest.com.proxy.library.vcu.edu/docview/304128764?accountid=14780.

Howe, M. G. (2009). *The effect of social support on depression in African American women diagnosed with systemic lupus erythematosus* (Order No. 3377912). Available from ProQuest Dissertations and Theses Global. Retrieved from http://search.proquest.com.proxy.library.vcu.edu/docview/305152883?accountid=14780.

Jack, D. C. (1984). *Clinical depression in women: Cognitive schemas of self, care, and relationships in a longitudinal study (inequality, marriage, communication)* (Order No. 8421187). Available from ProQuest Dissertations and Theses Global. Retrieved from http://search.proquest.com.proxy.library.vcu.edu/docview/303302763?accountid=14780.

Jones, A. L. (2010). *Phenomenological examination of depression in female collegiate athletes* (Order No. 1482540). Available from ProQuest Dissertations and Theses Global. Retrieved from http://search.proquest.com.proxy.library.vcu.edu/docview/762368795?accountid=14780.

Lazear, K. J., Pires, S. A., Isaacs, M. R., Chaulk, P., and Huang, L. (2008). Depression among low-income women of color: Qualitative findings from cross-cultural focus groups. *Journal of Immigrant and Minority Health, 10*(2), 127–133.

Marsach-Wood, R. (2008). *Exploring women's depression and the relationship of SSRI's and counseling as recommended treatments* (Order No. 3341605). Available from ProQuest Dissertations and Theses Global. Retrieved from http://search.proquest.com.proxy.library.vcu.edu/docview/275691682?accountid=14780.

Moreta, F. (2007). *The initial help seeking experiences of women with depression* (Order No. 1449042). Available from ProQuest Dissertations and Theses Global. Retrieved from http://search.proquest.com.proxy.library.vcu.edu/docview/304807582?accountid=14780.

Nicolaidis, C., Gregg, J., Galian, H., McFarland, B., Curry, M., and Gerrity, M. (2008). "You always end up feeling like you're some hypochondriac": Intimate partner violence survivors' experiences addressing depression and pain. *Journal of General Internal Medicine, 23*(8), 1157–1163.

Nicolaidis, C., Timmons, V., Thomas, M. J., Waters, A. S., Wahab, S., Mejia, A., et al. (2010). "You don't go tell white people nothing": African American women's perspectives on the influence of violence and race on depression and depression care. *American Journal of Public Health, 100*(8), 1470–1476.

Nicolaidis, C., Perez, M., Mejia, A., Alvarado, A., Celaya-Alston, R., Galian, H., et al. (2011). "Keeping things inside": Latina violence survivors' perceptions of depression. *Society of General Internal Medicine, 26*(10), 1131–1137.

Perez, L. (2013). *The lived experience of hope in women recovering from major depression* (Order No. 3574442). Available from ProQuest Dissertations and Theses Global. Retrieved from http://search.proquest.com.proxy.library.vcu.edu/docview/1448794755?accountid=14780.

Pieters, H. C., and Heilemann, M. V. (2010). "I can't do it on my own": Motivation to enter therapy for depression among low income, second generation Latinas. *Issues in Mental Health Nursing, 31*(4), 279–287. http://doi.org/10.3109/01612840903308549.

Poleshuck, E., Cerrito, L., Leshoure, B., Finocan-Kaag, N., and Kearney, G. (2013). Underserved women in a women's health clinic describe their experiences of depressive symptoms and why they have low uptake of psychotherapy. *Community Mental Health Journal*, 49(1), 50–60.

Poslusny, S. (2000). Street music or the blues? The lived experience and social environment of depression. *Public Health Nursing, 17*(4), 292–299.

Schneider, C. K. (1991). *Etiology and phenomonology of depression in women: An ethnographic approach* (Order No. 9200964). Available from ProQuest Dissertations and Theses Global. Retrieved from http://search.proquest.com.proxy.library.vcu.edu/docview/303979657?accountid=14780.

Soto, G. L. (2011). *The role of religion and spirituality for Latina women coping with depression* (Order No. 3509767). Available from ProQuest Dissertations and Theses Global. Retrieved from http://search.proquest.com.proxy.library.vcu.edu/docview/1020133328?accountid=14780.

Steen, M. J. (1991). *The essential structure and meaning of recovery from clinical depression for middle-adult, white, high school educated, employed, women in the United States in the late 1980's: A phenomenological study* (Order No. 9128365). Available from ProQuest

Dissertations and Theses Global. Retrieved from http://search.proquest.com.proxy.library.vcu.edu/docview/303950141?accountid=14780.

Waite, R., and Killian, P. (2008). Health beliefs about depression among African American women. *Perspectives in Psychiatric Care*, *44*(3), 185–195.

Waite, R., and Killian, P. (2009). Perspectives about depression: Explanatory models among African-American women. *Archives of Psychiatric Nursing*, *23*(4), 323–333.

Weathersby, J. H. (2008). *Transcending the now: A grounded theory study of depressive symptoms in African American women with breast cancer* (Order No. 3336636). Available from ProQuest Dissertations and Theses Global. Retrieved from http://search.proquest.com.proxy.library.vcu.edu/docview/304685223?accountid=14780.

Webster, D. W. (2005). *What women aged 30–50 who have received inpatient care for major depression reported learning from their experience about coping with life's difficulties and challenges* (Order No. 3186547). Available from ProQuest Dissertations and Theses Global. Retrieved from http://search.proquest.com.proxy.library.vcu.edu/docview/305027707?accountid=14780.

Part III

Disorders in older adults

9 The lived experience of adults with intellectual disabilities

Health, sexuality, and aging

Matthew Bogenschutz and Jacqueline Corcoran

People with intellectual and developmental disabilities (IDD) have seen many advances in how their supports are provided since the 1960s, when the move toward community services began. Along with this transition, a number of pressing questions have emerged, including how to meet the often complex healthcare needs of people with disabilities in the community, how to support responsible sexual activity, and how to plan for the needs of people with IDD in older age. While a growing body of research has emerged on these topics in recent years, the voices of people with IDD and their caregivers have seldom been represented. This chapter honors their voices by providing meta-syntheses of qualitative research about the health, sexuality, and aging of adults with IDD.

Context and current literature

Community living movement

Examination of our current knowledge of health, sexuality, and aging of people with IDD should be prefaced with an understanding of the trend toward community living that has been ongoing for people with IDD since the 1960s. The way in which people with IDD live has changed dramatically in the past five decades, and the community living movement has increasingly directed the structure of services and supports. One of the primary shifts is in where people with IDD live. Prior to the beginning of the community living movement, people with IDD who did not live with family mainly lived in large institutions, which have slowly phased out over time. In fact, recent estimates suggest that the vast majority of people with IDD who do not live with family now live in individualized settings (own or lease their own home, or in group homes with six people or less), while the proportion of people living in nursing facilities or institutions with seven or more people has steadily declined (Larson et al., 2014). These trends from the United States are generally mirrored in other developed countries, such as Australia, the United Kingdom, Ireland, Sweden, and the Netherlands, all of which have contributed significantly to our understanding of community living and supports for people with IDD.

In the United States, community inclusion of people with IDD is strongly supported by policy, which has been vital in pushing states toward more community options for people with disabilities. The Americans with Disabilities Act of 1990 (as amended; ADA) set the tone for the shift to community living, as the Act affirmed the right of people with IDD and other disabilities to have access to employment, housing, and education without discrimination based on their disability. The Olmstead Decision (Olmstead vs. LC and EW. 527 U.S. 581. 1999) stipulated that people with IDD and other disabilities should receive supports in the "most integrated setting" possible, effectively providing legal footing upon which to enforce elements of the ADA, the Americans with Disabilities Education Act, and other legislative acts. Taken together, these legal acts have set the tone for ongoing improvements in the American disability services system, which aim to support people with IDD in all areas of community life, including health, sexual expression, and aging with a disability.

Current literature

Though this chapter will present meta-syntheses of qualitative studies, the emergent literature on the health, sexuality, and aging of people with IDD also contains a variety of quantitative and theoretical studies that are important for situating an understanding of the qualitative findings to be presented later in this chapter. This section will briefly outline major quantitative findings to assist readers to gain a general overview of the current state of knowledge in the areas of focus.

Health and healthcare

Access to healthcare and health outcomes for people with IDD have been hot topics in the professional literature for the past decade. While the scope of information on this topic is quite large, it can broadly be broken down to concerns about healthcare access and disparities in health outcomes.

In terms of access to quality healthcare, a large-scale meta-analysis of 64 studies found that people with IDD had far worse access to preventative healthcare services, such as routine health screenings and immunizations, than the members of the general population (Larson et al., 2005). Individuals with disabilities also have fewer health maintenance visits for known health conditions than would be expected in the general population (Fisher, 2004). In their wide-ranging meta-analysis, Krahn et al. (2006) found a "cascade of disparities" related to the health status of people with IDD. Inattention to health needs by direct support workers, disparities in preventative health service utilization and a lack of health promotion activities were all among the disparities noted in this work. Such difficulties in access likely play a role in poor health outcomes for individuals with IDD.

A lack of general knowledge about the health system and how to access services may hinder quality medical care among people with IDD and their family supporters, especially among members of cultural minority groups (Choi and Wynne, 2000). Additionally, research has indicated major shortages of general practitioners and medical specialists who are adequately trained on disability-related issues (Iacono et al., 2003; Ward et al., 2010).

Poor health outcomes were noted by Fisher (2004), who found deficiencies in dental care and women's health outcomes in her meta-analysis of nursing literature. Specific health-related disparities have been noted in overall nutrition (Humphries et al., 2009), obesity (Melville et al., 2007), coronary heart disease (Sohler et al., 2009), and diabetes (McVilly et al., 2014), among a multitude of other conditions.

Intimacy and sexuality

Much attention has also turned to the sexuality of individuals with IDD in recent years, focusing both on understanding the sexual knowledge and engagement of individuals with IDD and on ethical issues regarding consent, rights, and exploitation.

Feelings of love have been found to be similar among people with and without IDD (Arias, Ovejero, and Morentin, 2009), and love is often accompanied by desire for physical intimacy. Healy et al. (2009) found that people with IDD are generally knowledgeable about sexual anatomy and pregnancy, although this finding has been challenged in other studies (Cheng and Udry, 2002; Galea et al., 2004) which suggests major gaps in sexual knowledge.

Despite sexual interest on the part of many people with IDD, many barriers to their participation in sexual relationships exist. For instance, family members tend to have restrictive attitudes about the sexual participation of their sons and daughters with IDD (Cuskelly and Bryde, 2004; Healy et al., 2009). In fact, parents of people with IDD had more conservative attitudes about the sexuality of their children with IDD than did paid support staff or members of the general community (Cuskelly and Bryde, 2004). In fact, 80 percent of parents of children with IDD in an Irish sample preferred low levels of physical intimacy for their adult children (Evans et al., 2009). Abbott and Howarth (2007) found that low levels of support were given for same-sex intimate relationships among people with IDD by parents, paid support workers, and community members alike.

Ethical debates about the capacity of some people with IDD to give sexual consent (Curtice et al., 2012; McGuire and Bayley, 2011) have given rise to efforts to enhance sexual decision making and delivery of sex education. For instance, Dukes and McGuire (2009), in an Irish study, saw notable improvement in both sexual knowledge and safety-oriented decision making among their small sample of adults with IDD who participated in an individually administered training program on sexuality. In a similar study in Japan, Hayashi, Arakida, and Ohashi (2011) found that their social skill-based sex education program for people with IDD yielded significant effects in increased social skills related to sexuality.

Aging

Life expectancy for people with disabilities has improved markedly in recent decades across many different disability groups (Coppus, 2013), with the most recent overall estimate putting the average lifespan of an individual with IDD at 66.1 years (Janicki et al., 1999). The effects of aging among adults with IDD depend, to some degree on the type of disability in question, as people with Down syndrome, for example, are particularly prone to cataracts and hearing loss, while musculoskeletal decline appears especially common among people with cerebral palsy (Perkins and Moran, 2010). Haverman and colleagues (2010), in their international review of literature on health of older adults with IDD, found that health conditions associated with aging largely corresponded to health problems in the general aging population, although increased prevalence of obesity and other risk factors may relate to earlier onset of chronic health conditions among people with IDD.

In addition to the health risks of older age, recent studies have also looked at social inclusion for older adults with IDD. In one small-scale study in Australia, 62 percent of older people with IDD did not have anybody outside the service system who checked up on them regularly, and patterns of social interaction did not change after relocation from an institutional setting to a community residence (Bigby, 2008). McCausland and colleagues (2009) found the inability to independently manage one's finances and inactivity to be among the top concerns among a sample of individuals with IDD aged 50 and over. People with IDD generally lack awareness of the ways in which their lives, activity levels, and health might change as they age (Innes, McCabe, and Watchman, 2012).

Attention has also been placed on future planning for people with IDD in recent years, as parents and other aging caregivers often want to put plans in place for continuity of support once they are no longer able to provide it, a factor that is strong in a meta-analysis by Innes et al. (2012). Future planning has been found useful in helping families to think about alternate living arrangements, sibling roles in supports for people with IDD, and developing financial trusts to help with future expenses (Heller and Caldwell, 2006). Younger families tend to indicate a greater desire for assistance with futures planning than do older families, perhaps because older families tended to be farther along in their planning already (Hewitt et al., 2010). Siblings, who often take on primary caregiving duties after parents are no longer able to do so, report ongoing difficulties with navigating the disability service system and planning for the future (Burke et al., 2015).

Findings of meta-syntheses

Health and healthcare

A total of 14 studies were identified, accounting for the perspectives of 310 participants in total. Studies were conducted in the United States, the United

Kingdom, the Netherlands, and Taiwan, representing a strong diversity of lived experiences of people with IDD, their caregivers, direct support staff, and health service providers. A synopsis of the methodology of the selected articles may be found in Table 9.1.

While the studies covered a wide range of health-related topics, the meta-synthesis found that three recurrent themes emerged: (1) perceptions and knowledge of conditions; (2) quality of care; and (3) barriers to healthcare. Each of these central themes will be explored below, and is presented in Table 9.2.

Perception and knowledge of conditions

This theme concentrated specifically on the ways in which people with IDD and their supporters perceived and expressed knowledge about health conditions they encountered. For people with IDD who spoke on their own behalf, there was often a good deal of confusion present. Two studies about diabetes illustrated this point (Cardol et al., 2012; Dysch et al., 2012). Regarding diabetes management, Cardol and colleagues (2012) found frustration among individuals with IDD when they could not eat some of their favorite foods, while Dysch and colleagues suggested that some people with IDD lacked insight about the chronic nature of diabetes, as illustrated by a participant who said: "I'm not sure if I'm going to having this for the rest of my life" (Dysch et al., 2012, p. 4). Such insights may suggest that additional information sharing about health conditions may be necessary, and should be appropriately focused to the learning level of people with IDD.

When family members served as study subjects, they were often understanding of the fact that people with IDD had healthcare needs similar to those of people of the same age without disabilities. However, in some instances caregivers expressed paternalistic opinions about engaging in healthcare, especially when it concerned sexual health. For instance, negative perceptions emerged around breast and cervical cancer screenings, with one parent stating that such procedures were not necessary if the person with IDD was not sexually active or "doesn't wanted to be touched in that area" (Swaine et al., 2013, p. 7). Similarly, the two Taiwanese articles included in this meta-synthesis addressed the ethics of sterilization of people with IDD (which remains a legal option in Taiwan though it has been banned in many countries), to show how cultural considerations contribute to perspectives about healthcare options for people with IDD and their families.

Quality of care

The theme of quality of care explored some of the markers of quality health services that were identified by participants. Several studies concentrated on the relationship between physicians and people with IDD. For instance, Swaine and colleagues noted that prior preparation of women with IDD to increase familiarity with the process improved the implementation of cervical screening, based on parental perspectives. Likewise, women with IDD self-reported positive overall attitudes toward preventative mammography, especially when personnel were supportive, though a general feeling of nervousness about the procedure was summed up by one participant with IDD who stated: "Oh, if you see the machine it's very big oooh! It's a big brute of a thing, oh my God" (Truesdale-Kennedy et al., 2010, p. 1299). Participants noted that up-front information about the process could help to reduce the anxiety induced when confronting imposing medical equipment.

Another aspect of quality involved the notion of care standards for people with IDD being the same as they would be for people without a disability. People with IDD noted that communication was important, and that a physician should communicate with them directly, not to direct support workers, as noted by one of the study participants who expressed the frustration that "my doctor did not talk to me, but to my support worker" (Wullink et al., 2009). For their part, physicians in one study suggested that they are concerned about being able to communicate effectively with people with IDD in order to accurately assess, diagnose, and prescribe (Ziviani et al., 2004).

Among parents of immigrants and refugees with disabilities, Bogenschutz (2014) found that caregiver's perceptions of quality focused on cultural and linguistic competence, and placed particularly high priority on interpreters who had special training on disability-related language. Additionally, service integration, especially for allied health services, was particularly important, as illustrated in this translated statement from a Mexican immigrant mother: "There is special education in school, and a therapist, psychologist; he has various things like speech help. And all of that is within the school" (Bogenschutz, 2014, p. S68).

Barriers to healthcare

Barriers to healthcare was the final theme identified in the meta-synthesis, and was among the most prevalent themes. Transition from pediatric care to the adult healthcare system was a barrier identified by Pickler et al. (2011), as medical personnel tended to treat a person with IDD based on their assumed developmental age rather than their chronological age, and because finding a physician with experience treating people with IDD was difficult. Instances such as this led some people with IDD to feel that they are discriminated against within the health system (Ali et al., 2013).

Communication difficulties were often identified as barriers (e.g. Ali et al., 2013; Bogenschutz, 2014; Wullink et al., 2009; Ziviani et al., 2004). Difficulties with accessing linguistically appropriate information was identified by Bogenschutz (2014), while Ali and colleagues (2013, p. e70855) noted that even when practitioners and patients with IDD were language concordant, the language was not easy to understand for some people, as elucidated by one of their participants in the following quote: "They just said that I had to sign something … it was like a consent form. They gave me a little booklet beforehand but it wasn't like an easy read one."

Involving individuals with IDD as members of the care team informing their own healthcare was also identified as a subtheme. For instance, in their study on how people with IDD experience hospitals, Gibbs et al. (2008) suggested that they do not feel a part of the process of healthcare provision when physicians do not take account of their perspectives, as summarized by one of their focus group participants who said: "I feel better if they would give me more time to explain things, they done all the talking they wrote all the drawings on your file and all that they didn't sort of explain things properly" (p. 1066). Additionally, patronizing attitudes and approaches to people with IDD were noted by direct support workers in a study about inclusive primary care in Scotland (Jones et al., 2008), perhaps suggesting that people with IDD are not always taken seriously in healthcare settings, especially in the absence of a family member or paid support worker.

Sexuality

The meta-synthesis on sexuality among people with IDD included 10 articles that included the views of 186 participants. Participants were mainly people with IDD with some paid direct support workers also represented. Participants identified as both male and female, expressed multiple sexual orientations, and represented an age range between 16 and 69. Studies we conducted in the United States, the United Kingdom, Sweden, Australia, South Africa, and China. Several different methodologies were used, as summarized in Table 9.3. Three main themes emerged from the meta-synthesis: (1) relationships; (2) sexual encounters; and (3) barriers to sexual expression. These are summarized in Table 9.4.

Relationships

Many people with IDD who were represented in the studies informing this synthesis wanted relationships, often with other people with IDD. Lofgren-Martenson (2004) reported that people with IDD expressed a desire for love and partnership, and often attended social events in hopes of connecting with a partner. Though same-sex relationships are common, few individuals who identified as gay or lesbian spoke of a long-term relationship (Stoffelen et al., 2013). Some degree of physical intimacy was an expected element of relationships among people with IDD, as exemplified by this quote from a participant in one of the studies:

> I felt closer to William than I did, than I did to Ben ... because he used to, he used, he used to put his two arms around me ... instead of just one it was two ... It made me feel more secure.
>
> (Sullivan et al., 2013, p. 3462)

Although relationships were highly sought by many people with IDD who informed these studies, many also noted the potential pitfalls of relationships.

Difficulties finding private time and space was noted as a difficulty that impeded the formation of emotional intimacy for some people with IDD (McClelland et al., 2012; Sullivan et al., 2013). Internationally, sexuality of women with IDD was often ignored by parents and direct support workers in Taiwan (Chou and Lou, 2007) and in Australia (Wilson et al., 2013), while a South African study by Phasha and Nyokangi (2012) suggested that women with IDD may be at high risk of sexual mistreatment.

Sexual expression

Qualitative research has also shown that adults with IDD wish to engage in physical expression of intimacy. For example, one study suggested that individuals with IDD express intimacy in many different ways, but physical intimacy is often in the form of hugging or kissing (Lofren-Martenson, 2004). Others (McClelland et al., 2012; Wilson et al., 2013) indicated that among people with IDD, masturbation was a common form of sexual expression, but that people with IDD, especially women, often received pressure not to do so from direct support workers or parents. Nevertheless, Bernert (2010) found that women with IDD generally felt competent to engage in adult activity, in which an important element was the right to make one's own choices about engagement in sexual activity in ways that are satisfying to each individual, sentiments echoed by Yau and colleagues (2009) in the Chinese-Australian context.

Many studies focused attention on the knowledge that individuals with IDD had about safer sex practices and sexual health. McCarthy (2009) found that women with IDD had very limited knowledge of basic reproduction or of contraception, and that none of the women in her study had been provided with accessible information about contraception choices, suggesting that medical professionals may not consider the sexual health needs of women with IDD. Likewise, knowledge about HIV was poor among a sample of gay and lesbian individuals with IDD in the Netherlands, and only five of the 18 male participants reported regular use of condoms for HIV prevention (Stoffelen et al., 2013).

Barriers to relationships and sexuality

Among all of the main themes identified in this meta-synthesis on disability and sexuality, barriers to free sexual expression were certainly the most salient, appearing prominently in nine of the 13 studies included. Often, barriers involved restricted rights to engage sexually due to the policies of group homes. Bernert (2010) found that most women in her study experienced limitations on their sexual expression and autonomy, mainly because of protective policies and programs that sought high degrees of protection of potentially vulnerable women, without balances for safe sexual activity. Men also had their right to sexuality restricted at times, as suggested by McClelland and colleagues, whose informants told them that others (parents or direct support workers) often had control over their ability to sexual activity, including both interpersonal intimacy and masturbation. In McClelland's study, participants tended to prefer sex in their own homes. However, restrictions often led them to engage in sex elsewhere, even though participants knew it was risky to do so, as summarized by one individual who said: "At my house at least you know that you have condoms" (McClelland et al., 2012, p. 815).

Restrictive attitudes toward the sexuality of adults with IDD also came from participants' parents. One study mentioned that fear of punishment by one's parents served as a deterrent to sex, as summarized by a lesbian-identified study informant who said: "I said to my mother, um, I'm going to invite her to stay at my house and she turned around and said well if you're going to do that don't come back to the house" (Sullivan et al., 2013, p. 69). Another study (Stoffelen et al., 2013) noted that parents of people with IDD prefer not to discuss issues of sexuality with their adult children, even when the individual with IDD wants to get accurate sexual information.

It is also worth mentioning that the lack of knowledge noted in the above section on sexual expression certainly qualifies as a barrier as well. Without adequate knowledge of safer sex practices, pregnancy, preventative health, and sexually transmitted infections, people with IDD cannot be expected to express their sexuality with optimal responsibility. This apparent lack of knowledge about sexuality among people with IDD led Swango-Wilson (2010) to suggest a sex education training program for people with IDD that included development of relationships in general, development of lasting relationships in particular, and safe intimacy.

Aging and future planning

The final meta-synthesis was about aging with IDD. This synthesis included 12 studies involving 448 participants in total. Findings from studies conducted in the United States, United Kingdom, Canada, Australia, Ireland, and Belgium were included. Again, three main themes emerged from the analysis: (1) the need for autonomy; (2) making community connections; and (3) issues related to being a caregiver for an aging adult with IDD, and the associated future planning to assume continuity of caregiving after the death of a parent. It is worth noting that many of the studies in this section elicited perspectives of parents or other caregivers, not people with IDD directly, and that much discussion focused on future planning for people with IDD as they age, not simply the experiences of older adults. A brief overview of each study's methods may be viewed in Table 9.5, and a thematic summary is present in Table 9.6.

Autonomy

Many aging adults with IDD and their caregivers focused on the importance of autonomy in the studies informing this meta-synthesis. The right to self-determination, always a major theme in IDD literature and practice, was highlighted strongly by Hole et al. (2013), whose participants shared frustration about limited choice making opportunities afforded to their children with IDD regarding where to live as they aged. Bekkema et al. (2014) found that familiarizing people with IDD about upcoming life transitions, and providing new knowledge about changing support needs and important decisions assisted older adults with IDD to understand and participate in planning for their future supports. In an Australian study, Bigby and Knox (2009) concluded that adults with IDD felt that others often made choices for them, and that decisions were focused on services, rather than their individual support needs as they aged.

Hole and colleagues (2013) noted that many people with IDD had fears about their futures once their family members died, and what this would mean for their choices, autonomy, and lifestyle. These sentiments are summarized by one of their participants in this quote:

> My mom died of a heart attack.... It was hard for me to take.... I didn't have any choice [I had to move] ... so I found it was too far for me.... It was just terrible.
>
> (p. 576)

Community connections

Finding meaningful ways to connect with the community is a challenge for people with IDD of all ages, but especially so for older adults. Hole and colleagues (2013) found that opportunities for meaningful social activity were more important to older individuals with IDD than were work or educational activities. Likewise, participants in another study (Taggart et al., 2012) suggested that community support is a protective factor against other life challenges, underscoring the centrality of connectedness in healthy aging.

In some studies, both people with IDD and their caregivers suggested concern about support options available to individuals with disabilities to help them participate in their communities (Taggart et al., 2012; Weeks et al., 2009); other studies have found innovative solutions. In one recent example, Wilson, Bigby, and colleagues (2013) reported on their efforts in Australia to link retirees without disabilities to individuals with IDD who were beginning the transition into retirement. This Transition to Retirement program was successful in building understanding and friendship between older adults with and without disabilities, as exemplified in this quote from one of the study's participants without a disability: "It's amazing to see a person in this kind of situation, how well she adjusted and I think it's great, we enjoyed having her ... I hope she stays with us for a very long time" (Wilson et al., 2013, p. 349).

Caregiving and future planning

The perspectives of aging caregivers on the futures of their children with IDD, and the future planning that is often associated with such transitions is also a prevalent theme in the recent literature. Planning for continuing supports for a person with IDD after parents are no longer able to do so was seen as essential by many parents who participated in qualitative studies that informed this synthesis (Hole et al., 2013; Taggart et al., 2012; Weeks et al., 2009). However, only a small number of participants indicated that they had begun any type of future planning (Shaw et al., 2011; Young, 2005), though many aspired to do so (Taggart et al., 2012).

The fact that many families want to engage in future planning for their sons and daughters, but that so few of them actually do, suggests that many barriers to such planning are in place. This meta-synthesis of qualitative studies indicates that these barriers are both personal and structural. Personally, many caregivers felt challenged in doing future planning because it was difficult to consider their own mortality, and what might happen to their adult child with IDD after their passing (Bigby and Knox, 2009; Taggart et al., 2012). Bekkema and colleagues (2014) suggested that challenges exist when eliciting the support preferences of people with severe IDD, reinforcing the importance of planning alongside caregivers when they are "healthier and better able to communicate" (p. 377). For their part, people with IDD also think about what may happen to them when their parents are no longer able to provide daily support, sometimes ruminating on their own mortality when thinking about their parents' potential passing (Todd and Read, 2010). The concerns of people with IDD regarding their future living situations are well-summarized by a participant in Shaw et al.'s study (2011, p. 899), who said: "I would like to live with my friends one day but not right now. My dad is old. If anything happens to dad, mum will be by herself."

Structural barriers also play a role in reducing participation in futures planning. Costly planning processes (Weeks et al., 2009), service waitlists, and a general lack of confidence in the paid supports system (Hole et al., 2013) all served as barriers to parents who were thinking about how to structure supports for their adult children in the future. After leaving home, adults with IDD often felt there was little continuity of care between their parent's caregiving approach and the methods used by paid support workers who helped them live in the community (Bigby, 1997).

Discussion

Summary of main findings

The findings from this series of meta-syntheses portray important facets of community living from the perspectives of people with disabilities, their families, and their paid direct support workers. When viewed from the perspective of the advance of community living, these syntheses suggest many positive advances. In each of the meta-syntheses above, people with IDD were able to take part in community life: seeking health services from typical community clinics, pursuing relationships and sexual intimacy, and aging in the community. While it is positive that people with IDD are beginning to have such experiences, these syntheses, consistent with other published research findings, also illustrate the depth of challenge that people with IDD face when living in community settings.

Each of this chapter's meta-syntheses identified barriers as a key component. In line with findings from previous meta-analyses (Krahn et al., 2006; Larson et al., 2005), this study identified inequitable access to health services a salient factor in the healthcare of people with IDD, findings that were reinforced by the work of Ali and colleagues (2013) and Gibbs and colleagues (2008), who pointed out that feelings of discrimination and exclusion for health-related decision making promoted mistrust between people with IDD and their health providers. Likewise, barriers to sexual expression were often expressed by participants in the studies informing this analysis (McClelland et al., 2012; Sullivan et al., 2013), just as in Cuskelly and Bryde's (2004) quantitative work, which identified restrictive attitudes about sexuality from parents and direct support staff to be influential in restraining sexual intimacy among people with IDD. While barriers to full community participation were also noted in the aging-related studies in this synthesis, promising practices were also apparent, particularly in the work of Wilson, Bigby, and colleagues (2013), who thoughtfully sought ways to integrate aging adults with and without disabilities in social activities. It is this sort of intervention that can help to overcome barriers to create a much more true sense of social inclusion for people with IDD.

The final theme overarching all three qualitative meta-syntheses in this chapter was that of support needs. While the need for competent, person-centered support is present in much of the extant literature (e.g. Choi and Wynne, 2000; Dukes and McGuire, 2009; Innes et al., 2012; Ward et al., 2010), the meta-syntheses often punctuated the point that progress in independent living cannot be made when supports are inadequate. This synthesis indicated gaps in educating, training, and supporting people with IDD that posed serious challenges to their ability to adequately participate in their own healthcare (Dysch et al., 2012; Pickler et al., 2011), engage in safe sexual practices (McCarthy, 2009; Swago-Wilson, 2010), and understand their own process of aging and the transitions it would bring (Bigby and Knox, 2009; Taggart et al., 2012).

Limitations

Inherent in any qualitative research is the inability to generalize findings beyond the researcher's sample. Despite the fact that similarities in expressed experiences uncovered in these meta-syntheses serve to enhance generalizability, and their concordance with quantitative literature, caution must be exercised not to take any of the qualitative findings presented here as being representative of people with IDD in general.

In addition, as is the case in much of the current research on people with IDD, relatively little diversity in race or socioeconomic status is evident in many of these qualitative studies. In fact, only the studies by Bogenschutz (2014) and

Ali and colleagues (2013) purposefully sampled from communities of color in order to elucidate the complex intersections between disability, race, ethnicity, and culture that are inherent in the human experience. This is a major shortcoming of not only the studies represented in these analyses, but in the field of IDD research more globally.

A final limitation of note is the international scope of the articles included in these meta-syntheses. While inclusion of international perspectives may certainly be considered a strength of this work, caution in interpretation is warranted, since service structures, public policies, and attitudes toward IDD vary dramatically throughout the world. What people with IDD and their supporters think is important in one country, may not apply at all in a neighboring country.

Practice and policy implications

Overarching all three syntheses was a call from people with IDD and their supporters for person-centeredness in the supports provided to them by medical professionals, residential and day services providers, and paid direct support workers. People with IDD were generally eager to engage as central participants in designing their supports, planning their medical care and retirements, and directing their own intimate relationships. Service providers would do well to honor these wishes by integrating person-centered thinking, planning, and practice into every facet of their work with people with IDD. By doing so, practitioners respect each person's right to individuality, rather than taking outdated and disrespectful institutional approaches to support.

Practitioners working with individuals with IDD may also look to these meta-syntheses to remind themselves that supports begin "where the person is." Supporting people with IDD to understand their medical conditions, prepare for aging, and safely engage in sexual relationships is fundamental to assisting an individual to lead a self-determined life in the community. This basic level of training should be considered an essential part of a practitioner's job, since higher-level community living is not possible without first helping people with IDD to build such understanding.

From a policy perspective, the meta-synthesis results suggest that community living movements have been successful, but should still be considered early in development. Much more work needs to be done, from the perspectives of people with IDD and their supporters, to support true community inclusion, expression of self, and integration in everyday life. Policy revisions should continually strive to support community living, and the infrastructure needed to support it. Policy makers should also consider community living not only a moral obligation, but a wise fiscal investment, since up-front investment in training on health promotion, safe sexual practice, and successful aging may pay dividends in the form of savings from eventual chronic illness treatment, additional direct support staffing needs, and increased self-sufficiency for people with IDD.

Directions for future research

There are ample opportunities to pursue future research based on the findings of these meta-syntheses. First, some exciting interventions were found in some of these qualitative studies, and future research may investigate ways to scale up such promising practices. For instance, the transition to retirement program piloted by Wilson, Bigby, and colleagues (2013) showed great promise for building greater social inclusion for people with IDD with their peers without IDD. Likewise, the sex education program used by Swago-Wilson (2010) showed promise as an intervention to help people with IDD to engage responsibly in sexual activity, and should be used on larger scale in order to demonstrate more generalizable efficacy.

Additionally, future research may benefit for deeper explorations about the intersections between IDD and race, ethnicity, sex, age, and other factors in order to more fully understand the experiences of people with IDD in the context of their full identities. Additionally, intersections at the systems level are important to understand more deeply. For instance, people with IDD may use a variety of residential service options to support their community living needs, and it is important to recognize how such differentials in supports may influence outcomes in health, sexual expression, and successful aging.

Table 9.1 Data extraction of studies of people with ID: overview

Author and purpose	*Design*	*Sample*	*Findings*
Ali et al. (2013) "To examine the extent to which adults with mild or moderate intellectual disability and carers believe that their needs are being accommodated by health services."	Semi-structured interviews were conducted with patients and carers. Thematic analysis.	$N = 29$. 14 dyads of individuals with ID and carers, and one single carer. Participants had mild or moderate ID, between ages 18 and 65. Both carer and individual with ID agreed to participate in study.	*Themes* Problems with communication. Problems with accessing help in a timely manner. Problems with how health professionals relate to carers. Challenges in negotiating complex healthcare systems. Problems with medical staff attitudes, knowledge, and behavior. Suggestions for improving care including accessible information, clinician education.
Barelds et al. (2010) To identify quality aspects of trajectories that are considered important by people with intellectual disabilities and their parents/relatives.	An attitude study using focus groups (8 groups – 4 with people with intellectual disabilities, split by ages). Miles and Huberman's data analysis approach.	$N = 46$. 21 parents/caregivers. 25 people with mild to moderate IDs. Participants recruited through nationwide interest group for parents and relatives of people with intellectual disabilities.	People with ID and their families differ in their perceptions of quality care. The focus group quality aspects fit closely into the different domains of two prominent models for quality assessment: the structure-process-outcome model and the SERVQUAL skeleton.

continued

Table 9.1 Continued

Author and purpose	*Design*	*Sample*	*Findings*
Bogenschutz (2014) To understand experiences of immigrant and refugee families in navigating the American healthcare system for their child with a disability.	Multi-case case study. Conducted two semi-structured interviews with each participant regarding their experiences accessing healthcare. Also did observation of each participant as they went to a health appointment. Conventional content analysis.	Purposive sampling. $N = 9$. 3 informants from each of the Hmong, Mexican, and Somali communities in one large metropolitan area. Wide range of disabilities and ages represented.	Participants showed strong resilience in navigating complex and confusing system. Facilitators of healthcare access included linguistically and culturally competent service providers, integration of services in common location, and using cultural reference points. Challenges to access included finding access to information, lack of service coordination, and limited availability of culturally appropriate services.
Cardol et al. (2012) To explore diabetes perceptions of people with ID.	Interviews of persons with ID. Grounded theory.	$N = 17$. Convenience sample. Recruited from 'Living Together' Panel, a national panel in the Netherlands of people with mild to moderate ID.	*Themes* • Majority feel loss with regard to food intake choices and control over daily life. • Most are familiar with the test and injections but do not like them. Were not bothered by pills. • Most were not feeling ill. • Most had unanswered questions. • Most relied on others for help. • There is relationship between better understanding and self-management. • There is relationship between confidence and self-management.

Chou and Lu (2012) To identify needs of individuals with ID and their caregivers in terms of menstruation.	Interviews of women living in Taiwan. Inductive analysis with constant comparison.	*N* = 12 mother caregivers of 13 daughters with ID. All subjects lived in Taiwan.	• Alternatives to sanitary pads. • Laundry as daily chore. • Isolation, inability to talk to others about experiences. • Menstrual management assistance as motherhood task. • Herbal medicines to regulate menstruation.
Chou et al. (2013) To gather information about experience of women with ID and their caregivers as they transition into perimenopause and postmenopause.	Semistructured interviews to determine attitudes and experiences of participants and cultural interpretations of those experiences and attitudes.	*N* = 14. All participants were from Taiwan.	Perceptions of menopause in women with ID did not differ from those of their caregivers. Women with ID had not been given knowledge about menopause. Female carers used HRT for their symptoms, women with ID did not and lacked access to regular healthcare or check-ups.
Dysch et al. (2012) "To explore the subjective experiences and perceptions of people with ID and diabetes" (p. 40).	Interviews with people with ID. Phenomenological analysis.	*N* = 4. Convenience sample. Participants were white. 3 female, 1 male. Recruited from diabetes clinic and ID team in UK city.	Participants expressed confusion about diabetes: • frustration with regimen, struggle with adherence; • diabetes was unwanted but tolerated; • support from others was helpful; • concurrent other health difficulties increases confusion.
Gibbs et al. (2008) To describe experiences of adults with ID and their caregivers in general hospital settings.	Focus group methodology. Grounded theory.	*N* = 25. Everyone with an ID had hospital visits. Participants with IDs recruited from day centers and group homes. Caregivers recruited using various sources.	*Themes* Feelings of anxiety and fear. Communication difficulties. Practicalities of being in or attending hospitals. Discrimination and negative comments. Behavior problems.

continued

Table 9.1 Continued

Author and purpose	*Design*	*Sample*	*Findings*
Jones et al. (2008) To identify barriers for people with ID in accessing healthcare.	Qualitative focus groups and individual interviews. Thematic analysis approach.	$N = 25$. Participants selected from service users and supporting social care staff groups.	Identified barriers: • accessing surgery; • communication problems; • time spent waiting; • feelings about seeing doctor; • health education; • making changes.
Pickler et al. (2011) To identify barriers and preferences of youth, their families and physicians when transitioning youth with IDs from pediatric to adult health care.	Focus group study (9 groups in three locations, urban, suburban and rural communities, each location hosted 3 focus groups 1 for youth, 1 for professionals and 1 for caregivers). Grounded theory approach.	$N = 48$. 16 youths 18–23 years, 15 professionals, 17 caregivers. Participants recruited either directly by researchers or through invitations from group of which they were part.	*Themes* • Pediatricians expressed that it was easier to continue care of ID patients in pediatric system. • Failure of medical system to distinguish between biological and developmental age. • Unavailability of adult health care providers and specialists to transition. • Perception that adult physicians are not equipped to treat adults with ID.
Swaine et al. (2013) To assess perception of female familial caregivers on barriers to women with ID receiving breast and cervical cancer screenings.	Interviews were conducted of women from a randomized controlled trial. Stratified by race and ethnicity. Convenience sample of those whose caregivers consented.	$N = 32$ caregivers. 78% were mothers of person with ID.	Barriers to person with ID receiving screenings for cervical and breast cancer: • caregiver did not believe it was needed due to hysterectomy, non-sexually active, or test not recommended by physician; • negative feelings of person with ID toward exam (pain/awkward/invasive); • clients more likely to feel comfortable with more knowledge, female physician, and physician they are familiar with.

Truesdale-Kennedy et al. (2010) To describe understanding of breast cancer and experiences of breast mammography among women with ID.	4 focus group interviews. Each group discussed 3 topics: breast cancer, experiences of mammography, and potential barriers for women with ID to attend breast screenings. Thematic content analysis.	$N = 19$. All female. Participants recruited through residential facility managers who identified potential participants.	*Themes* • Limited knowledge of what cancer is. • Women's experiences of breast mammography. • Confusion in breast screening process caused increased stress and anxiety, but helpful staff can lessen this.
Wullink et al. (2009) To compare and contrast preferences of individuals with ID seeking healthcare with professional requirements of general practitioners.	Qualitative focus groups and individual interviews.	$N = 12$ individuals with ID. Participants all members of client council of a residential facility and had been member of council for at least 1 year.	*Themes* • Allow patient to verbalize symptoms. • Doctor should listen carefully to patient. • Doctor should take patient seriously. • Doctor should explain and show what they are going to do before exam. • Doctor should ask permission before speaking to patient's support worker.
Ziviani et al. (2004) To understand factors that impact success in communication between individuals with ID and general practitioners (GPs) during medical consultations.	Qualitative interviews and observations. Thematic analysis with constant comparison.	$N = 17$. General practitioners. Individuals with ID. Care providers. Advocates.	ID perspectives: • communication difficulties with GPs; • want trustworthy GP; • annoyance with inappropriate communication. GP perspectives: • professional difficulties when communication is compromised; • difficulties in communication lead to time issues; • want advocates to attend all consultations. Advocates' perspectives: • concerned that ID individuals do not receive quality care; • want GPs to keep in mind the emotional needs of ID individuals.

Table 9.2 Themes from studies of people with ID: overview

Author	*Perceptions and knowledge of condition*	*Quality of care*	*Barriers*
Ali et al. (2013)		• Caregivers expressed issues with healthcare system and substandard care their loved ones received in terms of continuity of care. • When providers were accommodating and understanding more satisfaction was reported.	• Caregivers had difficulty receiving services for their loved one, and lack of information for services available. • Language barriers. • Individuals with ID felt ignored by their clinicians and the clinicians did not adapt their communication style to their needs. • Caregivers were not privy to clinicians' information or consulted. • Individuals with ID reported having clinicians being rude, disinterested, or insulting.
Barelds et al. (2010)	• Perceptions of quality of care differ significantly between individuals with ID and their caregivers/parents. • Individuals with ID were concerned with day-to-day aspects of medical care. • Caregivers' concerns more broad.		• Caregivers were concerned with access to support and other more broad barriers.
Bogenschutz (2014)	• Disability sometimes attributed to factors derived from culture of faith.	• Difficulties existed in finding quality care and in coordinating care between providers.	• Transportation to appointments was difficult. • Communication and translation barriers abounded.

Cardol et al. (2012)	• Theme of lack of control over food choice. • Theme of loss of control in social setting. • Theme of discomfort with injection but not as much with pills. • Feelings of sadness about having condition. • Theme of not feeling ill and therefore not concerned with illness. • Theme of minimal understanding of cause or prognosis of condition.	• Involving caregiver aids communication between client with ID and medical professional.	• Lack of self-management is related to lack of understanding condition. • Lack of self-management is related to lack of confidence.
Chou and Lu (2012)	• Mothers did not have ability to communicate knowledge regarding menstruation to their daughters. • Caregivers experienced feelings of isolation. • Mothers thought it was their responsibility or "fate" to help their daughters with menstruation.	• All mothers involved in this study were told by professionals (doctors, social service agents) to have their daughters' uteruses removed. • Use of seizure or psychiatric medication was thought to reduce length of cycle of woman with ID.	• Financial stressors of purchasing sanitary products or diapers. • Women were not given access to information or resources to help manage their daughters' menstruation. • Mothers reported doing laundry was daily chore.
Chou et al. (2013)	• Women with ID had not been provided knowledge about menopause. • Caregivers assumed their loved one with ID experienced similar symptoms as themselves during menopause.	• Most female caregivers who had experienced menopause had received medical care during menopause. • Most women with ID had not been offered HRT to help with symptoms.	• Most women in this study with ID had not received regular healthcare checkups (though article did not address reasons why this might be the case). • Male caregivers had hard time accessing information about menopause.

continued

Table 9.2 Continued

Author	*Perceptions and knowledge of condition*	*Quality of care*	*Barriers*
Dysch et al. (2012)	• Frustration with physical fluctuating state. • Frustration with regime, preparation, and planning. • Socially undesirable. • Dislike feeling different than others. • Dislike social impact. • Confusion about cause and prognosis of illness. • Confusion with language related to diabetes.		• Support from others is helpful. • Need for support from others is frustrating. • Multiple health difficulties add confusion.
Gibbs et al. (2008)	• Experiences of adults with ID and their caregivers in receiving services at a general hospital overall help to identify barriers to care.		• Feelings of fear and anxiety. • Communication difficulties. • Discrimination and negative comments. • Access. • Behavior problems.
Jones et al. (2008)			• Communication issues. • Access. • Wait time. • Attitudes and beliefs of medical care staff.
Pickler et al. (2011)		• Physicians believe it is easier to care for individuals with ID in pediatric setting.	• Failure of medical system to distinguish between chronological and developmental age. • Lack of specialists. • Perception that physicians for adults are not equipped to serve ID individuals.

Swaine et al. (2013)	• Little caregiver knowledge of necessity for breast cancer and cervical cancer screening for persons with ID.	• Enhanced communication to caregiver improved receipt of services. • Increased knowledge of person with ID improved patient comfort level. • Familiar physician increased comfort for patient with ID.	• Carrier misconception that screening not necessary due to hysterectomy, lack of sexual activity, previous trauma or physical discomfort. • Unfamiliar physician. • Male physician.
Truesdale-Kennedy et al. (2010)	• Lack of understanding what cancer and breast cancer is.	• Less anxiety was associated with more knowledge about screening done in an accessible way, or having a conversation. • Providers' positive attitude and reassurances made positive experience more likely.	• Embarrassment of taking off their clothes. • Confusion about mammograms led to increased fear about going.
Wullink et al. (2009)		• Physician should ask patient about symptoms. • Physicians should ask permission before speaking to support worker.	• Patients should be able to verbalize for themselves.
Ziviani et al. (2004)	• Support staff wants physicians to keep in mind emotional state of individuals with ID. • Support staff does not believe that individuals with ID receive same quality of care as those without ID.	• Physicians should ask permission before speaking to support worker. • Want physicians who are warm and trustworthy and interested in the individual. • Physicians desire better record keeping of medical history of individuals with ID.	• Communication difficulties with physician. • Informed consent. • Support staff are not attending all medical appointments for individuals with ID.

Table 9.3 Data extraction of studies of people with ID: sexuality

Author and purpose	*Design*	*Sample*	*Findings/themes*
Bernert (2010) To understand how women with ID experience sexuality.	Ethnographic study. Adapted grounded theory.	*N* = 14. Age 18–89 years. Referred from residential service providers in rural areas.	• Women expressed adult identities and expected sexual autonomy. • Structural barriers prevented free sexual expression for many women with ID.
Chou and Lu (2011) To examine process of decision making of sterilization of women with intellectual disabilities.	Semi-structured interviews. Phenomenological analysis.	*N* = 11. Purposive. Participants were women with ID who had experienced sterilization and their family members. Recruited from mini-census of women with ID who had undergone non-therapeutic sterilization.	• Sexuality of women with intellectual disabilities is ignored by their families and professionals. • Society views sterilization as a private, family matter. • Spouses and family members of women with intellectual disabilities make decisions for them regarding their reproductive choices.
Lofgren-Martenson (2004) To identify, describe, and understand opportunities and barriers to relationships and sexuality for young people with ID.	Qualitative interviews and participant observation at dances for people with ID.	*N* = 36 interview participants (youth, staff, parents). 14 participant observations. Study conducted in Sweden.	• Kissing, hugging, and French kissing are most common forms of physical intimacy. • Love and self-expression are desired and people with ID want to find a partner.

McCarthy (2009) To understand contraception use and knowledge of women with ID.	Exploratory study. Semi-structured interviews. Multi-stage narrative analysis.	$N = 23$. Ages 20–51 years. 12 lived independently.	• Knowledge about reproduction and contraception were both quite limited. • No informant had been provided with accessible information about contraception.
McClelland et al. (2012) To "explore the ways in which social and environmental conditions influence vulnerability to adverse sexual health outcomes" (p. 811) for LGBT people with intellectual disabilities.	10 semi-structured qualitative interviews and 2 focus groups. Community-based research approach. Relational analysis using NVivo version 8.	$N = 10$. Age 17–26 years. Labeled with ID and gay, lesbian, bisexual, questioning, or having fluid sexual orientations. Convenience sample from Toronto's ReachOUT program got feedback from a youth research advisory team.	• Themes identified included: living arrangements, rules, and autonomy; sex and sexual spaces.
Phasha and Nyokangi (2012) To "expos[e] violence among girls with intellectual disability."	Face-to-face interviews.	$N = 16$. Purposive sample recruited from two schools in South Africa for students with mild intellectual disabilities. Age 16–24 years. 5 males, 11 females.	• Touching: male students with ID touched females with ID against their will. • Intimidation: common when females with ID refused sexual demands/advances of males with ID.
Stoffelen et al. (2013) To "gain insight into the lives of a specific cohort of people with an ID who are homosexually active or who identify themselves as gay or lesbian and are living in the Netherlands" (p. 258).	Semi-structured interview, with topic list of interview questions following 2 pilot interviews. Exploratory.	$N = 21$. Purposive sample recruited through Dutch Gay, Lesbian, Bisexual, and Transgender Organization (COC).	• Themes identified included: sexual experiences, gay or lesbian identity, support, family, partner.

continued

Table 9.3 Continued

Author and purpose	*Design*	*Sample*	*Findings/themes*
Sullivan et al. (2013) To "explore the experiences and perceptions of close and sexual relationships of people with an intellectual disability" (p. 3456).	Semi-structured interviews. Exploratory. Interpretive phenomenological analysis.	$N = 10$. 6 male, 4 female. Recruited from nationwide advocacy organization for individuals with ID in Scotland.	• Themes identified by participants were: "relationships feeling safe and being useful"; "who's in charge?"; "struggling for an ordinary life"; "hidden feelings"; and "touching people in relationships." • Touching is wrong, touching is unsafe to talk about, "there is no freedom or fun."
Wilkinson et al. (2011) "Women with intellectual disabilities have equal rates of breast cancer but they have lower rates of mammography. No research to date has explored potential barriers to mammography for these women by involving the women themselves as participants" (p. 142).	Semi-structured interviews. Grounded theory.	$N = 27$ women with intellectual disabilities. Purposive sample.	• General level of independence. • Relationship with her physicians. • Participant's medical experience. • Experience with mammogram; medical knowledge, medical screenings; physician relationship, lack of accurate medical information.
Wilson et al. (2013). To explore situation of men and adolescent boys with moderate to profound intellectual disability.	Semi-structured interviews, participant observation, artifact collection. Grounded theory.	$N = 18$ caretakers to interview, observation of following 5 men and adolescents: Location 1 housed 1 man, Location 2 housed 2 adolescent boys, Location 3 housed 1 adolescent boy, 1 younger man; all residents of suburban Australia.	• No single masculinity, but various masculinities; masculinity is a changeable construct geographically, culturally and historically; sexual health, masculinity, gender role, caretaker gender role and relationship.

Table 9.4 Themes from studies of people with ID: sexuality

Author	*Sexuality*	*Relationship experiences*	*Barriers to healthy and safe sexual experiences*
Bernert (2010)	• Most women expressed an adult identity that resulted in their expectations of sexual autonomy.		• Most women experienced sexual limitations because of protective policies and programs.
Chou and Lu (2011)	• Sexuality of women with intellectual disabilities is ignored by their families and professionals they work with. • Individuals with intellectual disabilities do not have knowledge of their rights regarding sterilization.	• Spouses and family members of women with intellectual disabilities make decisions for them regarding their reproductive choices.	• Society views sterilization as a private, family matter, not as an ethical and human rights issue.
Lofgren-Martenson (2004)	• For people with intellectual disabilities, most common form of sexual expression is kissing, hugging, and sometimes French kissing.	• Need for love and self-expression was identified among this population. • Many people with intellectual disabilities attend dances in hopes of finding a partner.	
McCarthy (2009)			• Few women attended medical appointments alone. • Approximately half the women lacked basic knowledge about reproduction. • Knowledge of contraception found to be very limited. • None had been given accessible information about contraception.

continued

Table 9.4 Continued

Author	*Sexuality*	*Relationship experiences*	*Barriers to healthy and safe sexual experiences*
McClelland et al. (2012)	• Most reported others have some control over their sexuality. • Some were not allowed to masturbate, forbidden from having sex at all, or not in their residence. • Most were sexually active and expressed desire to have sexual and romantic relationships. • Prefer to have sex in their own homes. • Many participants have sex in public spaces.	• Participants cited adults who had control over their lives (parents, group home staff, social workers, partners, etc.). • Structured expectations (curfews, behavior, eating right, not damaging property, etc.). Some found these annoying, while others found them supportive/helpful.	• Participants saw several barriers to healthy sexual relationships: their environments, adults in their lives, access to condoms (most stated they use condoms more in their houses vs. when they have to have sex in a public space because of rules at home/group home, etc.).
Phasha and Nyokangi (2012)		• Coercive sex or rape reported by female students with ID who were in arranged relationships with male students with ID. • Touching: male students with ID touched female students with ID against their will. • Intimidation common when female students with ID refused sexual demands/advances of male students with ID.	• Concealment of sexual violence by schools promotes sexual violence. • Arranged relationships of male and female students with ID promotes sexual violence in schools.

Stoffelen et al. (2013)	• 9/21 participants had heterosexual sex at some points and few spoke of a long-term relationship. • All participants except one spoke of seeking a homosexual relationship after their first heterosexual experiences. • 9/21 indicated having a homosexual experience at a young age (12 or younger). • Violence against homosexuals reported by 10 participants. • Positive experiences were discussed by 10 participants. • 12 participants reported they had to hide their sexual relations.	• Few participants spoke of a long-term relationship. • 19 participants brought up "coming out" reactions from their families. • 2/21 participants reporting living with their partner; 7 reported being in a long-term relationship; 6/21 reported being treated badly or abused by their partner.	• 5/18 male participants reported always having a condom to prevent HIV, 3/18 sometimes, 2/18 unsure, and 2/18 no protective measures. • 6/18 men reported getting an HIV test once a year. • 6/21 reported being treated badly or abused by their partner. • 9/21 hoped to find a partner at meeting places offered by COC while many do not know how to find a new partner. • Difficulty with privacy in their living environments. • Specific training programs on socially acceptable sexual behavior and meeting places would be beneficial according to participants' responses.
Sullivan et al. (2013)	• People with intellectual disabilities found touching was seen as wrong by their family members. • People with intellectual disabilities think they do not have any freedom or fun to participate in sexual behaviors. • Sexual relationships are for people in marriages.	• Touching (such as holding hands) is important in relationships to people with intellectual disabilities.	

continued

Table 9.4 Continued

Author	*Sexuality*	*Relationship experiences*	*Barriers to healthy and safe sexual experiences*
Wilkinson et al. (2011)		• Limited relationships with medical professional. • Medical professionals did not develop relationship to provide support and medical information.	• Limited knowledge and understanding of preventative care. • Limited information provided to clients about self-care.
Wilson et al. (2013)	• Masturbation for men and boys was more a sensory and normal thing. • They liked to masturbate regularly.	• Most caretaker relationships mimic mothering; female caretakers. • Masculinity more comfortably identified with male caretakers. • Concept of masculinity influenced by presence and relationship with other males.	• Need for supportive staff to provide access for self-sexual acts. • Profound handicaps and need for 24/7 support limit sexual identity development. • Clear defined sense of masculinity and male identity is limitedly developed or supported.

Table 9.5 Data extraction of studies of people with ID: aging

Author and purpose	*Design*	*Sample*	*Findings*
Bekkema et al. (2014) To describe how caregivers and relatives shape respect for autonomy in end-of-life care for people with intellectual disabilities (ID).	Face-to-face semi-structured interviews.	*N* = 47 relatives and caregivers of 12 deceased (6 males, 6 females) individuals with ID. Individual interviews. Convenience sampling.	Themes identified: • challenges in respecting autonomy. If relatives and caregivers better respect autonomy there will be increased attention to maintaining an open, active, and reflective attitude; • caregivers should be appropriately educated regarding and individuals end-of life care needs.
Bigby (1997) To understand strengths and vulnerabilities of adults with ID in old age	Inductive analysis Interviews with each participant	*N* = 52 Adults aged 55 and over Living in the community	• Some participants felt they had better control of their lives in older age. • Participants were able to develop interpersonal relationships and seek social activities.
Bigby and Knox (2009) To understand perceptions of ID services from people with ID and their supporters	Social constructivism Analysis guided by Miles and Huberman	*N* = 16 triads (person with ID, unpaid supporter, paid supported) Ages 52–80 Residence across 2 Australian states	• People with ID were disappointed that decisions were often made for them, not with them. • Service providers are important for facilitating social opportunities for older adults with ID. • People with ID and their supporters were disappointed not to have more opportunity and input about future planning.
Buys et al. (2008) To explore meanings of active aging for older adults with lifelong intellectual disabilities.	Face-to-face semi-structured interviews.	*N* = 48. 16 family/friends or others in at least 3-year non-paid relationship with the adult with ID. 16 service providers. Purposeful sampling from two Australian states.	Themes identified: • being empowered; being actively involved; having a sense of security; maintaining skills and learning; having congenial living arrangements; having optimal health and fitness; being safe and feeling safe; having a satisfying relationship and support. • Older adults with lifelong ID wanted to continue activities that they found pleasurable even into their old age.

continued

Table 9.5 Continued

Author and purpose	*Design*	*Sample*	*Findings*
Dew et al. (2006) To better comprehend the experience of aging from the point of view of women with intellectual disabilities.	Structured narrative interview. Narrative data analysis.	*N* = 13. Participants recruited from two agencies that provide services to people with intellectual disabilities.	Significant number of participants said they: • were aging well; • had positive outlooks; • felt that people cared that they were accepted by community members; • were happy with their lives and could not identify anything in need of changing; • were in good health; • felt they needed more money to cover necessities.
Hole et al. (2013) To explore the concerns of adults with intellectual disabilities and their family members about the aging process.	Focus groups. Individual, semi-structured interviews.	*N* = 22 (11 individuals with ID, 11 family members). Convenience. Age 50+ years.	Themes identified: • For individuals with intellectual disabilities: future plans and hopes, future concerns. • For family members of individuals with intellectual disabilities: lack of peace/concern about future, need for proactive planning, complexity of planning process.
Judge et al. (2010) To gain insight into experiences of people with ID as they retire.	Semi-structured interviews. Phenomenological analysis.	*N* = 16. Age: 41 to 64 years. Gender: 5 male, 11 female. Participants recruited from 3 day programs in Scotland.	• Participants value being active. • Participants use day programs as their main means for socialization. • Participants either have no understanding of retirement, or feel that they have no part of decision making process. • Participants do not want their routines to change. • Participants want their independence to continue after retirement.

Shaw et al. (2011) To explore housing and old-age support preferences of people with IDs and their caregivers.	Focus groups and individual interviews. Thematic analysis.	$N = 25$ total from two groups, people with ID (15) and caregivers (10). People with ID were clients of an Australian supported employment provider. Ages: 19–55 years.	• Both groups discussed two shared themes, *living arrangements* and *housing preferences*; both groups predominantly preferred that the people with ID live near friends in their old age, and that the people with ID not live alone or in small groups but rather in large communities comprised of individuals with various disabilities.
Taggart et al. (2012) To explore impact on aging parents who are caregiving for an adult child with ID.	Mixed methods: questionnaire and semi-structured in-depth interviews.	Questionnaire: $N = 112$. Individual interview: $N = 19$. Convenience. Majority were female, caregiving alone.	• Majority of respondents reported very high stress levels and depression. • Biggest theme was apprehension about future, as most caregivers wanted adult child to stay in family and not live in an institution.
Todd and Read (2010) To understand experiences of people with ID in regards to death and dying and to use this information to help people with ID manage their fears about this topic.	Focus groups.	$N = 28$. Participants recruited from England and Wales.	• Participants understood that death is inevitable. • Participants were impacted by deaths of loved ones and thought about their own deaths as result. • Participants believe in an afterlife. • Participants felt that they may have been responsible for their caregivers' deaths, because they are difficult to care for, due to their disability.
Weeks et al. (2009) To explore challenges that older parents of children with ID experience and their wishes for their future care.	Screening pilot interviews, then in-depth interviews. Thematic analysis.	$N = 132$. Families in Prince Edward Island, Canada with parents over age of 50 years. 65.9% of families – two-parent households, 30.3% – single-mother households, 3.8% – single-father households.	Parents expressed concern about five themes: • availability of housing and provision of day-to-day care; • funding for services; • lack of choice in care provision and housing; • lack of caregiver's understanding of needs; • child's assistance provision in becoming a functional and productive member of society.

continued

Table 9.5 Continued

Author and purpose	*Design*	*Sample*	*Findings*
Young Olson (2005) To explore views of adults with IDs and their families about end-of-life planning and decision making, and to identify factors which impact opportunities of adults with IDs to participate in that planning.	Interview, focus groups, and record reviews. Thematic coding.	*N* = 30. 16 client participants and 14 participant families. Participants had to be able to communicate verbally.	• Caregivers often referred to their adult children as having child-to-teen level abilities, while respondents with ID saw themselves as mature. • Caregivers have a great deal of experience with making health care decisions, but respondents with ID have little experience with decision making. • Respondents had a clear understanding of death and experiences of loss. • Caregivers and their ID adult children both worry about what will happen when the caregivers die. • Client participants and caregivers see need for planning ahead, but many had done little or no planning before the study.

Table 9.6 Themes from studies of people with ID: aging

Author	*Autonomy*	*Community connections*	*Future planning*
Bekkema et al. (2014)	• Caregivers/relatives discussed both the challenges in respecting autonomy and the important qualities for respecting autonomy for those with ID. • Caregivers respect autonomy of persons with ID (help familiarize with transitions: changing care needs and wishes and important decisions).		• Caregivers found it hard to identify information needs and uncover wishes in people with severe ID. • Provide earlier attention to those with ID regarding their wishes and preferences. • It is important that caregivers/relatives keep an eye out for current needs and wishes as they change at end of life.
Bigby (1997)	• Some participants felt they had better control of their day-to-day life.	• Participants developed increased interpersonal relationships and social and domestic activities.	
Bigby and Knox (2009)	• Many adults with ID felt family and service providers made decisions for them without their input and were focused on services and less about them and their needs.	• Study found that the adults with ID found service facilities important in facilitating social relationships with other adults and staff.	• Adults with ID and their service providers felt frustrated by lack of focus on client's thoughts about future by management or policies.
Buys et al. (2008)	• Adults with ID wanted to have more control of important areas of their lives and wanted meaningful roles.	• Older adults with lifelong ID wanted to continue activities that they found pleasurable even into their old age. • The group also valued having companionship and maintaining contact with friends.	
Dew et al. (2006)		• Participants felt they were accepted by people in the community.	

continued

Table 9.5 Continued

Author	*Autonomy*	*Community connections*	*Future planning*
Hole et al. (2013)	• Adults with ID shared frustration about lack of choice they had following death of caregivers. • Family members highlighted importance of choice and self-determination for adults with ID.	• Adults with ID expressed desire to continue participating in leisurely activities they currently enjoy (travelling, shopping, etc.). For some, this included work. • Loneliness was an issue expressed by many adults with ID; there is a lack of community connections and social networks.	• Family members overwhelmingly expressed lack of peace and concern with respect to future. • Several formal and informal barriers resulting in lack of future planning: complexities of family networks, dissolving support networks, funding, systemic issues. • Family members all spoke of value and importance of proactive planning. • As caregivers age, need to organize legal affairs, formalize residential agreement.
Judge et al. (2010)	• Some participants feel they have no part in decision making process with regard to what will happen after retirement.	• Participants use their day programs as their main means for socialization.	• Some participants say that they have no understanding of retirement.
Shaw et al. (2011)		• People with ID and their caregivers predominantly preferred that the people with ID live near friends in their old age.	• None of the caregivers had planned for their disabled child's support outside the home.

Taggart et al. (2012)		• Most caretakers were not confident in community services. • Lack of community services was identified as a barrier to future planning.	• Many caregivers identified a consistent apprehension about future planning. • Small number of participants identified that they had definitive future plans. • Most future planning was aspirational. • Most acceptable future arrangements included moving in with other family (siblings).
Todd and Read (2010)	• Participants reported that they would like to be told that they, themselves, are going to die if this information is available.		
Weeks et al. (2009)	• Parents expressed concern about their child's assistance provision in becoming a functional and productive member of society.		• Parents expressed five thematic concerns about future planning for their children with intellectual disabilities.
Young and Olson (2005)	• Caregivers have great deal of experience with making health care decisions, but respondents with ID have little experience with any decision making; some are determined to participate in their own health care decisions and others do not want to participate at all.		• Client participants and caregivers see need for planning ahead, but many had done little or no planning before the study. • There was a lack of communication between families, future surrogates, clients, and service providers.

References

Abbott, D., and Howarth, J. (2007). Still off-limits? Staff views of supporting gay, lesbian and bisexual people with intellectual disabilities to develop sexual and intimate relationships? *Journal of Applied Research in Intellectual Disabilities*, *20*, 116–126.

Ali, A., Scior, K., Ratti, V., Strydom, A., King, M., and Hassiotis, A. (2013). Discrimination and other barriers to accessing health care: perspectives of patients with mild and moderate intellectual disability and their carers. *PLoS ONE*, 8(8), e70855.

Americans with Disabilities Act of 1990, Pub. L. No. 101–336, 104 Stat. 328 (1991).

Arias, B., Ovejero, A., and Morentin, R. (2009). Love and emotional well-being in people with intellectual disabilities. *The Spanish Journal of Psychology*, *12*, 204–216.

Barelds, A., de Goor, L., Heck, G., and Schols, J. (2010). Quality of care and service trajectories for people with intellectual disabilities: Defining the aspects of quality from the client's perspective. *Scandinavian Journal of Caring Sciences*, *24*(1), 164–174.

Bekkema, N., De Veer, A. J. E., Hertogh, C. M. P. M., and Francke, A. L. (2014). Respecting autonomy in the end of life care of people with intellectual disabilities. *Journal of Intellectual Disability Research*, 58(4), 368–380.

Bernert, D. (2010). Sexuality and disability in the lives of women with intellectual disabilities. *Sexuality and Disability*, 29(2), 129–141.

Bigby, C. (1997). Later life for adults with intellectual disability: A time of opportunity and vulnerability. *Journal of Intellectual and Developmental Disability*, *22*, 97–108.

Bigby, C. (2008). Known well by no-one: Trends in the informal social networks of middle-aged and older people with intellectual disability five years after moving to the community. *Journal of Intellectual and Developmental Disability*, *33*(2), 148–157.

Bigby, C., and Knox, M. (2009). "I want to see the Queen": Experiences of service use by ageing people with an intellectual disability. *Australian Social Work*, *62*, 216–231.

Bogenschutz, M. (2014). "We find a way": Challenges and facilitators for health care access among immigrants and refugees with intellectual and developmental disabilities. *Medical Care*, 52(10), S64–S70.

Burke, M., Fish, T., and Lawton, K. (2015). A comparative analysis of adult siblings' perception toward caregiving. *Intellectual and Developmental Disabilities*, *53*(2), 143–157.

Buys, L., Boulton-Lewis, G., Tedman-Jones, J., Edwards, H., and Knox, M. (2008). Issues of active ageing: Perceptions of older people with lifelong intellectual disability. *Australasian Journal on Ageing*, *27*, 67–71.

Cardol, J., Rijken, M., and van Schrojenstein Lantman-deValk, H. (2012). People with mild to moderate intellectual disability talking about their diabetes and how they manage. *Journal of Intellectual Disability Research*, 56(4), 351–360.

Cheng, M. M., and Udry, J. (2002). How much do mentally disabled adults know about sex and birth control? *Adolescent and Family Health*, *3*, 28–38.

Choi, K., and Wynne, M. (2000). Providing services to Asian Americans with developmental disabilities and their families: Mainstream service providers' perspective. *Community Mental Health Journal*, 36(6), 589–595.

Chou, Y., and Lu, Z.-Y. J. (2011). Deciding about sterilisation: Perspectives from women with an intellectual disability and their families in Taiwan. *Journal of Intellectual Disability Research*, 55(1), 63–74. doi:10.1111/j.1365-2788.2010.01347.x.

Chou, Y.-C., and Lu, Z.-Y. J. (2012). Caring for a daughter with intellectual disabilities in managing menstruation: A mother's perspective. *Journal of Intellectual and Developmental Disability*, *37*(1), 1–10.

Chou, Y.-C., Lu, X.-Y. J., and Pu, C.-Y. (2013). Menopause experiences and attitudes in women with intellectual disability and in their family carers. *Journal of Intellectual and Developmental Disability*, 38(2), 114–123.

Coppus, A. (2013). People with intellectual disability: What do we know about adulthood and life expectancy? *Developmental Disabilities Research Reviews*, 18(1), 6–16.

Curtice, M., Mayo, J., and Crocombe, J. (2012). Consent and sex in vulnerable adults: A review of case law. *British Journal of Learning Disabilities*, 41(4), 280–287.

Cuskelly, M., and Bryde, R. (2004). Attitudes towards the sexuality of adults with an intellectual disability: Parents, support staff, and a community sample. *Journal of Intellectual and Developmental Disability*, 29, 255–264.

Dew, A., Llewellyn, G., and Gorman, J. (2006). Having the time of my life: An exploratory study of women with intellectual disability. *Health Care for Women International*, 27, 908–929.

Dukes, E., and McGuire, B. (2009). Enhancing capacity to make sexuality-related decisions in people with an intellectual disability. *Journal of Intellectual Disability Research*, 53(8), 727–734.

Dysch, C., Chung, M., and Fox, J. (2012). How do people with intellectual disabilities and diabetes experience and perceive their illness? *Journal of Applied Research in Intellectual Disabilities*, 25(1), 39–49.

Evans, D. S., McGuire, B. E., Healy, E., and Carley, S. N. (2009). Sexuality and personal relationships for people with an intellectual disability. Part II: staff and family carer perspectives. *Journal of Intellectual Disability Research*, 53, 913–921.

Fisher, K. (2004). Health disparities and mental retardation. *Journal of Nursing Scholarship*, 36(1), 48–53.

Galea, J., Butler, J., and Iacono, T. (2004). The assessment of sexual knowledge in people with intellectual disability. *Journal of Intellectual and Developmental Disability*, 29, 350–365.

Gibbs, S. M., Brown, M. J., and Muir, W. J. (2008). The experiences of adults with intellectual disabilities and their carers in general hospitals: A focus group study. *Journal of Intellectual Disability Research*, 52(12), 1066–1077.

Haverman, M., Heller, T., Lee, L., Maaskant, M., Shhoshtari, S., and Strydom, A. (2010). Major health risks in aging persons with intellectual disabilities: An overview of recent studies. *Journal of Policy and Practice in Intellectual Disabilities*, 7(1), 59–69.

Hayashi, M., Arakida, M., and Ohashi, K. (2011). The effectiveness of a sex education program facilitating social skills for people with intellectual disability in Japan. *Journal of Intellectual and Developmental Disability*, 36(1), 11–19.

Healy, E., McGuire, B. E., Evans, D. S., and Carley, S. N. (2009). Sexuality and personal relationships for people with an intellectual disability. Part I: service-user perspectives. *Journal of Intellectual Disability Research*, 53, 905–912.

Heller, T., and Caldwell, J. (2006). Supporting aging caregivers and adults with developmental disabilities in future planning. *Mental Retardation*, 44(3), 189–202.

Hewitt, A., Lightfoot, E., Bogenschutz, M., McCormack, K., Sedlezky, L., and Doljanic, R. (2010). Parental caregivers' desires for lifetime assistance planning for future supports for their children with intellectual and developmental disabilities. *Journal of Family Social Work*, 13(5), 420–434.

Hole, R. D., Stainton, T., and Wilson, L. (2013). Ageing adults with intellectual disabilities: Self advocates' and family members' perspectives about the future. *Australian Social Work*, 66(4), 571–589.

Humphries, K., Traci, M. A., and Seekins, T. (2009). Nutrition and adults with intellectual or developmental disabilities: Systematic literature review results. *Intellectual and Developmental Disabilities*, *47*(3), 163–185.

Iacono, T., Davis, R., Humphreys, J., and Chandler, N. (2003). GP and support people's concerns and priorities for meeting the health care needs of individuals with developmental disabilities: A metropolitan and non-metropolitan comparison. *Journal of Intellectual and Developmental Disability*, *28*(4), 353–368.

Innes, A., McCabe, L., and Watchman, K. (2012). Caring for older people with an intellectual disability: A systematic review. *Maturitas*, *72*(4), 286–295.

Janicki, M., Dalton, A., Henderson, M., and Davidson, P. (1999). Mortality and morbidity among older adults with intellectual disability: Health services considerations. *Disability and Rehabilitation*, *21*, 284–294.

Jones, M. C., Mclafferty, E., Walley, R., Toland, J., and Melson, N. (2008). Inclusion in primary care for people with intellectual disabilities: Gaining the perspective of service user and supporting social care staff. *Journal of Intellectual Disabilities*, *12*(2), 93–109.

Judge, J., Walley, R., Anderson, B., and Young, R. (2010). Activity, aging and retirement: The views of a group of Scottish people with intellectual disabilities. *Journal of Policy and Practice in Intellectual Disabilities*, *7*, 295–301.

Krahn, G., Hammond, L., and Turner, A. (2006). A cascade of disparities: Health and health care access for people with intellectual disabilities. *Mental Retardation and Developmental Disabilities Research Reviews*, *12*, 70–82.

Larson, S., Anderson, L., and Doljanac, R. (2005). Access to health care. In W. Nehring (Ed.). *Health promotion for persons with intellectual/developmental disabilities: The state of scientific evidence* (pp. 124–189). Washington, D.C.: American Association on Mental Retardation.

Larson, S., Hallas-Muchow, L., Hewitt, A., Pettingell, S., Anderson, L., Moseley, C. R. et al. (2014). *In-home and residential long-term supports and services for persons with intellectual and developmental disabilities: Status and trends through 2012*. Minneapolis: University of Minnesota, Research and Training Center on Community Living, Institute on Community Integration.

Lofgren-Martenson, L. (2004). "May I?" about sexuality and love in the new generation with intellectual disabilities. *Sexuality and Disability*, *22*(3), 197–207.

McCarthy, M. (2009). Contraception and women with intellectual disabilities. *Journal of Applied Research in Intellectual Disabilities*, *22*, 363–369.

McCausland, D., Guerin, S., Tyrell, J., Donohoe, C., O'Donoghue, I., and Dodd, P. (2009). Self-reported needs among older persons with intellectual disabilities in an Irish community-based service. *Research in Developmental Disabilities*, *31*(2), 381–387.

McClelland, A., Flicker, S., Nepveux, D., Nixon, S., Vo, T., Wilson, C., et al. (2012). Seeking safer spaces: Queer and trans young people labeled with intellectual disabilities and the paradoxical risks of protection. *Journal of Homosexuality*, *59*(6), 808–819.

McGuire, B., and Bayley, A. (2011). Relationships, sexuality and decision-making capacity in people with an intellectual disability. *Current Opinion in Psychiatry*, *24*(5), 398–402.

McVilly, K., McGillivray, J., Curtis, A., Lehmann, J., Morrish, L., and Speight, J. (2014). Diabetes in people with an intellectual disability: A systematic review of prevalence, incidence and impact. *Diabetic Medicine*, *31*(8), 897–904.

Melville, C. A., Hamilton, S., Hankey, C., Miller, S., and Boyle, S. (2007). The prevalence and determinants of obesity in adults with intellectual disabilities. *Obesity Reviews*, *8*(3), 223–230.

Perkins, E. A., and Moran, J. A. (2010). Aging adults with intellectual disabilities. *Journal of the American Medical Association*, *304*(1), 91–92.

Phasha, T., and Nyokangi, D. (2012). School-based sexual violence among female learners with mild intellectual disabilities in South Africa. *Violence Against Women*, *18*(3), 309–321.

Pickler, L., Kellar-Guenther, Y., and Goldson, E. (2011). Barriers to transition to adult care for youth with intellectual disabilities. *International Journal of Child and Adolescent Health*, 3(4), 575–584.

Shaw, K., Cartwright, C., and Craig, J. (2011). The housing and support needs of people with an intellectual disability into older age. *Journal of Intellectual Disability Research*, *55*(9), 895–903.

Sohler, N., Lubetkin, E., Levy, J., Soghomonian, C., and Rimmerman, A. (2009). Factors associated with obesity and coronary heart disease in people with intellectual disabilities. *Social Work in Health Care*, *48*(1), 76–89.

Stoffelen, J., Kok, G., Hospers, H., and Curfs, L. (2013). Homosexuality among people with a mild intellectual disability: An explorative study on the lived experiences of homosexual people in the Netherlands with a mild intellectual disability. *Journal of Intellectual Disability Research*, *57*(3), 257–267.

Sullivan, G., Bowden, K., McKenzie, K., and Quayle, E. (2013). "Touching people in relationships": A qualitative study of close relationships for people with an intellectual disability. *Journal of Clinical Nursing*, *22*, 23–24.

Swaine, J. G., Dababnah, S., Parish, S. L, and Luken, K. (2013). Family caregivers' perspectives on barriers and facilitators of cervical and breast cancer screening for women with intellectual disability. *Intellectual and Developmental Disabilities*, *51*(1), 62–73.

Swango-Wilson, A. (2010). Systems theory and the development of sexual identity for individuals with intellectual/developmental disability. *Sexuality and Disability*, *28*(3), 157–164. doi:10.1007/s11195-010-9167-3.

Taggart, L., Truesdale-Kennedy, M., Ryan, A., and McConkey, R. (2012). Examining the support needs of ageing family carers in developing future plans for a relative with an intellectual disability. *Journal of Intellectual Disabilities*, *16*(3), 217–234.

Todd, S., and Read, S. (2010). Thinking about death and what it means: The perspectives of people with intellectual disability. *International Journal of Child Health and Human Development*, *2*, 207–213.

Truesdale-Kennedy, M., Taggart, L., and McIlfatrick, S. (2010). Breast cancer knowledge among women with intellectual disabilities and their experiences of receiving breast mammography. *Journal of Advanced Nursing*, *67*(6), 1294–1304.

Ward, R. L., Nichols, A. D., and Freedman, R. (2010). Uncovering health care inequalities among adults with intellectual and developmental disabilities. *Health and Social Work*, *35*(4), 280–290.

Weeks, L. E., Nilsson, T., Bryanton, O., and Kozma, A. (2009). Current and future concerns of older parents of sons and daughters with intellectual disabilities. *Journal of Policy and Practice in Intellectual Disabilities*, 6(3), 180–188.

Wilkinson, J., Deis, C., Bowen, D., and Bokhour, B. (2011). "It's easier said than done": Perspectives on mammography from women with intellectual disabilities. *Annals of Family Medicine*, 9(2), 142–147.

Wilson, N., Bigby, C., Stancliffe, R., Balandin, S., Craig, D., and Anderson, K. (2013). Mentors' experiences of supporting older adults with intellectual disability to participate in community groups. *Journal of Intellectual and Developmental Disability*, 38, 344–355.

Wilson, N., Parmenter, T., Stancliffe, R., and Shuttleworth, R. (2013). From diminished men to conditionally masculine: Sexuality and Australian men and adolescent boys with intellectual disabilities. *Culture, Health and Sexuality*, *15*(6), 738–751.

Wullink, M., Veldhuijzen, W., Lantman-de Valk, H. M., Metsemakers, J. F. M., and Dinant, G. J. (2009). Doctor-patient communication with people with intellectual disabilities: A qualitative study. *BMC Family Practice*, *10*(82), 82–91.

Yau, M. K., Ng, G. S., Lau, D. Y., Chan, K. S., and Chan, J. S. (2009). Exploring sexuality and sexual concerns of adult persons with intellectual disability in a cultural context. *British Journal of Developmental Disabilities*, *55*, *Part 2*(109), 97–108. Retrieved from http://search.ebscohost.com.proxy.library.vcu.edu/login.aspx?direct=true&AuthType=ip,url,cookie,uid&db=ccm&AN=105422447&site=ehost-live&scope=site.

Young Olson, S. (2005). *End-of-life planning and decision-making: Implications for adults with mental retardation* (Doctoral dissertation). Retrieved from UMI Microform (UMI Number 3198339).

Ziviani, J., Lennox, N., Allison, H., Lyons, M., and Del Mar, C. (2004). Meeting in the middle: Improving communication in primary health care consultations with people with an intellectual disability. *Journal of Intellectual and Developmental Disability*, *29*(3), 211–225.

10 The lived experience of adult child caregivers of parents with Alzheimer's disease

Heeyhul Moon and Jacqueline Corcoran

In 2013, 15.4 million informal caregivers – including immediate family members, other relatives and friends – provided 17.7 billion hours of care with a value of over $220.2 billion for persons with Alzheimer's disease (AD) and other dementias (Alzheimer's Association, 2014). Eighty percent of the care given to persons with neurocognitive disorders is provided by family members (Horvath et al., 2013). Approximately one-third of these informal caregivers, who belong to mainly the baby boomer generation (born between 1946 and 1964), are "sandwich generation caregivers" who provide care simultaneously for both dependent children and aging parents (Alzheimer's Association, 2013; National Alliance for Caregiving, 2009).

Previous research has examined the positive aspects of dementia caregiving, such as experiences, appraisal, emotions, and the strengths and resources to maintain care (Zarit, 2012). However, the literature also has documented that providing care for AD and other dementia patients is extremely stressful and results in negative impacts on emotional, psychological, physical, financial, and social well-being, compared to caregiving work for older adults with other diseases (Pinquart and Sörensen 2003; Sörensen and Conwell 2011). For instance, those who provide dementia care were 3.5 times more likely to report great difficulty associated with caregiving than those who provide non-dementia care. Such care provision resulted in an estimated $9.1 billion due to increased caregiver healthcare costs in 2012. In 2013, the Alzheimer's Association published figures (based on a 2004 study) showing that half of unpaid non-spouse caregivers of people with Alzheimer's and other dementias have caregiving-related out-of pocket expenses averaging $300 per month. In particular, many current sandwich generation caregivers may face multiple roles and strains due to providing personal and financial care for their families including children, aging parent, sibling, spouse, and themselves (Fingerman et al., 2012; Moon and Dilworth-Anderson, 2014).

Behavioral and psychological symptoms of dementia (BPSD) are major sources of a dementia caregiver's burden, but the caregivers will face difference care challenges depending on types of dementia such as Alzheimer's dementia (AD), vascular dementia (VaD), frontotemporal dementia (FTD), and others (de Vugt et al., 2006; Wong et al., 2012). For instance, according to De Vugt et al. (2006), caregivers of people with AD reported higher levels of depression and anxiety and feeling more competent than caregivers of FTD. Thus, a greater understating of the impact of specific types, such as AD (constituting roughly 60–80 percent of dementia cases; Alzheimer's Association, 2014) on caregiving stress and coping experience may be beneficial to develop more specific caregiver intervention.

There is also reason to believe that differences exist between spouse and adult child caregivers. A number of studies recognize differences in caregiving provision and in effects on caregiver stress depending on the kin relationship of the caregiver (i.e., adult children, children-in-law, spouse (Deimling et al., 2001; Pearlin et al., 1990; Pinquart and Sörensen, 2003; Suitor and Pillemer, 1993). In a meta-analysis by Pinquart and Sörenson (2011), spouse caregivers reported providing more care and using less informal support than adult children and children-in-law caregivers, which may worsen the psychological wellbeing of spouse caregivers. On the other hand, adult-child caregivers may face challenges that are different than the challenges reported by spouses, such as multiple role conflicts as mother, wife, and employee as well as caregiving. Further, interventions on caregivers of patients with AD may have different effects on spouses and adult children caregivers (Brodaty et al., 2003; Sörenson and Conwell 2011). In some studies (e.g. Singe and Elmståhl, 2008), spouses are more likely to benefit from psycho interventions compared to adult children caregiver in burden, depression, or delayed nursing home placement (Brodaty et al., 2003; Sörenson and Conwell 2011) although spouse caregivers reported higher level of burden or distress at the point of intake.

To develop a more in-depth view of the AD caregiving experience, qualitative research has also been conducted. Qualitative research can enhance our understanding of the underlying meaning that children attribute to their parent's disease and their caregiving role. Due to the increase in the numbers of people with AD living in the community and being cared for by their adult children caregivers, it is important to integrate this qualitative research to understand the caregiver experience and to provide interventions tailored to improve their well-being and to maintain their caregiver role.

Before presenting the results of the meta-synthesis on adult child caregiving experience with Alzheimers Disease, the prior meta-syntheses will be reviewed. Yong and Price (2014) conducted a meta-synthesis of the qualitative literature on "the human occupational impact" of partner and close family caregiving of people with dementia. Altogether they included 20 studies and found five themes: (1) family caregivers had to adapt and change as the condition of their family member deteriorated; (2) staying motivated and in control, which included being able to complete practical tasks, taking breaks, getting support, and connecting with spirituality and religion; (3) preserving occupational balance and well-being, meaning striking a balance between over-functioning for their family members and allowing them dignity and respect by allowing them to do previously enjoyed activities; (4) gaining meaning from the caregiving role, which involved familial obligation to care for the person with dementia, with women deriving more of a sense of identify from caregiving and men providing practical support; and (5) occupational impact from care demands and losses, which included the demands of constant caregiving and loss of relationship with the person with dementia, as well as loss of personal and social activities.

Another meta-synthesis was conducted with a specific emphasis on grief in caregivers of persons with dementia (Large and Slinger, 2015). Eleven studies were included with different types of family caregivers. Themes were as follows: (1) challenges of caregiving, including feelings of burden and strain and having to give up other activities; (2) losses and changes in the relationship, which depended on the progression of the dementia, but often included the loss of the person that was known; (3) the long-term nature of the disease and the slow deterioration means that caregivers may remain in a "state of grieving" without closure; (4) striving despite dementia, which translated into the development of coping mechanisms; these often included accentuating the positives and detaching from the person with dementia; (5) utilizing social support, which included informal and formal support; there were mixed reviews about formal support, complaining about professionals lacking information and providing contradictory information; and (6) death as a relief from caregiving.

As opposed to the various types of caregiving studied in previous meta-syntheses, the purpose of this chapter is to conduct a meta-synthesis of the qualitative studies on experiences of informal adult child caregivers for persons with AD only. Synthesis of only one population (child adult caregivers) and problem (caregivers of Alzheimers disease) involves a more homogenous process (Sandelowski and Barroso, 2006). Separating out types of caregivers allows us to explore more fully the experience and needs of adult children caregivers that may experience different stress coping process compared to that of spouse caregivers (Gaugler et al., 2015).

Themes

After a comprehensive search (the general process is described in Chapter 2), seven studies were located that had a total of 180 participants. There were slightly more female participants than male. A majority of participants were Caucasian, but African-Americans, Latinos, and Israelis were also included. Four studies were conducted in the United States, one was conducted in Israel, and three did not specify a geographic location. The age of participants ranged from 28 and 67; however, the average age in most studies was around 52 years. The majority of participants were recruited from hospitals or clinics with some recruited from the Alzheimer's Association through convenience or purposive sampling. For more detail on studies, see Table 10.1.

Two major themes, each comprised of several elements, emerged from the child caregivers' perspective: (1) positive aspects of care, including people's motivations for caregiving, the benefits they receive from caregiving, and the ways they have found to cope with caregiving; and, more prominently,

(2) negative aspects of care, which included the impact on relationships, difficult emotions, and lack of access to services and resources. See Table 10.2.

Positive aspects

Motivations for caregiving

People often discussed an obligation to care based on reciprocation of the person with Alzheimer's previous care of themselves. As an example, one participant said: "She had cared for me when I was sick. I owed this to her" (Sanders and McFarland, 2002, p. 69). Participants found caregiving a way to "pay back" for what had been done for them. This positive motivation made people go through with the ordeal required in caregiving.

Benefits from caregiving

Another subtheme involved the benefits derived from caregiving, which included spending time with the parent, getting to know a parent more, developing compassion, and appreciating each other. One participant discussed how spending time with her parent was beneficial: "Yes, this illness caused daily stress, chaos, uncertainty and sadness, but it also fostered something totally unexpected and most precious – time to get to know my [parent with Alzheimer's disease]. Would I do it again? Absolutely!" (Montano, 2011, p. 458). A few participants also explained how caregiving strengthened their interpersonal skills, their patience, and their compassion (Sanders and McFarland, 2002).

Coping strategies

Two studies explicitly focused on coping strategies. The findings of these studies indicated that participants principally used three different strategies: humor, utilizing community resources, and self-care. One participant stated that "Reminiscing about something – that's a big thing for humor. If you start reminiscing about crazy things you've done together or things you've laughed over ... that's the most fun" (Tan and Schneider, 2009, p. 401), and another participant agreed with this, saying that "[humor is] my way of coping" (Tan and Schneider, 2009, p. 401).

One of the community resources that participants mentioned using was support groups. Some participants, in fact, had more than one support group:

> I have a couple different support groups and ... keeping those friendships strong have been important to me ... as far as being able to get through it ... they fill in for everything ... when life does get overwhelming, they're the first people that are here to pitch in.
>
> (Schumacher, MacNeil, Mobily, Teague, and Butcher, 2012, p. 52)

Self-care was a main coping strategy for these children caregivers. One participant reported:

> Well, I was so stressed that sometimes physically you just have to, like maybe my taking care of myself was going for a walk just because you had so much anxiety you had to do something, if you don't move you would jump out of your skin.... I just had to.
>
> (Schumacher et al., 2012, p. 52)

Negative aspects of care

Participants in all seven studies reported experiencing negative aspects of care, including the impact on relationships, experiencing difficult emotions, and lack of access to resources.

Impact on relationships

The studies' findings related to relationships had two aspects: one of these was the direct impact on personal relationships (with the parent, a spouse, their own children and their friendships) in terms of time and commitment caused by caregiving for their parent with AD; another aspect involved the reversal of caregiving roles when the child cared for the parent. Dealing with difficult emotions and a lack of time for tasks and activities due to caring for a parent were reported by many participants, together with the effects on their other relationships and immediate family. For instance, one participant commented that "In some cases [spouse] has to be number 2 depending on what is going on that week" (Montano, 2011, 464). Another participant mentioned that "by having her along we aren't actin as ... a regular family ... changes ... the way that my husband and I talk to each other" (Schumacher et al. 2012, p. 49).

Participants also reported conflicts in time commitments, responsibilities, and priorities (and difficulty resolving the conflicts) between their families and caring for their parents, and some participants said that they felt that they had to put their other responsibilities and priorities aside in order to care for their parent. One participant stated: "Maybe you should look at life in a different way and you have different anxieties that merge and come to the fore, and maybe you should be spending more time with the family" (Globerman, 1996, p. 42). Another participant reported: "Basically you just put things aside. And you do what has to be done" (Tan and Schneider, 2009, p. 401). Participants in three studies mentioned experiencing a lack of spontaneity and a loss of privacy after beginning to care for their parent. One participant explains: "I miss travel; we traveled a lot before, and it's just something that we haven't been able to do..." (Schumacher et al., 2012, p. 53). There was also mention of how caregiving impacted professional responsibilities and participants' ability to move vertically within their company. One participant explained that "Well from a professional standpoint, it was very difficult to balance all of my responsibilities with her and then of course, all of the unwritten professional development expectations, and still give attention to my mom" (Sanders and McFarland, 2002, p. 71). The caregiving role made it challenging to balance priorities and prioritize tasks after taking on the role in the same way they had used prior to starting to provide care, and other daily activities and life choices were often put on hold in order to complete their duty as a caregiver.

Difficult emotions

Difficult emotions (in addition to that experienced in relationships with others) was another subtheme reported by participants in all seven studies. Participants remarked that they felt many different emotions while caregiving for their parent, including shame, embarrassment, frustration, isolation, guilt, sorrow, grief, fear, and being overwhelmed. One participant commented that "sometimes I feel like I just want to scream. You feel like you are in all by yourself" (Habermann et al., 2013, p. 186). Another participant reported guilt at excluding the parent with AD from family functions: "And so for Patrick's [wedding] we did not have her [come] and that just about broke my heart" (Schumacher et al., 2012, p. 50). Another participant described feeling shame at the behavior of their parent with AD: "I take her with me to the synagogue … and then she starts talking during prayer time and she starts saying again and again, 'I will not talk,' but she does not stop talking. I feel so humiliated" (Werner et al., 2010, p. 162). Grief at losing (either mentally or physically) the parent they loved and remembered, was also reported by participants; one said: "You're losing bits and pieces of your loved one all the time…" (Tan and Schneider, 2009, p. 404).

Lack of access to resources

A subtheme of negative aspects of care involved lack of access to information, resources, and services. Participants reported difficulties in obtaining timely and appropriate answers to their questions and in getting resources to assist them and their parent with their needs. One participant stated:

> We sought help, several times, mainly from the Long-term Care Law of the National Insurance Institute. But it took a long time until we received any answer, although we showed certificates which confirmed that she needed help around the clock.
>
> (Werner et al., 2010, p. 165)

Other interactions were described as problematic with people having to advocate heavily to get their family member's needs met. An example of a lack of help was described by one participant who said:

> My mother had hallucinations. I told her family physician about it and she answered that there was nothing to be done. Finally, only after I pressured

her, she gave a medicine that helps, but her treatment was rude and unprofessional.

(Werner et al., 2010, p. 165)

Another example in the same study involved a problem with nurses unable to do an assessment: "I heard that persons with AD who are in a terrible condition don't get the benefit because the nurse does not understand their needs. They have to lie and overact to receive what they deserve by law" (p. 165).

Discussion

In keeping with previous work on the negative effects of dementia caregiving (e.g., Pinquart and Sörensen 2003; Sörensen and Conwell, 2011), participants in all seven studies analyzed in our meta-synthesis reported various stressors including decreased relationship quality, emotional distress, and lack of access to resources. In a systematic review of 10 studies, caregivers of people with dementia were found to have elevated rates of depression (Cuijpers, 2005). Possibly, as the care receivers (CRs) lose their cognitive functions, the responsibility of spouses and adult daughters of patients with mild cognitive impairment is increased and caregivers were more inclined to engage in assessing the CRs' needs and making decisions. Such increased involvement negatively impacted the caregivers' emotions (Adams, 2006), as well as their relationship quality. It is also possible that adult-child or other non-spouse caregivers are distressed because they are juggling multiple role responsibilities.

Similar to the quantitative studies (Pinquart and Sörensen, 2011), the adult children caregivers in the source studies for this meta-synthesis reported multiple role strains, including family and work conflicts and limited social life. While several quantitative studies have indicated substantial need for services for these reasons among these caregivers of people with dementia, they are less likely to use the services (e.g., Sun et al., 2014; Brodaty et al., 2005). As identified by the current study, there also may be frustration with services not meeting their own or the CR's needs.

Simultaneously, adult children caregivers reported positive aspects of care, including motivations for care and benefits of caring. Possibly adult children caregivers experience gain or gratification from dementia caregiving, which corroborated the results documented by previous research (Cohen et al., 2002; Peacock et al., 2010). Adult caregivers in the meta-synthesis were able to employ coping strategies to meet the challenges of care. In a meta-analysis of 35 studies, coping styles that were predictive of positive outcomes (less anxiety and depression), included acceptance of the role (Li et al., 2012). Those that saw benefits to the role as described in the meta-synthesis may be more accepting of the caregiving role.

An enriched relationship is also one of the potential benefits identified in the meta-synthesis. To corroborate this emergent finding was a review of 15 studies looking at relationship quality between caregivers and the person with dementia (Quinn et al., 2009). A positive relationship was associated with greater caregiving wellbeing and the ability to maintain the caregiver role.

Unlike previous meta-synthesis studies (Large and Slinger, 2009; Yong and Price, 2014) that included all types of family caregivers with different kinds of dementia, not just Alzheimer's, our meta-synthesis concerned itself solely with child caregivers. Between all three meta-syntheses, many themes overlapped, lending credence to emergent experiences that caregivers might often feel. These included the adaptations that were necessary to care for a family member with dementia, as well as the grief involved in losing the person that was known previously and other negative emotions. Our meta-synthesis uncovered benefits of caring, while in Yong and Price (2014), they were subsumed under the process of finding meaning in caregiving, and Large and Slinger (2009) also discussed the development of coping skills.

Shared themes between Large and Slinger (2009) and our meta-synthesis were the social support that was discussed as a separate theme in their study, even though we had it under coping mechanisms. Part of Langer's social support involved seeking professional support, and there were some negative comments about accessing professional services that seemed in our study to warrant a separate category of its own.

Limitations and implications

A limitation is a possible lack of generalizability due to a lack of variation in source study information regarding location, participant gender, and participant socioeconomic status. Those studies that included such information indicated that most participants were Caucasian and were middle class. Due to the lack of diversity, the findings of this meta-synthesis cannot necessarily be generalized to all child caregivers of a parent with Alzheimer's disease.

Despite these limitations, several implications can be drawn from our results. Service providers may need to assess the benefits from caregiving and the coping strategies reported here and strive to optimize these positive aspects to caregiving. As Pearlin and colleagues (1990) postulated, inner growth during such a difficult time may have a positive impact on perceived well-being, as well as health. Regardless of the individual differences in duration and severity of AD and the resulting variations in the demands of caregiving, such focus on inner growth through caregiving might be helpful for adult children caregivers to maintain their roles.

Findings of this meta-synthesis can also be shared by providers when presenting psychoeducation to adult children caregivers to help them become aware of potential strengths in the caregiving role, normalize reactions, and to act as a basis of discussion about their own experience. In the meta-analysis of coping styles, emotional support was found to be a predictor of less anxiety and depression in caregivers (Li et al., 2011). Practitioners can provide emotional support as part of their role, assist caregivers in accessing emotional support through their informal network, and make referrals to support and education programs.

The latter have shown to be effective in reducing caregiver burden (Marim et al., 2013).

Our findings additionally highlight the need to provide appropriate and individualized services for the adult children caregivers, especially those belonging to the "sandwich generation." The adult children caregivers in our analysis reported difficulties in balancing their own lives and the care they were providing, with resulting impacts on the relationship quality with their parents with the disease and their other family members, social life/leisure time and employment. Depending on an individual's needs, appropriate information and assistance or social support (e.g., adult day care, care respite, home aides, intervention services) might reduce caregiver stress and improve caregiving quality by providing time for caregivers and alleviating care burdens (Gaugler et al., 2003; Mossello et al., 2008).

Finally, there should be strong support systems for caregivers of people with AD, in particular, the adult children caregivers for Alzheimer's disease who may have multiple roles in and external to their families. Due to limited funding and policy-related issues, local agencies have a hard time providing appropriate services for the family (Family Caregiver Alliance, 2014). However, since our society mainly relies on family caregivers, federal and state governments should provide support and educational, practical, adequate, and affordable services for these caregivers as well as their parents with AD (Feinberg and Newman. 2004; Rose et al., 2015).

Table 10.1 Data extraction of studies of adult child caregivers of parents with Alzheimer's disease

Author and purpose	*Design*	*Data analysis*	*Sample information*	*Major findings*
Globerman (1996) To find motivations of daughters- and sons-in-law for caring for relatives of Alzheimer's Disease.	Face-to-face interviews, open-ended questions.	Ethnography.	$N = 97$. No geographic information provided (Toronto, Canada). Majority female. No age range specified. Participants recruited from geriatric clinic.	*Four themes* • Role of caregiver: reactive versus proactive. • Obligation to caregiving: doing so because it is the right thing to do, personal and connection with caretaker. • Reasons behind caregiving: to keep stress off spouse to care for parent, assisting in relationships between caregiver and family. • Impact of caregiving involvement: putting lives on hold.
Habermann et al. (2013) To explore positive experiences children have when caring for their parents who have a neurodegenerative disease.	Semi-structured face-to-face interviews.	Conventional content analysis.	$N = 34$. Southeastern United States. Mean age: 52 years. Gender: 82% female. Race: 53% Caucasian, 47% African American. Participants recruited from larger randomized clinical trial.	*Three themes for relationships* • Spending and enjoying time together. • Giving back care. • Appreciating each other and getting closer.

Montano (2011) To understand family relationships of daughter taking care of her parent with Alzheimer's Disease.	Face-to-face interview (semi-structured), observations, participant journals.	Cross-case analysis (compare each study).	$N = 9$. San Diego, CA, US. Age range: 28–54 years. Gender: all females. Race: 4 Caucasian, 4 Latino, 1 African American. Participants recruited from local chapter of Alzheimer's Association and various centers.	*Themes* • Sense of inclusion. • Family unity. • Emotional strain, emotional stress. • Sense of unity and solidarity. • Grief. • Sacrifice of time for traditional family care (young children). • Increased marital stress. • Relationship issues with parent.
Sanders and McFarland (2002) Perceptions of son caring for his parent who has Alzheimer's.	Face-to-face interviews.	Open coding to develop common concepts and themes.	$N = 18$. United States (northern rural areas) (Pennsylvania). Age range: 35–67 years. Gender: all male. Race: all Caucasian. Participants recruited from volunteer participation in local Alzheimer's Association chapter and word of mouth.	• Sense of commitment to parent (obligation to care). • Role reversal/role changes. • Strengthen interpersonal skills (patience and compassion). • Conflicts: interpersonal (primary caregiver, guilt for own children) and professional (jeopardizing employment, taking off work). • Emotional and psychological strain (embarrassment for parent's behavior). • Access to services.

continued

Table 10.1 Continued

Author and purpose	*Design*	*Data analysis*	*Sample information*	*Major findings*
Schumacher et al. (2012) To understand lived experience of leisure for adults who have minor child living in home and who are caring for their parent with AD.	Semi-structured face-to-face interviews.	Hermeneutic. Phenomenology, study of lived experience.	$N = 6$. Iowa City, Iowa, US. Age range: 37–54 years. Gender: majority female. Race: all Caucasian. Participants recruited from placing information in newspapers regarding study.	*Six themes* • Reconciling life transitions: overwhelming, stress, discovering memory loss, integrating parent demands and family needs, juggling multiple life challenges, balancing guilt and grief. • Succumbing to infinite obligations: crushing time and emotional pressure, acknowledging inequities. • Time shifts: nursing home alters time, longing for spontaneity, evaluating time for self-care. • Constructing a foundation: partners grant a reprieve, gathering support. • Revisit control: positive power, humor as a stabilizer, balanced perspective. • Freedom to recreate: yearning for old leisure, structured relief, modifying leisure.

Tan and Schneider (2009) Adult-child caregivers using humor as a coping strategy for caring for parent who has Alzheimer's.	Semi-structured, face-to-face interviews.	Phenomenological analysis (themes).	$N = 6$. No geographic area specifically listed (Canada). Age range 30–60 years. Gender: 5 female, 1 male. Participants recruited from local support group.	*Four themes* • Overall experience of caregiver (prioritizing/balancing commitments, stress, role reversal). • Humor in caregiving (witnesses to humor, timing, topic). • Factors of using humor (coping, perspective on life, family upbringing). • Benefits of humor (escape, stress relief).
Werner et al. (2010) Experience of family stigma of child caregivers of persons with AD.	Semi-structured face-to-face interview.	Open coding, Axial coding, integration.	$N = 10$. Northern Israel. Mean age: 52.9 years. Gender: 8 female, 2 male. Participants recruited from support groups by Israeli Alzheimer's Association.	*Three themes* • Caregivers' stigma (function of parent, emotional reactions, positive and negative: shame, embarrassment, disgust, compassion, sorrow, guilt). • Stigma from public (function of parent, positive and negative emotions: pity, fear). • Stigma from social structures: function of parent, insufficient knowledge, lack of resources or access to services, flawed health system.

Table 10.2 Themes from studies of adult child caregivers of parents with Alzheimer's disease

Themes		*Findings*	*Studies*
Positive aspects of care.	Motivation for caregiving.	• Obligation to care for parent. • To keep stress off spouse to care for parent.	Globerman (1996) Habermann et al. (2013) Montano (2011) Sanders & McFarland (2002)
	Benefits from caregiving.	• Getting to know parent more. • Personal growth. • Spending time with parent/family unity. • Appreciating each other. • Giving back care. • Strengthen interpersonal skills (patience, compassion).	Habermann et al. (2013) Montano (2011) Werner et al. (2010) Sanders & McFarland (2002)
	Coping strategies.	• Humor and humor as a stress relief. • Utilizing community resources (adult day care, respite, home aids, intervention services). • Self-care.	Schumacher et al. (2012) Tan & Schneider (2009)
Negative aspects of care.	Impact on relationships.	• Role reversal (child now taking care of parent). • Stress (over healthy parent staying healthy, lack of knowledge of disease, immediate family). • Relationship issues with parent. • Sacrifice of time with immediate family (caregiver's own children/spouse). • Putting life on hold. • Family stress. • Balancing/prioritizing commitments.	Globerman (1996) Habermann *et al.* (2013) Montano (2011) Sanders & McFarland (2002) Schumacher et al. (2012) Tan & Schneider (2009) Werner et al. (2010)

Difficult emotions.	• Shame/embarrassment. • Overwhelming. • Emotional pressure/burden. • Fear of losing parent (mentally and physically). • Frustration. • Loss and complicated grief. • Sorrow (pain for self not parent). • Guilt for not being able to change/slow down progression. • Urgency to take control over decisions.	Globerman (1996) Habermann et al. (2013) Montano (2011) Sanders & McFarland (2002) Schumacher et al. (2012) Tan & Schneider (2009) Werner et al. (2010)
Lack of resources.	• Professional responsibilities/ability to progress with employment (taking time off). • Limited access to/lack of services. • Flawed health system. • Lack of social life/spontaneity/privacy.	Sanders & McFarland (2002) Schumacher et al. (2012) Werner et al. (2010)

References

Alzheimer's Association. (2013). 2013 Alzheimer's disease facts and figures. *Alzheimer's and Dementia*, 9(2), 208–245. doi:10.1016/j.jalz.2013.02.003.

Alzheimer's Association. (2014). 2014 Alzheimer's disease facts and figures. *Alzheimer's and Dementia*, *10*(2), e47–e92. doi:10.1016/j.jalz.2014.02.001.

American Psychiatric Association (2013). *Desk reference to the diagnostic criteria from DSM-5*. Arlington, VA: Author.

Boise, L., Neal, M. B., and Kaye, J. (2004). Dementia assessment in primary care: Results from a study in three managed care systems. *The Journals of Gerontology Series A: Biological Sciences and Medical Sciences*, 59(6), M621–M626.

Brodaty, H., Green, A., and Koschera, A. (2003) Meta-analysis of psychosocial interventions for caregivers of people with dementia. *Journal of the American Geriatrics Society*, *51*(5), 657–664.

Brodaty, H., Thomson, C., Thompson, C., and Fine, M. (2005). Why caregivers of people with dementia and memory loss don't use services. *International Journal of Geriatric Psychiatry*, *20*(6), 537–546.

Cohen, C. A., Colantonio, A., and Vernich L. (2002) Positive aspects of caregiving: Rounding out the caregiver experience *International Journal of Geriatric Psychiatry*, *17*, 184–188.

Cuijpers, P. (2005). Depressive disorders in caregivers of dementia patients: A systematic review. *Aging and Mental Health*, 9, 325–330.

De Vugt, M. E., Riedijk, S. R., Aalten, P., Tibben, A., Van Swieten, J. C., and Verhey, F. R. J. (2006). Impact of behavioural problems on spousal caregivers: A comparison between Alzheimer's disease and frontotemporal dementia. *Dementia and Geriatric Cognitive Disorders*, *22*(1), 35–41. doi:10.1159/000093102.

Deimling, G. T., Smerglia, V. L., and Schaefer, M. L. (2001). The impact of family environment and decision-making satisfaction on caregiver depression: A path analytic model. *Journal of Aging and Health*, *13*(1), 47–71.

Family Caregiver Alliance. (2014). Caregiving. Retrieved from https://caregiver.org/caregiving.

Feinberg, L. F., and Newman, S. L. (2004). A study of 10 states since passage of the National Family Caregiver Support Program: Policies, perceptions, and program development. *The Gerontologist*, *44*(6), 760–769.

Finfgeld, D. L. (2003). Metasyntheses: The state of the art – So far. *Qualitative Health Research*, *13*, 893–904.

Fingerman, K. L., Pillemer, K. A., Silverstein, M., and Suitor, J. J. (2012). The baby boomers' intergenerational relationships. *Gerontologist*, *52*(2), 199–209.

Gallagher, D., Mhaolain, A., Crosby, L., Ryan, D., Lacey, L., Coen, R., et al. (2011). Self-efficacy for managing dementia may protect against burden and depression in Alzheimer's caregivers. *Aging and Mental Health*, *15*(6), 663–670.

Garcia-Alberca, J. M., Cruz, B., Lara, J. P., Garrido, V., Gris, E., Lara, A., et al. (2012). Disengagement coping partially mediates the relationship between caregiver burden and anxiety and depression in caregivers of people with Alzheimer's disease. Results from the MALAGA-AD study. *Journal of Affective Disorders*, *136*(3), 848–856.

Gaugler, J. E., Reese, M., and Mittelman, M. S. (2015). Effects of the Minnesota adaptation of the NYU caregiver intervention on depressive symptoms and quality of life for adult child caregivers of persons with dementia. *American Journal of Geriatric Psychiatry*, *23*(11), 1179–1192. doi:10.1016/j.jagp.2015.06.007.

Gaugler, J. E., Jarrott, S. E., Zarit, S. H., Stephens, M. P., Townsend, A., and Greene, R. (2003). Adult day service use and reductions in caregiving hours: Effects on stress and psychological well-being for dementia caregivers. *International Journal of Geriatric Psychiatry*, *18*, 55–62.

Globerman, J. (1996). The case of daughters-in-law and son-in-law in the care of relatives with Alzheimer's disease. *Family Relations*, *45*(1), 37–45.

Habermann, B., Hines, D., and Davis, L. (2013). Caring for parents with neurodegenerative disease: A qualitative description. *Clinical Nurse Specialist*, *27*(4), 182–187.

Hayes, J., Boylstein, C., and Zimmerman, M. (2007). Living and loving with dementia: Negotiating spousal and caregiver identity through narrative. *Journal of Aging Studies*, *23*, 48–59.

Hayslip Jr., B., Han, G., and Anderson, C. (2008). Predictors of Alzheimer's disease caregiver depression and burden: What noncaregiving adults can learn from active caregivers. *Educational Gerontology*, *34*, 945–969.

Henry, J. D., Rendell, P. G., Scicluna, A., Jackson, M., and Phillips, L. H. (2009). Emotion experience, expression, and regulation in Alzheimer's disease. *Psychology and Aging*, *24*(1), 252–257.

Hooyman, N. R., and Kiyak, H. A (2005). *Social gerontology: A multidisciplinary perspective*. Boston, MA: Pearson/Allyn and Bacon.

Horvath, K. J., Trudeau, S. A., Rudolph, J. L., Trudeau, P. A., Duffy, M. E., and Berlowitz, D. (2013). Clinical trial of a home safety toolkit for Alzheimer's disease. *International Journal of Alzheimer's Disease*, *2013*, 1–11.

Jones, M. L. (2004). Application of systematic review methods to qualitative research: Practical issues. *Journal of Advanced Nursing*, *48*, 271–278.

Large, S. and Slinger, R. (2013). Grief in caregivers of persons with Alzheimer's disease and related dementia: A qualitative synthesis. *Dementia*. *14*(2), 164–183. doi:10.1177/1471301213494511.

Li, R., Cooper, C., Bradley, J., Shulman, A., and Livingston, G. (2012). Coping strategies and psychological morbidity in family carers of people with dementia: A systematic review and meta-analysis. *Journal of Affective Disorders*, *139*(1), 1–11. doi:10.1016/j.jad.2011.05.055.

Light, E., and Lebowitz, B. (1990). *Alzeimer's disease treatment and family stress: Directions for research*. New York: Hemisphere.

Lott, L., and Klein, D. T. (2003). Psychotherapeutic interventions. In D. P. Hay, D. T. Klein, L. K. Hay, G. T. Grossman, and J. S. Kennedy (Eds.), *Agitation in patients with dementia: A practical guide to diagnosis and management. Clinical practice series* (pp. 103–118). Arlington, VA: American Psychiatric Publishing.

Lou, V. W., Lau, B. H. P., and Cheung, K. S.-L. (2014). Positive Aspects of Caregiving (PAC): Scale validation among Chinese dementia caregivers. *Archives of gerontology and geriatrics*, *60*(2), 299–306.

Mannion, E. (2008). Alzheimer's disease: The psychological and physical effects of the caregiver's role. Part 1. *Gerontological Care and Practice*,*20*(4), 27–32.

Marim, C. M., Silva, V., Taminato, M., and Aparecida Barbosa, D. (2013). Effectiveness of educational programs on reducing the burden of caregivers of elderly individuals with dementia: A systematic review. *Revista Latino-Americana de Enfermagem*, *21*, 267–275.

Meade, M. O., and Richardson, W. S. (1997) Selecting and appraising studies for a systematic review. *Annals of Internal Medicine*, *127*, 531–537.

Montano, R. (2011). *Living with Alzheimer's disease: Daughter caregivers and their contemporary families* (Doctorial Dissertation). Retrieved from ProQuest Dissertations and Thesis Full Text (3454482).

Moon, H., and Dilworth-Anderson, P. (2014). Baby boomer caregiver and dementia caregiving: findings from the National Study of Caregiving. *Age and Ageing, 44*(2), 300–306.

Mossello, E., Caleri, V., Razzi, E., Di Bari, M., Cantini, C., Tonon, E., et al. (2008) Day care for older dementia patients: Favorable effects on behavioral and psychological symptoms and caregiver stress. *International Journal of Geriatric Psychiatry, 23*, 1066–1072.

Napoles, A. M., Chadiha, L., Eversley, R., and Moreno-John, G. (2010). Reviews: Developing culturally sensitive dementia caregiver interventions: Are we there yet? *American Journal of Alzheimer's Disease and Other Dementias, 25*(5), 389–406.

National Alliance for Caregiving. (2009). *Caregiving in the U.S.: Executive summary*.

Noblit, G. W., and Hare, R. D. (1988). *Meta-ethnography: Synthesizing qualitative studies*. Newbury Park, CA: Sage Publications.

Paterson, B., Thorne, S., Canam, C., and Jillings, C. (2001). *Metastudy of qualitative health research*. Thousand Oaks, CA: Sage Publications.

Peacock, S., Forbes, D., Markle-Reid, M., Hawranik, P., Morgan, D., Jansen, L., et al. (2010) The positive aspects of caregiving journey with dementia: Using a strengths-based perspective to reveal opportunities. *Journal of Applied Gerontology, 29*, 640–659.

Pearlin, L. I., Mullan, J. T., and Semple, S. J. (1990). Caregiving and the stress process: An overview of concepts and their measures. *Gerontologist, 30*, 583–594.

Pinquart, M., and Sörensen, S. (2003). Differences between caregivers and noncaregivers in psychological health and physical health: A meta-analysis. *Psychology and aging, 18*(2), 250.

Pinquart, M., and Sörensen, S. (2005). Ethnic differences in stressors, resources, and psychological outcomes of family caregiving: A meta-analysis. *Gerontologist, 45(1)*, 90–106.

Pinquart, M., and Sörensen, S. (2011). Spouses, adult children, and children-in-law as caregivers of older adults: A meta-analytic comparison. *Psychology and Aging, 26*(1), 1–14. doi:10.1037/a0021863.

Quinn, C., Clare, L., and Woods, B. (2009). The impact of the quality of relationship on the experiences and wellbeing of caregivers of people with dementia: A systematic review. *Aging and Mental Health, 13*, 143–154.

Rosa, E., Lussignoli, G., Sabbatini, F., Chiappa, A., Di Cesare, S., Lamanna, L., et al. (2010). Needs of caregivers of the patients with dementia. *Archives of Gerontology and Geriatrics, 51*, 54–58.

Rose, M. S., Noelker, L. S., and Kagan, J. (2015). Improving policies for caregiver respite services. *The Gerontologist, 55*(2), 302–308.

Sandelowski, M. (2004). Using qualitative research. *Qualitative Health Research, 14*, 1366–1386.

Sandelowski, M., and Barroso, J. (2006). *Handbook for synthesizing qualitative research*. New York: Springer Publishing.

Sanders, S., and McFarland, P. (2002). Perceptions of caregiving role by sons caring for a parent with Alzheimer's disease: A qualitative study. *Journal of Gerontological Social Work, 37*(2), 61–76.

Schumacher, L., MacNeil, R., Mobily, K., Teague, M., and Butcher, H. (2012). The leisure journey for sandwich generation caregivers. *Therapeutic Recreation Journal, 46*(1), 42–59.

Scott, C. B. (2013). Alzheimer's disease caregiver burden: Does resilience matter? *Journal of Human Behavior in the Social Environment, 23*(8), 879–892.

Signe, A., and Elmståhl, S. (2008). Psychosocial intervention for family caregivers of people with dementia reduces caregiver's burden: Development and effect after 6 and 12 months. *Scandinavian Journal of Caring Sciences, 22*, 98–109. doi:10.1111/j.1471-6712.2007.00498.x.

Sörensen, S., and Conwell, Y. (2011). Issues in dementia caregiving: Effects on mental and physical health, intervention strategies, and research needs. *The American Journal of Geriatric Psychiatry: Official Journal of the American Association for Geriatric Psychiatry, 19*(6), 491.

Suitor, J. J., and Pillemer, K. (1993). Support and interpersonal stress in the social networks of married daughters caring for parents with dementia. *Journal of Gerontology, 48*, S1–S8.

Sun, F., Mutlu, A., and Coon, D. (2014). Service barriers faced by Chinese American families with a dementia relative: Perspectives from family caregivers and service professionals. *Clinical Gerontologist, 37*(2), 120–138. doi:10.1080/07317115.2013.868848.

Tan, T., and Schneider, M. A. (2009). Humor as a coping strategy for adult-child caregivers of individuals with Alzheimer's disease. *Geriatric Nursing, 30*(6), 397–408.

Waldemar, G., Dubois, B., Emre, M., Georges, J., McKeith, G., Rossor, M., et al. (2007). Recommendations for the diagnosis and management of Alzheimer's disease and other disorders associated with dementia: EFNS guidelines. *European Journal of Neurology, 14*, 1–26.

Werner, P., Goldstein, D., and Buchbinder, E. (2010). Subjective experience of family stigma as reported by children of Alzheimer's disease patients. *Qualitative Health Research, 20*(2), 159–169.

Wong, C., Merrilees, J., Ketelle, R., Barton, C., Wallhagen, M., and Miller, B. (2012). The experience of caregiving: Differences between behavioral variant of frontotemporal dementia and alzheimer disease. *American Journal of Geriatric Psychiatry, 20*(8), 724–728. doi:10.1097/JGP.0b013e318233154d.

Yong, A. S. L., and Price, L. (2014). The human occupational impact of partner and close family caregiving in dementia: A meta-synthesis of the qualitative research, using a bespoke quality appraisal tool. *The British Journal of Occupational Therapy, 77*(8), 410–421.

Zarit, S. H. (2012). Positive aspects of caregiving: More than looking on the bright side. *Aging and Mental Health, 16*(6), 673–674. doi:10.1080/13607863.2012.692768.

11 The lived experience of older adults with depression

For older adults, DSM-IV diagnosable depression rates range from 0.8 to 8 percent (Kraaij, Arensman, and Spinhoven, 2002). Although their depression rates may be lower than other age groups, they are more likely to die by suicide (Centers for Disease Control and Prevention, 2005). The literature commonly presents that older adults are less likely to complain of affective symptoms, such as sadness, anxiety, or hopelessness (Agency for Health Care Policy and Research, 1993; Bird and Parslow, 2002; Fiske et al., 2009); they may speak instead of physical ailments and show more physical signs, such as weight loss, insomnia, and fatigue, as well as cognitive disturbances, such as memory impairment and difficulty concentrating.

A meta-analysis of 13 studies was undertaken to determine the risk factors for depression in older adults living in the community (Cole and Dendukuri, 2003). Biological factors included insomnia and female gender. The gender gap in the prevalence of depression in females starting in adolescence and persisting into old age (Barry et al., 2008; Kessler, 2003) has been well-documented. Psychological factors included bereavement and having experienced prior depression (Cole and Dendukuri, 2003). Interestingly, no social factors, including lack of social support, appeared to be associated with depression. A more recent review of the literature identified curtailment of daily activities as a major risk factor for depression, as well as self-critical thinking (Fiske et al., 2009). Protective influences involved having obtained higher education and socioeconomic status, involvement in meaningful activities, and religious and/or spiritual engagement.

Themes

The inclusion criteria produced a total of 13 studies published between 2001 and 2009 with 356 participants total. A majority of these participants were women and either Caucasian or African-American. Most studies were conducted in the United States; however, Sweden and Australia were also represented. All participants were over the age of 60 and samples were typically in their seventies. The majority were recruited from either primary care physicians or inpatient hospital treatment settings. See Table 11.1.

Results revealed four major themes dealing with the participants' depression: (1) experiences; (2) causes; (3) recovery; and (4) barriers to treatment. The data from the studies were organized around these broad themes.

Experiences

Participants described their experiences with depression in various ways. See Table 11.2. Eight studies discussed the emotional experience of depression. Negative feelings toward oneself, including lack of self-worth and self-blame, emerged as a common occurrence among depressed older adults. One participant reported: "Mostly just that – feeling like you are not good for anything … I am not worth – why bother" (Wilby, 2008, p. 102). Another participant responded: "I haven't lived the way you're supposed to, I haven't been of use in the way I ought to have been earlier" (Hedelin and Strandmark, 2001, p. 412). Persistent sadness emerged as another feeling experienced by participants in three studies. One person commented: "It's just I'm sad. And I think it's just because there's a lot of sad stuff. It's just been really hard" (Dekker et al., 2009, p. 313). Other participants anchored their sadness to specific situations, such as getting old, feeling alone, experiencing family problems, and grieving. For example, one participant stated: "I do feel sad. I've lost my sister a couple of months ago … and it's sad because I'm alone" (Hostetter, 2003, p. 114).

Hopelessness was also described by participants in three studies. Feelings of hopelessness existed around the ability to get better: "I'm dying of depression and I am not going to make it" (Ugarriza, 2002, p. 26), and the meaninglessness of life. One participant expressed this powerful despair by stating:

> It's like I'm in a pit trying to climb up, but I haven't got the strength, and if I then get medicines, which perhaps don't help, then I feel as if I'm stuck in that pit.… Then it gets even blacker, and I think now I'm finished…
>
> (Hedelin and Strandmark, 2001, p. 410)

Other subthemes focused on the emotional experiences of depression include fear (two studies), powerlessness (two studies), and isolation (two studies).

Physical symptoms of depression were further experienced by participants in five studies. These physical symptoms can be divided into declining wellness, pain or illness; decreased energy level; and changes in sleep habits and appetite. One participant, noting a decline in their energy and increased sleep, stated: "Sometimes I just come in the room, shut the door and go to, and just go to sleep, just lay here" (Dekker et al., 2009, p. 313). Comments such as "sometimes the whole body is in pain" (Hedelin and Strandmark, 2001, p. 412) refer to the physical pain present in the experience of the depression.

Finally, a subtheme of denial was expressed in myriad ways. Some participants did not call what they were experiencing depression or were unable to see it as a clinical problem. They did not tell others what they were feeling.

Others talked about it in ways that were depersonalized; for instance, they didn't talk about their own experience, but kept using second-person pronouns to describe their depression.

Causes

Eight of the 13 studies explored participants' attributions for the causes of their depression (see Table 11.3). Biological/medical explanations and grief and loss were each cited in five studies. Biological or medical causes included conditions such as chronic health problems, pain, chemical imbalance, and loss of function. One participant described her depression with regard to her physical ailments: "A lot of worries ... a lot of problems.... I have fungus on my feet and toes ... I cannot control my urine ... I have a lot of difficulties that made me depressed" (Ugarriza, 2002, p. 25).

Experiences of grief and loss, particularly death of family members, were especially significant. Statements like "Well actually I think I was alright until I started losing my family, you know, just like one behind the other" (Bayer, 2007, p. 76) and "I lost my husband. I wound up in [inpatient treatment] two days after he died" (Ugarriza, 2002, p. 26) were common among participants. Related themes having to do with relationships involved conflict or perceived neglect, particularly by family members (three studies), and the experience of loneliness (two studies) as leading to depression.

Three studies discussed how participants were baffled as to the cause of their depression. One participant commented: "I don't really know. I don't know where the [depression is] coming from, I really don't. I just get like that sometimes and I don't know why. I can't tell you why" (Proctor et al., 2008, p. 672).

Financial hardship (four studies) was considered a contributor to depressed mood. When asked specifically what causes depression, one participant simply replied: "Being poor" (Wilby, 2008, p. 77). Other mentions of finances included lifelong poverty, living on fixed income, and bankruptcy. Another participant stated:

> We didn't have money to go to school when we were coming up. We had to work on the farm. And we didn't have the proper food, like milk. See, you must eat to support your body and be strong in your head. If you don't have that strength, things like suffering might get the best of you.
>
> (Black et al., 2007, p. S395)

Recovery

Recovery from depression was a major theme of nine studies (see Table 11.5). More studies reported people relying on their own coping resources (eight studies) than professional services (six studies). Various coping methods were endorsed in studies: spirituality, social support, distraction, and personal qualities (represented in four studies each). Many elder participants found their spirituality helpful; they believed their faith had the power to resolve depression or to give them the strength to get through the experience. One participant stated: "You got to put your faith in the Lord. If you don't you're going to feel bad and you're going to get up and do anything but just lay there and complain" (Wittink et al., 2008, p. 404). Another commented: "My sister will pick me up and we will go to church on Sunday.... That helps me when I feel blue. The Lord uplifts me" (Bayer, 2007, p. 84).

In terms of social support, being able to share the depression with others and having social outlets and activities helped to relieve the symptoms of depression. One participant commented: "Sometimes when I feel bad I call my friend in Dubach. She listens and we talk for a long time. It helps to let it out" (Bayer, 2007, p. 84). Having distractions served as another coping strategy for depression. Participating in hobbies was a common way to handle the depression: "I like to do crafts. I like to work crosswords and do Sudoku. Other times that just gets my mind off things and just concentrating on that one thing" (Dekker et al., 2009, p. 314). Personal attributes, such as positive thinking and drawing on personal strength to fight the illness were further named as beneficial for alleviating depression. As one participant explained:

> The main thing I think that I've found is trying to keep my mind off of things that make me sad. If I find myself drifting that way, well then I know right away I've got to think of 2 positives. Because that's a negative. And like I said, when you've got a negative, you've got to come up with 2 positive things to replace that.
>
> (Dekker et al., 2009, p. 315)

When elders mentioned professional treatment, medication was the most frequent modality mentioned (three studies). One participant related: "I used to hate days like today where it was sunny. Like I couldn't stand to be in the sun and ever since I've been on antidepressants, I enjoy sunshine." Other forms of treatment named as beneficial by participants included electroconvulsive therapy, psychotherapy, and talking to medical doctors.

Barriers to treatment

A fourth theme involved barriers to intervention for depression (see Table 11.4). Five studies discussed why participants did not pursue more formal treatment for depressive symptoms. The foremost explanation was their fears and negative perceptions about treatment (three studies). Many participants feared taking antidepressants or had had a bad experience in the past with the medication. One participant stated: "I'm not interested in pills anymore. I get bad dreams. I mean, they gave me pills that left me waking up and not knowing where I was. I was still in a dream" (Givens et al., 2006, p. 148).

Another major barrier was participants' views of depression (three studies): they believed their symptoms were unimportant and minimized them; they claimed depression was a normal part of life; and/or they felt they should be able to deal with the depression themselves. One participant claimed: "At my age, I'll just live with it" (Wilby, 2008, p. 98), and another stated: "I doubt if I ever discuss [the depression] with [the physician]. I never felt it important enough to discuss it with him" (Wittink et al., 2006, p. 305). A final subtheme involved surrendering to the depression given people's despair and hopelessness about the prospect of recovering (two studies).

Implications for practice

The meta-synthesis of the qualitative literature related to older people's experience with depression yielded information with implications for practice with this population. Although the literature speaks to how older adults manifest and describe depression in more physical than emotional ways (Agency for Health Care Policy and Research, 1993; Bird and Parslow, 2002; Fiske et al., 2009), this meta-synthesis suggests that emotional symptoms, such as sadness, hopelessness, and negative feelings toward the self, were more prominent than physical symptoms, such as chronic pain, sleep, appetite, and change in energy. However, when making attributions about the causes of their depression, participants often pointed to physical illness, disability, and decline. An implication from this finding is that practitioners should ask about emotional symptoms as older adults seem to be able to articulate their pain in this way. Ensuring that elders receive appropriate medical care and pain management also appear important as in this study it came up as a reason for the onset of depression. Discussing ways that older patients can manage pain, whether it is experienced emotionally or physically is another emergent implication.

Similar to other literature, this meta-synthesis also found that certain beliefs about depression held by this cohort may present barriers. Sometimes older adults did not recognize their symptoms as fitting the clinical profile for depression or resigned themselves to live with it, considering it a normal part of aging. An implication is that practitioners can educate the elderly population that depression is a treatable clinical condition and can provide information on appropriate treatments, offering referrals. As well as educating, social workers should also explore perceptions and preferences about seeking intervention.

In the meta-synthesis, participants rarely discussed psychosocial treatments. Although they mentioned "talking to the doctor" as one of the treatments they had found helpful, they were typically referring to medical doctors and personnel, rather than social workers or psychotherapists. An implication is that psychosocial treatments, such as life review, psychodynamic or cognitive-behavioral therapy could be explained as options for treatment that have research evidence supporting them (Wilson et al., 2008).

As in the quantitative literature, bereavement emerged as a risk factor for depression in the elderly (Cole and Dendukuri, 2003). However, the metasynthesis broadened our understanding of depression as not only about relationship loss, but also about other relationship stressors and challenges, particularly in regard to family members. A clear implication is that practitioners, in order to help older clients, must be willing to actively involve family members and to work toward improved communication and the reparation of longstanding conflict. Additionally, those working with the elderly need to be skilled at grief and loss counseling so that depression is not necessarily an outcome of loss.

Older adults named a wide array of coping resources available to them. The studies revealed that while some older adults used formal treatment, particularly medication, they placed more emphasis on other strategies and resources. Another implication from these findings is that those who work with elderly depression must recognize the critical role that spirituality plays in helping people cope with and overcome depression. Practitioners can ask about and encourage those aspects of spirituality that are helpful to people suffering from depression.

Further, people reported that social activities and distraction improved their mood. An implication is that enrichment and social activities may be an important component of any services that are offered. Behavioral activation treatment, a specific type of cognitive-behavioral therapy, centering on activity scheduling and increasing pleasant activities, has been found beneficial for people suffering from depression (Cuijpers et al., 2007), even when compared to more complex therapies (Cuijpers et al., 2008). Therefore, behavioral activation treatment may be an important initial intervention and may serve to be sufficient for many sufferers of depression.

Limitations

Potential limitations of this study largely surround current controversy of qualitative research and more specifically, metasynthesis. Criticisms of metasynthesis include its heavy reliance on secondary interpretation of experiences, which is likely to differ according to the researcher. An additional criticism of the use of metasynthesis is its creation of abstract phenomenon rather than concrete evidence (Finlayson and Dixon, 2008).

Other limitations of this study exist as a result of the primary qualitative study available. While this metasynthesis encompasses all the available literature, studies were derived from developed countries, which excludes the experience of depression in older adults who live in less developed nations. The metasynthesis was also largely composed of majority female samples, which is consistent with gender discrepancies in depression consistently documented in the literature (Kessler, 2003), but lacks the important voice of older adult men with depression.

Other limitations involve the lack of definitive criteria for concepts such as depression and age. Studies used for this metasynthesis included individuals who were medically diagnosed with depression as well as those who complained of depressive symptoms but did not necessarily meet the DSM criteria for depression. The absence of uniform criteria for depression may have combined experiences that may have been heterogenous in nature.

Also, in primary studies, participants ranged in age from 60 to 91. Individuals within this large age range may experience depression differently. Further, there was no distinction made between those who were community dewelling (four studies) and those who were in long-term care facilities (two studies). In the remainder of studies, it is unknown if participants lived in the community or in assistive facilitites. It is likely that people who live in the community or in facilities may have different experiences and beliefs about depression, but we were not able to ascertain these differences.

Conclusion

Despite its limitations, this study offers a comprehensive understanding of older adults' perceptions of depression and its causes, experience, recovery, and barriers to treatment. This study also includes data from a variety of literature sources, countries, and qualitative methodologies in an attempt to encompass as many aspects of depression as possible and to increase generalizability. While the inclusion of various qualitative methodologies is sometimes seen as a limitation of metasynthesis, this inclusion also provides depth to the metasynthesis through various phenomenological insights (Paterson et al., 2001). As the population continues to age, practitioners will more often encounter possible depression in this population and will need to understand the experience and ways to be most helpful.

Table 11.1 Data extraction of studies of older adults with depression

Author and purpose	*Design*	*Data analysis*	*Sample information*	*Major findings*
Bayer (2007) To explore role of family relations in symptoms of depression in older adults receiving outpatient mental health services in a rural area.	In-depth interviews.	Ethnography.	N = 14. Louisiana, US. All living at poverty level in rural area, receiving outpatient mental health services. Average age: 73.5 years. Gender: 2 male, 12 female. Race: 6 Caucasian, 8 African American. Education: 3 High school, 9 less. Participants recruited at outpatient group meeting at hospital in rural Louisiana.	Four themes emerged from reasons for seeking mental health treatment: • long-term physical illness, such as chronic pain, heart conditions, arthritis, diabetes, and not being able to physically complete tasks once able to do (p. 74); • memory problems, such as losing bills/important documents, forgetting what to say, having to depend on others to remember for them; • grief from losing parents, spouses, children, and friends; anniversaries of deaths; • family problems, specifically isolation (not being visited or called by children or grandchildren); caregiving responsibilities for spouses, children, and grandchildren; children who want money or have substance abuse issues (pp. 79–80). Outlets for coping with depressive symptoms were also described: • having social outlets with loved ones, friends, supportive family; • hobbies such as fishing and quilting; • spirituality, going to church; • talking with others about depressive symptoms.

continued

Table 11.1 Continued

Author and purpose	*Design*	*Data analysis*	*Sample information*	*Major findings*
Black et al. (2007) To explore lived experience of depression, sadness, and suffering in elderly person aged 80 and older; to understand meaning of depression and how it is experienced and expressed.	Formal ethnographic interviews. Informal conversation.	A "bottom-up" theoretical framework. Social constructivist: 1 phenomenology and the sociology of knowledge; 2 conceptualizations from cultural anthropology; 3 African American religious studies and the psychology of religion.	$N = 20$. United States. All African American women. Split evenly (10 : 10) according to health status (excellent/good : fair/poor). Data collected from research funding by the National Institute on Aging ($N = 120$), this sample was stratified; this study used the stratified groups of women and health status.	Depression is linked to a diminishment of personal strength: • depression takes form of emotional, mental, or physical strength that is decreasing due to difficulties that occur throughout life; • one must fight depression with all strength that remains in their body. Depression is related to sadness and suffering: • lifelong poverty; • poor relationships; • early experiences of grief. Individuals with depression often have feelings of "no way out." Depression is prevented or resolved by personal responsibility: • primary means to prevent or resolve depression were religious beliefs; • faith in God convinced participants that negative situations would improve or they would have strength to bear them.

Dekker et al. (2009) To illustrate experience of depression in older adult patients with heart failure.	Semi-structured interviews.	Inductive Approach; ATLAS ti (version 5).	$N = 10$. United States All with heart failure. Gender: 5 female, 5 male. Mean age: 63 years. 20% minority. 70% married. 70% have some college education or greater. Purposeful sampling of outpatients in a clinical trial of biofeedback and cognitive therapy in patients with heart failure.	Participants described emotional symptoms of depression as: • sadness; • irritability; • anxiety. Depression also described in terms of somatic symptoms of changes in appetite, sleep, and energy (p. 313). All participants described negative thinking or self-critical thoughts. Participants identified stressors such as: • financial difficulties; • family problems; • health issues. Ways of coping: • involvement in activities; • distraction through spirituality/religion; • family and friends (social support); • taking antidepressants (medical intervention); • positive thinking to cope with depression (most often used).

continued

Table 11.1 Continued

Author and purpose	*Design*	*Data analysis*	*Sample information*	*Major findings*
Givens et al. (2006) To explore older adults' rationales for resisting use of antidepressants for treatment of depression.	Cross-sectional. Semi-structured interviews.	Constant comparative method; QSR N6.	*N* = 42. United States Gender: 64% female, 36% male. Race: 40% African American, 55% white, 5% Asian. Age: 24% 60–69, 50% 70–79, 26% over 80 years. Education level: 14% less than high school, 33% high school, 52% greater than high school. Marital status: 31% married, 69% not married. Purposeful sampling of participants recruited from primary care practices affiliated with University of Pennsylvania Health System and Philadelphia, VA.	Four themes were present in participants responses to not using anti-depressants: • fear of addiction; • resistance to view depression as medical illness (p. 148); • concern that natural sadness may be inhibited by antidepressants; • past negative experiences with medication to treat depression are an obstacle to treatment (p. 148).

Hedelin and Strandmark (2001) To gain deeper understanding of depression in elderly women through investigating and describing meaning of depression in their lives, as seen from a life-world perspective.	Interviews.	Phenomenological approach.	$N = 5$. Sweden. All women. Mean age: 81 years. Living situation: 3 lived alone, 1 with adult son, 1 with husband. Marital status: 2 widowed, 2 divorced, 1 married.	Depression was caused by specific life events or series of traumatic events. Depression associated with increased sensitivity to life events: • alienation and fear; • meaningless, emptiness, and hopelessness; • self-blame for their illness; • diminished vitality and physical pain; • state of tension between giving up/giving in and fighting illness.
Hostetter (2003) To explore experience of elderly living with subthreshold depression symptoms.	Semi-structured interviews; in-depth interviews.	Hermaneutic phenomenology.	$N = 10$. Rural Texas, United States. All community-dwelling. Gender: 8 female, 2 male. Mean age: 76.6 years. Marital status: 3 married, 5 widowed, 2 divorced. Convenience sample. Recruited from a parish ministry, investigator's practice, and a physician.	8 essential themes experienced by all: • feeling useless versus have to keep busy; • less energy and/or ability to motivate self; • not confiding in others about the depression; • feelings come and go and are distractible; • experience loneliness; • sadness; • sleep changes; • trying to figure out what the depression is about internally; • aggravation of feelings with chronic pain and/or decline in physical mobility.

continued

Table 11.1 Continued

Author and purpose	*Design*	*Data analysis*	*Sample information*	*Major findings*
Orr and O'Connor (2005) To explore experience of electroconvulsive therapy (ECT) in older adult women as well as their depression, self-concepts, and helping relationships in order to improve practice.	Interview.	Content-analysis; post-modernist idea of language; contrast-comparison of themes.	$N = 6$. Canada. All women receiving ECT and Caucasian. All women Caucasian. Age range: 71–89 years. Living arrangements: 4 alone, 2 private assisted-living facility. Education ranged from high school to college degree. Participants recruited with health of community health professionals.	Perceived powerlessness over the depression: • participants describe its unexpectedness; • they didn't see a cause behind the depression; • participants were disconnected from the depression experience, using "you" instead of "I" (p. 25); • participants developed alliances with doctors as way to control the depression, although they were turning over control to doctors. ECT was a substitute for medication. Participants did not remember a lot about the experience and they often stated what they "should" experience instead. Despite doubts/unhappiness with ECT, they would return if needed.

Pollitt and O'Connor (2008) To address gap in knowledge about subjective experience of older psychiatric patients admitted to hospital for depression.	Open-ended, semi-structured interviews.	Grounded theory.	*N* = 50. Australia. Mean age 77 years. 58% skilled or semi-skilled manual workers. Half were first-time admissions; 44% were involuntary patients; 20% had psychotic symptoms. 54% treated with ECT. 36% had been born outside Australia. Recruited sequentially from publicly funded aged psychiatry wards located in 3 hospitals in southeastern Melbourne, Australia.	*Themes* • Feeling misplaced, lonely, frightened, or helpless (in hospital) changed to more positive feelings as treatment took effect and surroundings became more familiar. • Participants viewed staff of hospital in high regard. • Some patients made friends in the hospital. • While they had been in a ward with difficult patients they were able to make the best of it. Coping strategies included being: • passive; • strategic; • assertive; • thinking positive; • aware of self. Respondents reported benefiting from feeling useful, being given or undertaking tasks such as gardening, sweeping floors, clearing tables, running errands for staff, helping other patients while in the hospital.

continued

Table 11.1 Continued

Author and purpose	*Design*	*Data analysis*	*Sample information*	*Major findings*
Proctor et al. (2008) To compare treatment priority of depression with other problem-solving priorities in older adults with comorbid problems.	Mixed-method. Semi-structured interviews.	Iterative content-analysis approach. NVivo (qualitative data analysis software).	N = 49. United States Long-term care clients with history of depression. Gender: 90% female, 10% male. Mean age: 74 years. Race: 61% Caucasian, 39% African American. Location: 51% urban, 49% rural. Mean years of education completed: 9.5. Purposeful sampling of long-term care adults living in their homes.	Depression is a normal part of life: • Participants had difficulty identifying their symptoms as depression. • Some participants did not know how depression was related to other aspects of their lives. • Others were able to make direct connections to health, expectations, loneliness, and financial difficulties (p. 673).

Ugarriza (2002) To understand role age and culture play, and beliefs older adults may have about depression and treatment.	Structured interviews.	Kleinman explanatory model.	$N = 30$. United States. All female. Mean age: 85 years. Birth country: 1 Germany, 2 Poland, 27 United States. Education: Majority had high school education. Recruited from in-patient treatment for depression at southeastern US private hospital.	Participant reasons for etiology/onset (pp. 25–26): • depression was a result of changes in their health; • loss of function contributed to depression; • death of family members (second most common reason), specifically husband (most common); • 6 could not give reason for depression. Problems with depression (p. 26): • problems depression caused were related to physical illness (pain, hurting, etc.) (41%); • said depression caused problems related to ADLs (32%). Severity of depression (pp. 26–27): • All but 5 stated depression was severe, deep, and of long duration; • Felt hopeless; • Experienced helplessness. Treatment preference: • use of medication (13 participants); • didn't know (5); • talking to psychiatrist/doctor (4); • therapy/group/occupational/movement/art (4). Fears about depression: • number one fear was that they would not recover the ability to accomplish things (11); • feared they would suffer physical damage or ill health because of poor appetite or eating habits (5); • feared depression was permanent (4).

continued

Table 11.1 Continued

Author and purpose	*Design*	*Data analysis*	*Sample information*	*Major findings*
Wilby (2008) To examine ways older adults cope, how their coping skills impact depression, and how they perceive effectiveness of coping skills.	Mixed method. In-depth interview.	NVivo software program.	$N = 25$. Utah, United States. All community dwelling. Random selection of elders from randomly selected voting precincts screened out for cognitive impairment and non-English speaking, $N = 91$, 25 were depressed. Demographics from depressed sample not described. Demographics for total sample: Gender: 44% male, 56% female. Race: 95% white, 1% Asian American, 0% Hispanic, 0% Native American, 0% African American, 3% other. Education: 3% middle school, 23% high school, 24% college, 32% graduate school. Income: 8% below $10,000, 46% $10,000–29,999, 19% $30,000–49,999, 25% $50,000 and above. Religion: 8% Catholic, 7% Protestant, 72% Latter Day Saints, 0% Jewish, 2% none.	Barriers to seeking treatment: • minimization of symptoms; • withdrawal and hopelessness – it's just the way things are; • dissatisfaction with prior treatment; • one should be able to solve the problem themselves; • other people caused the depression, therefore they saw no need for seeking treatment; • faith – no need for treatment; • need for privacy. Through interviews with depressed participants 9 main themes emerged about the causes of depression: • loss and complicated grief, specifically loss of spouse, friend, family members; • hopelessness, that one would not ever get better (p. 75); • history of childhood abuse including sexual and physical; • chemical imbalance – "Oh, they say … that it is hereditary" (p. 76); • loneliness, not being around others (p. 76); • lack of self worth, not being good for anything; • medical problems, feeling tired, having chronic conditions such as diabetes; • disappointment, specifically in inability to attain goals, meet expectations for one's self (p. 77); • poverty.

Wittink et al. (2006) To understand concordance and discordance between physicians and patients about depression status by assessing older patients' views of interactions with their physicians.	Semi-structured interviews.	Constant comparison model.	*N* = 48. United States. Demographics from depressed sample not described. Demographics for total sample: Majority women (75%). Mean age: 73 years. 46% African American. Education less than high school (37.5%). Recruited from offices of primary care physicians (as part of Spectrum Study).	*Four themes* • Patients express belief that their physicians are able to "pick up" on depression without patient being explicit about their emotions. • They perceived themselves as being well liked by physician and wanted to portray a positive image to physician. • Physicians focus mostly on physical issues and tend to ignore emotional ones. • Patients feel any discussion of emotional issues will lead to referral to a psychiatrist.
Wittink et al. (2009) To explore role of spirituality in the conceptualization of depression in older African Americans.	Cross-sectional. Semi-structured interviews.	Grounded theory. Constant-comparative method; QSR-N6.	*N* = 47 (1 identifiable as depressed). United States. All African American. Gender: female (79%). Mean age: 78 years. 70% attend church once a week. 70% engage in religious activity at least once/day. Participants recruited through primary care physicians' offices in Baltimore, MD.	Spirituality played active part in participant's experience of depression. Spirituality continued to be present in participant's description of antidepressants.

Table 11.2 Themes from studies of older adults with depression: experiences

Themes		*Findings*	*Studies*
Emotional.	Negative feelings towards self.	• Disappointment, specifically in inability to attain goals, meet expectations for one's self. • Negative thinking or self-critical thoughts. • Self-blame for their illness. • Lack of self-worth, not being good for anything. • Feeling useless.	Dekker et al. (2009) Hedelin and Strandmark (2001) Hostetter (2003) Wilby (2008)
	Sadness.	• Emotional symptoms of sadness. • Sadness and suffering.	Black et al. (2007) Dekker et al. (2009) Hostetter (2003)
	Hopelessness.	• Meaningless, emptiness. • Hopelessness, that one would not get better.	Hedelin and Strandmark (2001) Ugarriza (2002) Wilby (2008)
	Fear.	• Fear they would not recover the ability to accomplish things. • Feared depression was permanent. • Feared they would suffer physical damage or ill health.*	Hedelin and Strandmark (2001) Ugarriza (2002)
	Powerlessness.	• Perceived powerlessness over the depression. • They often have feelings of "no way out." • Diminishment of personal strength.	Black et al. (2007) Orr and O'Connor (2005)
	Isolation.	• Alienation. • Experience loneliness.	Hedelin and Strandmark (2001) Hostetter (2003)

Physical.	Declining overall wellness.	• Decline in physical mobility. • Physical strength that is decreasing due to difficulties that occur throughout life. • Depression also described in terms of somatic symptoms of changes in appetite, sleep, and energy. • Diminished vitality.	Black et al. (2007) Dekker et al. (2009) Hedelin and Strandmark (2001) Hostetter (2003) Ugarriza (2002)
	Pain/illness.	• Physical chronic pain. • Feared they would suffer physical damage or ill health.*	Hedelin and& Strandmark (2001) Hostetter (2003) Ugarriza (2002)

Note
* Double coded for subtheme.

Table 11.3 Themes from studies of older adults with depression: causes

Themes	*Findings*	*Studies*
Biological/medical.	• Most said depression was a result of changes in their health. • Depression caused problem related to ADLS. • Memory problems. • Loss of function contributed to depression. • Medical problems, feeling tired, having chronic conditions such as diabetes. • Problems related to physical illness and pain. • Chemical imbalance (hereditary).	Bayer (2007) Dekker et al. (2009) Proctor et al. (2008) Ugarriza (2002) Wilby (2008)
Grief/loss.	• Loss and complicated grief, specifically loss of spouse, friend, or family member. • Early experiences of grief. • Anniversaries of deaths.	Bayer (2007) Black et al. (2007) Dekker et al. (2009) Ugarriza (2002) Wilby (2008)
Financial.	• Financial difficulties. • Poverty.	Black et al. (2007) Dekker et al. (2009) Proctor et al. (2008) Wilby (2008)
Relationship issues.	• Family problems, specifically isolation (not being visited or called by children or grandchildren); caregiving responsibilities for spouse, children, and grandchildren; children who want money or have substance abuse issues. • Poor relationships.	Bayer (2007) Black et al. (2007) Dekker et al. (2009)
No cause.	• Some participants did not know how depression was related to other aspects of their lives. • They didn't see a cause behind the depression. • Could not give reason for depression.	Orr and O'Connor (2005) Proctor et al. (2008) Ugarriza (2002)
Trauma.	• Depression was caused by specific life events or series of traumatic events. • History of childhood abuse including sexual and physical.	Hedelin and Strandmark (2001) Wilby (2008)
Loneliness.	• Loneliness, not being around others.	Proctor et al. (2008) Wilby (2008)

Table 11.4 Themes from studies of older adults with depression: recovery

Themes		*Findings*	*Studies*
Coping strategies.	Spirituality.	• Spirituality continued to be present in participant's description of antidepressants.* • Faith in God convinced participants that negative situations would improve or they would have strength to bear them. • Primary means to prevent or resolve depression were religious beliefs. • Distraction through spirituality/religion.* • Going to church.	Bayer (2007) Black et al. (2007) Dekker et al. (2009) Wittink et al. (2008)
	Social support.	• Participants developed alliances with doctors as way to control the depression.* • Having social outlets with loved ones, friends, and supportive family. • Talking with others about depressive symptoms. • Some patients made friends in the hospital.	Bayer (2007) Dekker et al. (2009) Orr and O'Connor (2005) Pollitt and O'Connor (2008)
	Distractions.	• Respondents reported benefiting from feeling useful, being given or undertaking tasks. • Have to keep busy. • Involvement in activities. • Hobbies such as fishing and quilting. • Distraction through spirituality/religion.*	Bayer (2007) Dekker et al. (2009) Hostetter (2003) Pollitt and O'Connor (2008)
	Personal attributes.	*Positive thinking* • Positive thinking to cope with depression. • Able to make best of it. *Personal strength* • Fighting illness. • Coping strategies were being assertive. • One must fight depression with all strength that remains in their body. • Depression is prevented or resolved by personal responsibility.	Black et al. (2007) Dekker et al. (2009) Hedelin and Strandmark (2001) Pollitt and O'Connor (2008)

continued

Table 11.4 Continued

Themes	*Findings*	*Studies*
Formal treatment.	• Participants viewed staff of hospital in high regard. • 46% expressed overall favorable view of their hospital. • ECT was substitute for medication. • Despite doubts/unhappiness with ECT, they would return if needed. • Talking to psychiatrist/doctor. • Participants developed alliances with doctors as way to control the depression.* • Patients express belief that their physicians are able to "pick up" on depression without patient being explicit about their emotions. • Therapy/group/occupational/movement/art. • Best treatment is use of medication. • Participants used antidepressants most often. • Spirituality continued to be present in participants' description of antidepressants.*	Dekker et al. (2009) Orr and O'Connor (2005) Pollitt and O'Connor (2008) Ugarriza (2002) Wittink et al. (2006, 2008)

Note
* Double coded for subtheme.

Table 11.5 Themes from studies of older adults with depression: barriers to treatment

Themes	*Findings*	*Studies*
Fears and negative perceptions about treatment.	• Fear of addiction. • Patients feel any discussion of emotional issues will lead to referral to a psychiatrist. • Past negative experiences with medication to treat depression are obstacle to treatment. • Concern that natural sadness may be inhibited by antidepressants. • Dissatisfaction with prior treatment.	Givens et al. (2006) Wilby (2008) Wittink et al. (2006)
Minimization.	• Other people caused the depression, therefore saw no need for seeking treatment. • Physicians focus mostly on the physical issues and tend to ignore emotional ones. • Minimization of symptoms. • Depression is normal part of life. • Faith – no need for treatment. • One should be able to solve the problem oneself.	Proctor et al. (2008) Wilby (2008) Wittink et al. (2006)
Surrendering to depression.	• Withdrawal and hopelessness. • It's just the way things are.	Hedelin and Strandmark (2001) Wilby (2008)

References

Agency for Health Care Policy and Research. (1993). *Depression in primary care: Vol. 1. Detection and diagnosis clinical practice Guideline*. Retrieved April 9, 2004, from www.mentalhealth.com/bookah/p44-d1.html.

Barry, L. C., Allore, H. G., Guo, Z., Bruce, M. L., and Gill, T. M. (2008). Higher burden of depression among older women: The effect of onset, persistence, and mortality over time. *Archives of General Psychiatry*, *65*(2), 172–178.

Bird, M., and Parslow, R. (2002). Potential for community programs to prevent depression in older people. *Medical Journal of Australia*, *7*, 107–110.

Centers for Disease Control and Prevention. National Center for Injury Prevention and Control (2005). *Web-based Injury Statistics Query and Reporting System (WISQARS)*. Retrieved from www.cdc.gov/ncipc/wisqars.

Cole, M. G., and Dendukuri, N. (2003). Risk factors for depression among elderly community subjects: A systematic review and meta-analysis. *The American Journal of Psychiatry*, *160*(6), 1147–1156.

Cuijpers, P., van Straten, A., and Warmerdam, L. (2007). Behavioral activation treatments of depression: A meta-analysis. *Clinical Psychology Review*, *27*(3), 318–326.

Cuijpers, P., van Straten, A., Andersson, G., and van Oppen, P. (2008). Psychotherapy for depression in adults: A meta-analysis of comparative outcome studies. *Journal of Consulting and Clinical Psychology*, *76*(6), 909–922.

Finfgeld, D. L. (2003). Metasynthesis: The state of the art – so far. *Qualitative Health Research*, *13*(7), 893–904.

Finlayson, K. W., and Dixon, A. (2008). Qualitative meta-synthesis: A guide for the novice. *Nurse Researcher*, *15*(2), 59–71.

Fiske, A., Wetherell, J. L., and Gatz, M. (2009). Depression in older adults. *Annual Review of Clinical Psychology*, 5, 363–389.

Jones, M. L. (2004) Application of systematic review methods to qualitative research: Practical issues. *Journal of Advanced Nursing*, 48(3), 271–278.

Kessler, R. C. (2003). Epidemiology of women and depression. *Journal of Affective Disorders*, *74*(1), 5–13.

Kraaij, V., Arensman, E., and Spinhoven, P. (2002). Negative life events and depression in elderly persons: A meta-analysis. *Journals of Gerontology Series B – Psychological Sciences and Social Sciences*, *57B*(1), 87–94.

Meade, M. O., and Richardson, W. S. (1997). Selecting and appraising studies for a systematic review. *Annals of Internal Medicine*, *127*, 531–537.

Noblit, G. W., and Hare, R. D. (1988). *Meta-ethnography: Synthesizing qualitative studies*. Newbury Park, CA: Sage Publications.

Paterson, B., Thorne, S., Canam, C., and Jillings, C. (2001). *Metastudy of qualitative health research*. Thousand Oaks, CA: Sage Publications.

Sandelowski, M. (2004). Using qualitative research. *Qualitative Health Research*, *14*(10), 1366–1386.

Wilson, K., Mottram, P. G., and Vassilas, C. (2008). Psychotherapeutic treatments for older depressed people. *Cochrane Database of Systematic Reviews*, *1*, CD004853. doi: 10.1002/14651858.CD004853.pub2.

Included studies

Bayer, E. R. (2007). Impact of family and social interaction on depressive symptoms among older adults in a rural environment. *Dissertation Abstracts International*, 68, 08B (UMI No. 3277077).

Black, H. K., White, T., and Hannum, S. T. (2007). Lived experience of depression in elderly African American women. *Journal of Gerontology: Social Sciences*, *62B*(6), S392–S398.

Dekker, R. L., Peden, A. R., Lennie, T. A., Schooler, M. P., and Moser, D. K. (2009). Living with depressive symptoms: Patients with heart failure. *American Journal of Critical Care*, *18*(4), 310–318.

Givens, J. L., Datto, C. J., Ruckdeschel, K., Knott, K., Zubritsky, C., Oslin, D. W., et al. (2006). Older patients' aversion to antidepressants: A qualitative study. *Journal of General Internal Medicine*, *21*(2), 146–151.

Hedelin, B., and Strandmark, M. (2001). The meaning of depression from the life-world perspective of elderly women. *Issues in Mental Health Nursing*, *22*(4), 401–420.

Hostetter, C. M. (2003). Subthreshold depressive symptoms in elders: phenomenological exploration. UMI Dissertation Services, ProQuest Information and Learning, Ann Arbor, MI (UMI 3086769).

Orr, A., and O'Connor, D. (2005). Dimensions of power: Older women's experiences with electroconvulsive therapy (ECT). *Journal of Women and Aging*, *17*(1/2), 19–36.

Pollitt, P. A., and O'Connor, D. W. (2008). What was good about admission to an aged psychiatry ward? The subjective experiences of patients with depression. *International Psychogeriatrics*, *20*(3), 628–640.

Proctor, E. K., Haschle, L., Morrow-Howell, N., Shumway, M., and Snell, G. (2008). Perceptions about competing psychosocial problems and treatment priorities among older adults with depression. *Psychiatric Services*, *59*(6), 670–675.

Ugarriza, D. N. (2002). Elderly women's explanation of depression. *Journal of Gerontological Nursing*, *28*(5), 22–29.

Wilby, F. E. (2008). Coping and depression in community dwelling elders. *Dissertation Abstracts International*, 69, 02A (UMI No. 3302496).

Wittink, M. N., Barg, F. K., and Gallo, J. J. (2006). Unwritten rules of talking to doctors about depression: Integrating qualitative and quantitative methods. *Analysis of Family Medicine*, *4*(4), 302–309.

Wittink, M. N., Dahlberd, B., Biruk, C., and Barg, F. K. (2008). How older adults combine medical and experiential notions of depression. *Qualitative Health Research*, *18*(9), 1174–1183.

Wittink, M. N., Joo, J. H., Lewis, L. M., and Barg, F. K. (2009). Losing faith and using faith: Older African Americans discuss spirituality, religious activities, and depression. *Journal of General Internal Medicine*, *24*(3), 402–427. doi:10.1007/s11606-008-0897-1.

Index

www.ingramcontent.com/pod-product-compliance
Ingram Content Group UK Ltd.
Pitfield, Milton Keynes, MK11 3LW, UK
UKHW021021180425
457613UK00020B/1012